Evaluation and Management of Adiposity

Evaluation and Management of Adiposity

Editor: Jamie Churchill

MURPHY & MOORE
www.murphy-moorepublishing.com

www.murphy-moorepublishing.com

MURPHY & MOORE

Cataloging-in-Publication Data

Evaluation and management of adiposity / edited by Jamie Churchill.
p. cm.
Includes bibliographical references and index.
ISBN 978-1-63987-219-0
1. Obesity. 2. Body weight. 3. Metabolism--Disorders. 4. Nutrition disorders. I. Churchill, Jamie.
RC628 .E93 2022
616.398--dc23

Murphy & Moore Publishing,
1 Rockefeller Plaza,
New York City, NY 10020, USA

ISBN 978-1-63987-219-0 (Hardback)

Contents

Preface

Adiposity refers to the state of being severely overweight. It is associated with a growing risk of diseases. Body mass index is generally used as a measure for adiposity. It is calculated by dividing an individual's body weight by height. Adiposity is not regarded as a disease by many physicians and is considered as a sign of unhealthy lifestyle. This is due to its association with various secondary diseases such as high blood pressure, type 2 diabetes, fatty liver and disorders of adipose tissue. The fat distribution of the body is a major factor that determines the risk of development of these secondary diseases. Some of the factors which contribute to the development of adiposity are biological, genetic, neurobiological, social and psychological factors. It strives to provide a fair idea about this discipline and to help develop a better understanding of the latest advances within this field. Also included herein is a detailed explanation of the various ways of managing adiposity. The extensive content of this book provides the readers with a thorough understanding of the subject.

This book is a comprehensive compilation of works of different researchers from varied parts of the world. It includes valuable experiences of the researchers with the sole objective of providing the readers (learners) with a proper knowledge of the concerned field. This book will be beneficial in evoking inspiration and enhancing the knowledge of the interested readers.

In the end, I would like to extend my heartiest thanks to the authors who worked with great determination on their chapters. I also appreciate the publisher's support in the course of the book. I would also like to deeply acknowledge my family who stood by me as a source of inspiration during the project.

Editor

1

Prevalence of Metabolic Syndrome in Obese Pediatric Population: Relation to Serum Leptin Concentrations

Teodoro Durá-Travé, Fidel Gallinas-Victoriano, Leyre Lloreda-Martín, Alberto Ríos-Muñoz, Inés Niyubahwe and Ander Ernaga-Lorea

Abstract

Childhood obesity represents the most relevant nutritional disorder in our environment. This study examines the prevalence of metabolic syndrome in an obese pediatric population and its relation to serum leptin concentrations. A cross-sectional clinical and metabolic study was accomplished in a group of 106 obese children (47 males and 59 females). Patients were classified into prepubertal group (Tanner stage I) and pubertal group (Tanner stages II–V). Prevalence of insulin resistance [homeostasis model assessment (HOMA)], hypertriglyceridemia, low high-density lipoprotein (HDL) and arterial hypertension (HTA) was 38.7, 45.3, 28.3 and 33.8%, respectively. Metabolic syndrome prevalence (30.2%) was significantly higher in the pubertal group (38%) than the prepubertal group (23.2%). There was a positive correlation between leptin and body mass index (BMI) (r = 0.529), leptin and HOMA indexes (r = 0.562) and leptin and triglycerides (r = 0.314). In addition, there was a positive correlation between HOMA indexes and triglycerides (r = 0.596). Clinical and metabolic disorders associated with obesity and related to the so-called metabolic syndrome are already present in pediatric population. Leptin could play an important role in the etiopathogenesis of the metabolic syndrome.

Keywords: childhood obesity, insulin resistance, leptin, metabolic syndrome, triglycerides, blood pressure

1. Introduction

Childhood obesity represents the most relevant nutritional disorder in our environment [1, 2]. It usually initiates at early stages in life, when child feeding depends—almost exclusively—on feeding habits and preferences in a family setting; it is subsequently exacerbated (by the time of school attendance and/or adolescence), probably in relation to the adoption of unhealthy feeding habits and lifestyle [3, 4].

Study	Excess adiposity	Hypertension	Dyslipidemia	Abnormal glucose homeostasis
Cook et al. [12]	WC ≥ 90th percentile	SBP or DBP ≥ 90th percentile	Triglycerides ≥ 110 mg/dl or HDL-chol ≤ 40 mg/dl	Fasting glucose ≥ 110 mg/dl
De Ferranti et al. [13]	WC ≥ 75th percentile	SBP ≥ 90th percentile	Triglycerides ≥ 100 mg/dl HDL-chol ≤ 50 mg/dl	Fasting glucose ≥ 110 mg/dl
Weiss et al. [14]	BMI ≥ 97th percentile	SBP ≥ 95th percentile	Triglycerides ≥ 95th percentile or HDL-chol ≤ 5th percentile	OGTT: glucose at 120 min >140 and <200 mg/dl
Cruz et al. [15]	WC ≥ 90th percentile	SBP or DBP ≥ 90th percentile	Triglycerides ≥ 90th percentile or HDL-C ≤ 10th percentile	OGTT: glucose at 120 min >140 and <200 mg/dl
Viner et al. [16]	BMI ≥ 95th percentile	SBP ≥ 95th percentile	Triglycerides ≥ 150 mg/dl or HDL-chol ≤35 mg/dl or total-chol ≥ 95th percentile	Fasting glucose ≥ 110 mg/dl or OGTT: glucose >140 and <200 at 2 h or fasting insulin ≥15 mU/L (prepubertal) or ≥30 (pubertal)
Ford et al. [17]	WC ≥ 90th percentile	SBP or DBP ≥ 90th percentile	Triglycerides ≥ 110 mg/dl or HDL-chol ≤ 40 mg/dl	Fasting glucose ≥ 110 mg/dl
Lambert et al. [18]	BMI ≥ 85th percentile	SBP ≥ 75th percentile	Triglycerides ≥ 90th percentile or HDL-C ≤ 10th percentile	Fasting glucose ≥ 110 mg/dl or fasting insulin ≥ 75th percentile
Zimmet et al. [19]	WC ≥ 90th percentile	SBP ≥ 130 or DBP ≥ 85 mmHg	Triglycerides ≥ 75th percentile or HDL-chol ≤ 25th percentile	Fasting glucose ≥ 110 mg/dl

WC, waist circumference; BMI, body mass index; SBP, systolic blood pressure; DBP, diastolic blood pressure; HDL-chol, high-density lipoprotein cholesterol; OGTT, oral glucose tolerance test.

Table 1. Criteria for the diagnosis of the pediatric metabolic syndrome (all definitions considered a child as having the metabolic syndrome when three or more of the following characteristics were present).

Additional studies—except for uncommon situations such as endocrine, genetic or metabolic pathologies, which justify excess body weight—are used for the diagnosis and/or early detection of metabolic complications and, particularly, the metabolic syndrome. This syndrome is characterized by a cluster of symptoms associated with obesity, such as insulin resistance, arterial hypertension (HTA) and dyslipidemia, and its interest lies in the high predictive value for cardiovascular disease and type 2 diabetes in adulthood, especially when it is already present in school children and/or adolescents [5–11].

In the pediatric age, there are no clearly defined parameters for its diagnosis, being several different criteria proposed [12–19] (**Table 1**) on the basis of an extrapolation from clinical guides of adult populations: WHO [20], the National Cholesterol Education Program's Adult Treatment Panel III [21], the European Group for the Study of Insulin Resistance [22] and the International Diabetes Federation (IDF) [23]; this would explain the disparity in published data with respect to the applied criteria [12–16]. Even when the International Diabetes Federation (IDF) refers to the inability for diagnosis in school age, epidemiological data allow suspecting that metabolic syndrome or its components are already present at early stages [23–29].

Leptin is an adipocytokine that, in addition to multiple neuroendocrine functions, has a role in the regulation of energy balance as well as in carbohydrate and lipid metabolism and arterial pressure regulation. In this way, many authors have suggested that leptin might be involved in the etiopathogenesis of metabolic syndrome [30–32].

The aim of this work is to determine the prevalence of metabolic syndrome and its relation to serum leptin concentrations in a group of obese pediatric population.

2. Methods

2.1. Patients

A clinical assessment and metabolic study was accomplished in all patients diagnosed with obesity who attended follow-up consultation within the year 2014. Clinical evaluation was conducted in one of the three offices of the Pediatric Endocrinology Unit of the Navarra Hospital Complex. Pubertal stage was determined in each patient according to Tanner's criteria, and patients were classified into two different groups: prepubertal group (Tanner stage I) and pubertal group (Tanner stages II–V).

All those patients with personal history of endocrine disease, malformation syndromes or iatrogenic obesity (drug treatments) were excluded.

The metabolic syndrome was defined by modified Cook's criteria [12] as the manifestation of at least three of the following features: low HDL-cholesterol (<40 mg/dl), hypertriglyceridemia (TG > 110 mg/dl), obesity, arterial hypertension and insulin resistance.

2.2. Clinical assessment

The assessment of weight and height was accomplished in underwear and barefoot. Weight was measured using an Año-Sayol scale, with a reading interval of 0–120 kg and precision 100 g, and height was measured using a Holtain wall stadiometer ranging 60–210 cm and precision 0.1 cm. Body mass index (BMI) was calculated according to the corresponding formula: weight (kg)/height^2 (m). Values of Z score for BMI were calculated using a nutrition application (Aplicación Nutricional) program from the Spanish Society of Pediatric Gastroenterology,

Hepatology and Nutrition (available at http://www.gastroinf.es/nutritional/). The inclusion criterion was BMI (Z score) values exceeding +2.0 (97th percentile) by age and sex according to the growing charts from Ferrández et al. (Centro Andrea Prader, Zaragoza 2002) [33].

Blood pressure (BP) was measured in the right arm with the patient in the supine position using Visomat comfort 20/40 (Roche Diagnostics Inc.) digital blood pressure monitor, recording the lowest of three measurements. Arterial hypertension (HTA) was considered when systolic blood pressure (SBP) and/or diastolic blood pressure (DBP) was equal to or higher than 95th percentile by age, sex and height from the American reference charts (National high blood pressure Program in Children and Adolescents) [34].

The institutionalized program for Child Care in the Community of Navarre (Comunidad Foral de Navarra, Spain) includes periodic health examinations at ages 1, 2, 3, 4, 6, 8, 10 and 12 years. The anthropometric measurements (weight and height) are recorded in the corresponding clinical history. This record has allowed the registration of the age of onset for obesity and the time of evolution at the moment of the examination.

2.3. Metabolic study

Plasma concentrations for glucose, insulin, triglycerides, total cholesterol (total-chol), high-density lipoprotein cholesterol (HDL-chol), low-density lipoprotein cholesterol (LDL-chol) and leptin were measured under basal fasting conditions using standardized methodologies.

In order to determine insulin resistance, the homeostasis model-assessment (HOMA) indexes were calculated from fasting glucose and insulin concentrations (glucose levels in mmol × insulin in μUml/L/22.5). Insulin resistance was considered when HOMA value was equal to or higher than 3.8 [35].

2.4. Statistical analysis

Results are displayed as percentages (%) and means (M) with corresponding standard deviations (SDS). Statistical analysis (descriptive statistics, Student's *T*, chi-square test and Pearson's correlation) was done using the Statistical Packages for the Social Sciences version 20.0 (Chicago, IL, USA). Statistical significance was assumed when *p* value was lower than 0.05.

Parents and/or legal guardians were informed and provided verbal consent for the participation in this study in all cases. The study was approved by the Ethics Committee for Human Investigation at our institution.

3. Results

The sample of patients consisted of 106 patients (47 males and 59 females). The prepubertal group included 56 patients (22 males and 34 females) and the pubertal group included 50 patients (25 males and 25 females).

Clinical data	Prepubertal group	Pubertal group	Total
Age of onset (years)			
Males	3.50 ± 1.75	5.10 ± 3.22**	4.35 ± 2.73
Females	3.38 ± 1.36	7.89 ± 3.56**	5.29 ± 3.37
Total	3.43 ± 1.51*	6.50 ± 3.65*	4.88 ± 3.12
Age at examination (years)			
Males	8.78 ± 1.01	12.42 ± 1.43**	10.72 ± 2.21
Females	8.55 ± 1.26	13.22 ± 1.15**	10.53 ± 2.62
Total	8.64 ± 1.17*	12.82 ± 1.35*	10.61 ± 2.44
Evolution (years)			
Males	5.27 ± 1.49	7.95 ± 2.86	6.64 ± 2.64
Females	5.16 ± 1.85	6.65 ± 2.71	5.71 ± 2.23
Total	5.21 ± 1.71*	7.35 ± 2.84*	6.14 ± 2.49
BMI (Z score)			
Males	4.05 ± 1.13	3.95 ± 1.31**	4.00 ± 1.21**
Females	3.55 ± 1.27	2.60 ± 0.50**	3.14 ± 1.11**
Total	3.74 ± 1.23*	3.27 ± 1.20*	3.52 ± 1.23
Systolic BP (mmHg)			
Males	113.68 ± 11.55	120.09 ± 14.74	116.88 ± 13.48
Females	108.78 ± 16.94	121.17 ± 16.10	113.96 ± 17.56
Total	110.77 ± 15.05*	120.64 ± 15.29*	115.26 ± 15.87
Diastolic BP (mmHg)			
Males	67.22 ± 11.45	70.81 ± 17.08	69.02 ± 14.49
Females	67.59 ± 11.85	70.04 ± 12.27	68.61 ± 11.98
Total	67.44 ± 11.58	70.42 ± 14.65	68.79 ± 13.08

*$p < 0.05$ among age groups.
**$p < 0.05$ between sexes.

Table 2. Average values (M ± SD) for the clinical features in both age groups according to sex.

Table 2 lists and compares the clinical features in both groups according to pubertal stage and sex. Within the pubertal group, the average values for age of onset, age at examination, years of evolution and systolic blood pressure were significantly higher ($p < 0.05$); within the prepubertal group, BMI values (Z score) at examination were higher ($p < 0.05$). There were no statistically significant differences among the average values of diastolic blood pressure between the different groups. The average BMI values (Z score) in the pubertal group were significantly higher ($p < 0.05$) in males. Finally, within the pubertal group, the average values for age of onset (obesity) were significantly lower ($p < 0.05$) in males.

Biochemical data	Prepubertal group	Pubertal group	Total
Glycemia (mg/dl)			
Males	93.40 ± 10.58	92.92 ± 10.18	93.14 ± 10.39
Females	89.12 ± 7.55	90.16 ± 8.87	89.56 ± 8.08
Total	90.83 ± 9.17	91.54 ± 9.55	91.17 ± 9.31
Insulin (uU/ml)			
Males	17.48 ± 14.58	18.22 ± 10.49	17.86 ± 12.52
Females	13.58 ± 9.70	23.82 ± 15.58	17.57 ± 13.18
Total	15.14 ± 11.93*	20.89 ± 13.31*	17.70 ± 12.82
HOMA			
Males	3.50 ± 2.09	4.01 ± 1.64**	3.77 ± 1.86**
Females	3.17 ± 1.41	3.08 ± 1.25**	3.13 ± 1.34**
Total	3.30 ± 1.70	3.54 ± 1.52	3.42 ± 1.61
Total-chol (mg/dl)			
Males	165.04 ± 27.34	152.72 ± 21.77	158.48 ± 25.05
Females	160.84 ± 27.18	157.32 ± 22.62	159.32 ± 25.17
Total	162.52 ± 27.07	155.02 ± 22.10	158.95 ± 25.00
LDL-chol (mg/dl)			
Males	93.50 ± 27.51	87.86 ± 21.26	90.62 ± 24.40
Females	94.06 ± 27.58	87.50 ± 20.64	91.25 ± 24.85
Total	93.83 ± 27.29	87.68 ± 20.72	90.97 ± 24.53
HDL-chol (mg/dl)			
Males	51.90 ± 11.31	43.30 ± 8.57**	47.51 ± 10.80
Females	49.48 ± 12.37	50.08 ± 9.93**	49.73 ± 11.32
Total	48.73 ± 9.76	47.25 ± 9.01	48.75 ± 11.09
Triglycerides (mg/dl)			
Males	115.95 ± 65.88	126.36 ± 45.59	121.48 ± 55.62
Females	98.08 ± 42.87	104.32 ± 42.08	100.72 ± 42.29
Total	105.10 ± 53.27	115.34 ± 44.83	109.93 ± 49.50
Leptin (ng/ml)			
Males	30.14 ± 11.75	34.38 ± 17.01**	32.39 ± 14.78**
Females	29.11 ± 12.43	24.66 ± 8.72**	27.22 ± 11.15**
Total	29.51 ± 12.07	29.52 ± 14.25	29.51 ± 13.08

*$p < 0.05$ among age groups.
**$p < 0.05$ between sexes.

Table 3. Average values (M ± SD) for metabolic study in both age groups according to sex.

Table 3 displays and compares the average values for the results of blood tests among the different groups according to pubertal stage and sex. Within the pubertal group, average values for insulin were significantly higher ($p < 0.05$) than the prepubertal group. The average values for HDL-chol within the pubertal group were significantly higher ($p < 0.05$) in females, and the average values for HOMA and leptin within the pubertal group were significantly higher ($p < 0.05$) in males.

There was a significant positive correlation ($p < 0.05$) between leptin plasma levels and BMI values ($r = 0.529$; **Figure 1**). In addition, there was a significant positive correlation between leptin plasma levels and HOMA indexes ($r = 0.562$; **Figure 2**). There was also a significant positive correlation ($p < 0.05$) between HOMA indexes and plasma concentrations of triglycerides ($r = 0.596$; **Figure 3**) as well as with age at examination ($r = 0.207$). And there was also a significant positive correlation ($p < 0.05$) between leptin plasma levels and plasma concentrations of triglycerides ($r = 0.314$; **Figure 4**).

Table 4 presents and compares the percentage values for the different clinical and metabolic parameters used as constituents of the metabolic syndrome in both groups. The percentage of patients who showed systolic blood pressure values higher than 95th percentile for the applied reference was significantly higher in the pubertal group ($p < 0.05$). There were no statistically significant differences among both groups regarding the percentage of patients who present HOMA index values higher than 3.8, plasma triglycerides higher than 110 mg/dl, HDL-chol values lower than 40 mg/dl and diastolic blood pressure values higher than 95th percentile for the applied reference charts. Within the pubertal group, the metabolic syndrome prevalence (38%) was significantly higher ($p < 0.05$) than the prepubertal group (23.2%).

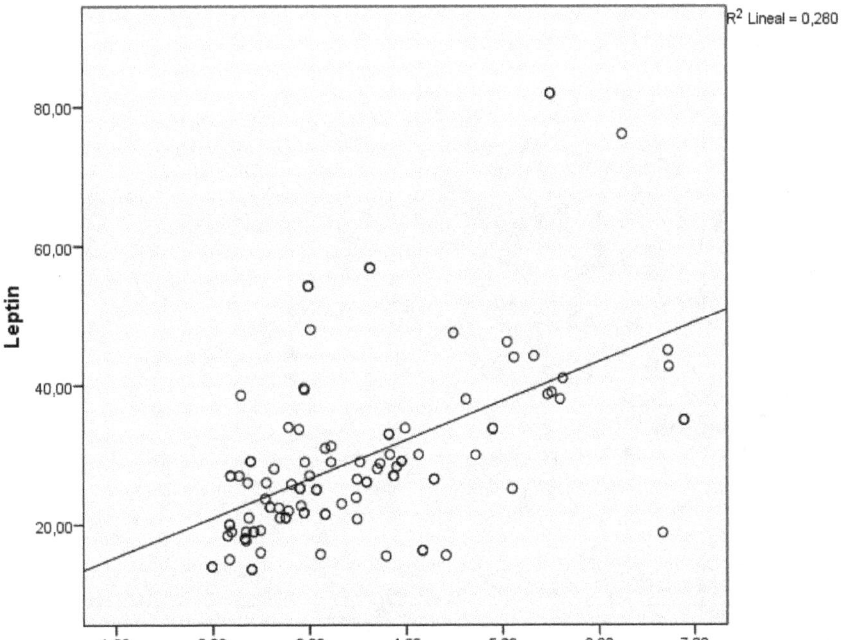

Figure 1. Leptin plasma levels (ng/ml) in relation to BMI (Z score).

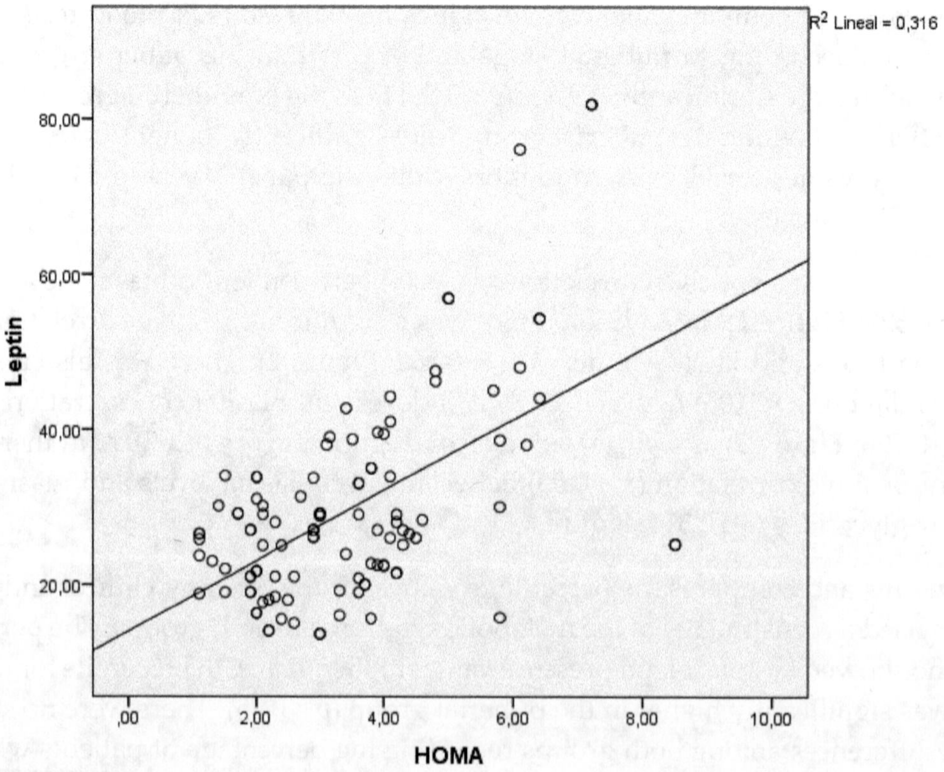

Figure 2. Leptin plasma levels (ng/ml) in relation to insulin resistance (HOMA).

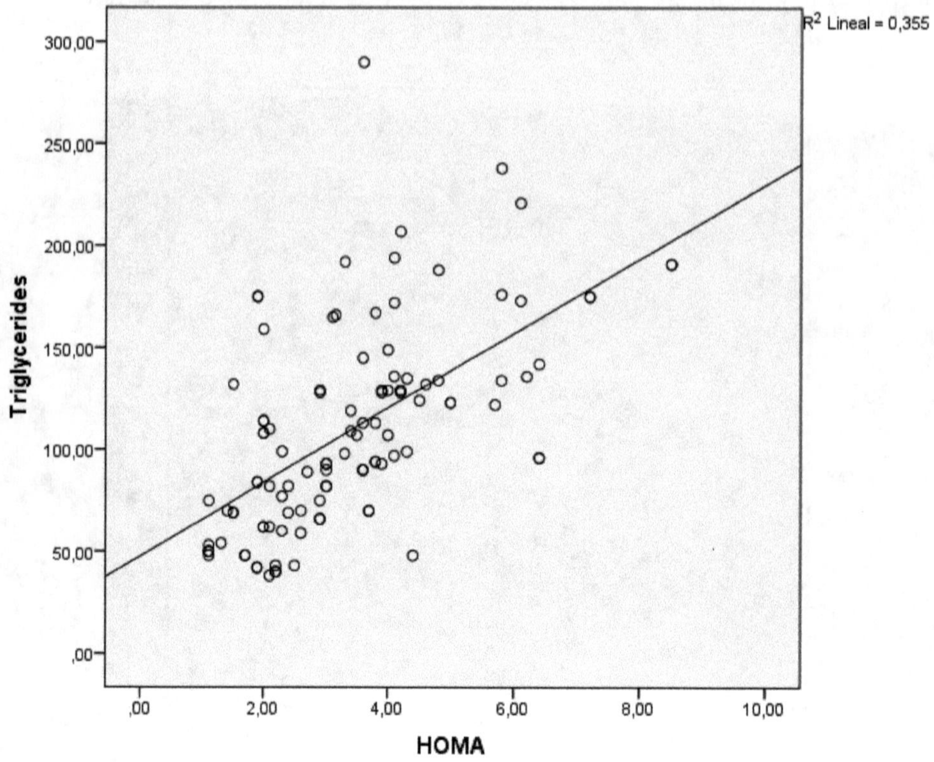

Figure 3. Triglycerides plasma concentrations (mg/dl) in relation to insulin resistance (HOMA).

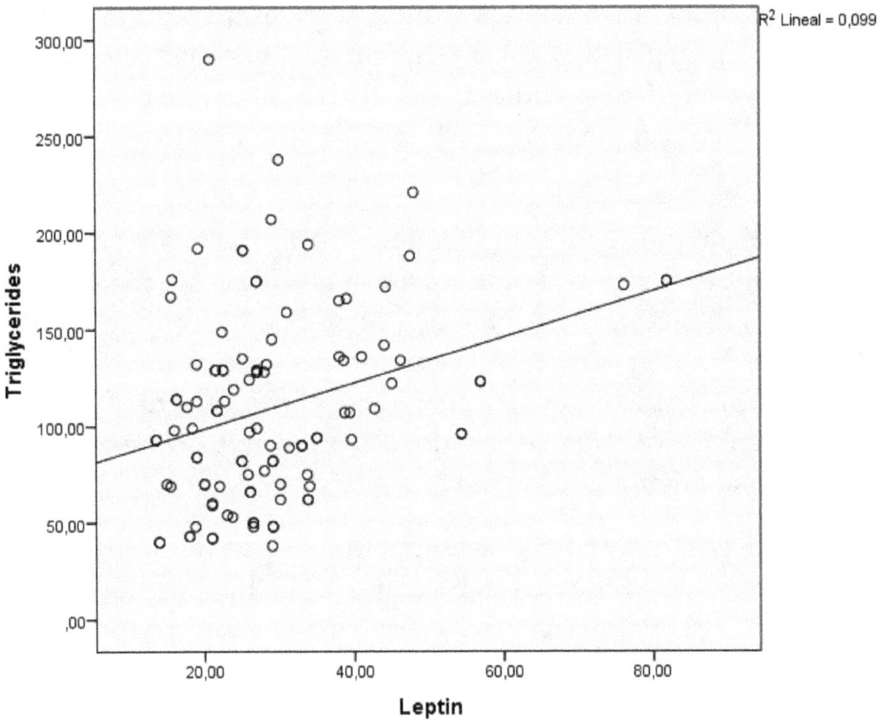

Figure 4. Triglycerides plasma concentrations (mg/dl) in relation to leptin plasma levels (ng/ml).

Diagnostic criteria	Prepubertal group *n* (%)	Pubertal group *n* (%)	Total *n* (%)
HOMA > 3.8	21 (37.5)	20 (40.0)	41 (38.7)
Triglycerides > 110 mg/dl	23 (41.1)	25 (50.0)	48 (45.3)
HDL-chol < 40 mg/dl	13 (23.6)	17 (36.2)	30 (28.3)
SBP > p95th*	14 (25.9)	21 (46.7)	35 (33.8)
DBP > p95th*	9 (16.7)	7 (15.6)	16 (15.1)
Metabolic syndrome*	13 (23.2)	19 (38)	32 (30.2)

*$p < 0.05$ among age groups.

Table 4. Prevalence of the different diagnostic criteria of metabolic syndrome in both groups.

4. Discussion

The prevalence of metabolic syndrome within the whole sample was 30.2%, being significantly higher in the pubertal group (38%) than the prepubertal group (23.2%). The comparison of these results with those described by the other authors reveals that the prevalence found is similar to references from Cook (28.7%) [12], De Ferranti (31.2%) [13], Weiss (38.7%) [14], Cruz (30%) [15] and Viner (30%) [16] in obese United Kingdom or American children and adolescents, although slightly higher than references from Lopez-Capapé (18%) [25], Tapia (18.6%) [27] and Olza (16.8%) [28] in Spanish obese pediatric population. Nevertheless, the contrast of the rate of prevalence from different studies has a relative value, since the criteria applied are different, and even different cut points for each component of metabolic syndrome are used [26, 28].

This study follows Cook modified criteria (abdominal perimeter has been replaced by BMI in the assessment of obesity, and fasting plasma glucose higher than 110 mg/dl has been replaced by HOMA index higher than 3.8). These criteria have gradually acquired clinical relevance in the assessment of metabolic syndrome in pediatric age and support from the scientific community [12, 25, 27, 28, 31]; this allows, on one side, the achievement of comparisons among the results of the different national and international studies and, on the other side, justifies its use as reference diagnosis criteria in this work.

The IDF considers fat distribution and, concretely, central or visceral obesity—which is defined by abdominal perimeter—as a "sine qua non" criterion for the diagnosis of metabolic syndrome due to its high predictive value for cardiovascular disease in adult life [36, 37]. However, there is some controversy regarding the adequacy of its use as a main and/or necessary diagnostic criterion [38]; in fact, recent studies conducted in pediatric population have used both abdominal perimeter [12, 13, 15, 39] and BMI [14, 16, 18, 25] interchangeably. In this case, the inclusion criterion was BMI value (Z-score) higher than +2.0 (97th percentile) by age and sex according to the growing charts from Ferrández et al. (Centro Andrea Prader, Zaragoza 2002) [33].

Insulin resistance, as several authors have highlighted [16, 25], has been a very frequently noted metabolic disorder in the population studied. It is worth indicating that, when Reaven [40] described the syndrome X, he considered insulin resistance as the determining pathophysiological factor and, in fact, the WHO included it as main and necessary criterion in order to diagnose the metabolic syndrome [20]. However, the diagnosed criteria subsequently proposed by the National Cholesterol Education Programs Adult Treatment Program III [21] and the IDF [23] opted for a "lipid centric" theory, with special focus on dyslipidemia and/or fat distribution.

Even though several criteria have been used to evaluate peripheral insulin sensitivity and/or alterations in glucose metabolism (fasting glucose, glycemia after an oral glucose tolerance test (OGTT), fasting insulin levels, etc.), the use of a mathematical model called *homeostasis model assessment* (HOMA) as a criterion for insulin resistance has been widely contrasted as an early disorder in glucose homeostasis (hyperinsulinemia with euglycemia). In this case, despite the application of a quite restrictive cut point [21], insulin resistance was already detected in 39% of the patients included in the study. In addition, the existing correlation between the HOMA indexes and the age of the patients at the moment of examination suggests that the onset of this metabolic comorbidity associated with obesity is related to hormonal changes concomitant with puberty rather than to the evolution time of obesity.

The situation of insulin resistance usually involves a disturbance in lipid profile by stimulating lipolysis and, therefore, an increase in plasma exchange of fatty acids that, at the same time, stimulate the hepatic triglyceride synthesis. This explains its correlation with the HOMA index of the patients. In addition, the concentration of low-density lipoproteins is usually in normal range while the concentration of high-density lipoproteins is usually low, being this considered as a side effect of hypertriglyceridemia [41–43]. Dyslipidemia observed in patients with insulin resistance corresponded with the situation expected in this metabolic condition. Furthermore, hyperinsulinemia causes water and sodium retention and activates the sympathetic nervous system, contributing to the development of hypertension.

Leptin participates directly in the regulation of energy homeostasis through an anorectic effect and an increase in thermogenesis. Plasma concentrations reflect the reserve of organic fat and are considered as a predictive factor for insulin resistance [44]. This would explain, on one hand, the existing correlation between plasma concentrations and BMI, and, on the other hand, the correlation with the HOMA index in the patients included in this work. In addition, leptin stimulates lipolysis in adipocytes and, consequently, contributes to dyslipidemia (there was a correlation with leptin plasma levels and triglycerides); it also stimulates angiogenesis and/or endothelial dysfunction and would explain, to a great extent, the development of hypertension, which is frequently associated with obesity [30]. Instead, it has been reported that adiponectin has a paradoxical effect. Adiponectin levels correlate negatively with insulin and triglyceride concentrations and BMI and positively with insulin sensitivity and high-density lipoprotein levels. Adiponectin increases fatty acid combustion and decreases triglyceride content in the liver and skeletal muscle and thus increases insulin sensitivity [45, 46]. Recently, several authors had suggested that leptin/adiponectin ratio could be a better biomark for metabolic syndrome [47–49].

As a conclusion, we remark the finding of clinical and metabolic disorders associated with obesity and related to the so-called metabolic syndrome, which, to a great extent, are already present in pediatric population. In the same way, the positive correlation between leptin plasma levels and BMI values, HOMA indexes and plasma concentrations of triglycerides suggests that leptin could play an important role in the etiopathogenesis of metabolic syndrome and/or comorbidities that are associated with obesity.

Author details

Teodoro Durá-Travé[1,2,3*], Fidel Gallinas-Victoriano[2], Leyre Lloreda-Martín[1], Alberto Ríos-Muñoz[2], Inés Niyubahwe[2] and Ander Ernaga-Lorea[2]

*Address all correspondence to: tduratra@cfnavarra.es

1 Department of Pediatrics, School of Medicine, University of Navarra, Pamplona, Spain

2 Department of Pediatrics, Navarra Hospital Complex, Pamplona, Spain

3 Navarra Institute for Health Research (IdisNa), Pamplona, Spain

References

[1] Odgen CL, Flegal KM, Carroll MD, Johnson CL. Prevalence and trends in overweight among US children and adolescents, 1999–2000. JAMA. 2002; 88:1728–32.

[2] Tzotzas T, Krassas GE. Prevalence and trends of obesity in children and adults of South Europe. Pediatr Endocrinol Rev. 2004; 1 Suppl 3:448–454.

[3] Durá-Travé T, Hualde-Olascoaga J, Garralda-Torres I, Grupo Colaborador de Navarra. Overweight among children in Navarra (Spain) and its impact on adolescence. Med Clin (Barc). 2012; 138:52–56.

[4] Durá-Travé T, Gallinas-Victoriano F, Grupo Colaborador de Navarra. Natural evolution of excess body weight (overweight and obesity) in children. An Pediatr (Barc). 2013; 79:300–6.

[5] Srinivasan SR, Myers L, Berenson GS. Predictability of childhood adiposity and insulin for developing insulin resistance syndrome (syndrome X) in young adulthood: the Bogalusa Heart Study. Diabetes. 2002; 51:204–9.

[6] Bao W, Srinivasan SR, Wattigney WA, Berenson GS. Persistence of multiple cardiovascular risk clustering related to syndrome X from childhood to young adulthood. The Bogalusa Heart Study. Arch Intern Med. 1994; 154:1842–7.

[7] Freedman DS, Khan LK, Dietz WH, Srinivasan SR, Berenson GS. Relationship of childhood obesity to coronary heart disease risk factors in adulthood: the Bogalusa Heart Study. Pediatrics. 2001; 108:712–8.

[8] Brambilla P, Lissau I, Flodmark CE, Moreno LA, Widhalm K, Wabitsch M, et al. Metabolic risk-factor clustering estimation in children: to draw a line across pediatric metabolic syndrome. Int J Obes (Lond). 2007; 31:591–600.

[9] Yusuf S, Hawkwn S, Ounpuu S, Dans T, Avezum A, Lanas F, et al. Effect of potentially modifiable risk factors associated with myocardial infarction in 52 countries (the INTER-HEART study): case-control study. Lancet. 2004; 364:937–52.

[10] Goodman E, Dolan LM, Morrison JA, Daniels SR: Factor analysis of clustered cardiovascular risks in adolescence: obesity is the predominant correlate of risk among youth. Circulation. 2005; 111:1970–77.

[11] Freedman DS, Dietz WH, Srinivasan SR, Berenson GS. The relation of overweight to cardiovascular risk factors among children and adolescents: the Bogalusa Heart Study. Pediatrics. 1999; 103:1175–82.

[12] Cook S, Weitzman M, Auinger P, et al. Prevalence of a metabolic syndrome phenotype in adolescents. Findings from the third National Health and Nutrition Examination Survey, 1988–1994. Arch Pediatr Adolesc Med. 2003;157:821–7.

[13] De Ferranti SD, Gauvreau K, Ludwig DS, et al. Prevalence of the metabolic syndrome in American adolescents: findings from the third National Health and Nutrition Examination Survey. Circulation. 2004;110:2494–7.

[14] Weiss R, Dziura J, Burgert TS, et al. Obesity and the metabolic syndrome in children and adolescents. N Engl J Med. 2004;350:2362–74.

[15] Cruz ML, Weigensberg MJ, Huang TT, Ball G, Shaibi GQ, Goran MI. The metabolic syndrome in overweight Hispanic youth and the role of insulin sensitivity. J Clin Endocrinol Metab. 2004; 89:108–113.

[16] Viner RM, Segal TY, Lichtarowicz-Krynska E, et al. Prevalence of the insulin resistance syndrome in obesity. Arch Dis Child. 2005; 90:10–4.

[17] Ford ES, Ajani UA, Morkdad AH. The metabolic syndrome and concentration of C-reactive protein among U.S. youth. Diabetes Care. 2005; 28: 878–81.

[18] Lambert M, Paradis G, O′Loughlin J, Delvin EE, Hanley JA, Levy E. Insulin resistance syndrome in a representative sample of children and adolescents from Quebec, Canada. Int J Obes Relat Metab Disord. 2004; 28:833–41.

[19] Zimmet P, Alberti KG, Kaufman F, Tajima N, Silink M, Arslanian S, et al. IDF Consensus Group: The metabolic syndrome in children and adolescents – an IDF consensus report. Pediatr Diabetes. 2007; 8:299–306.

[20] Alberti KG, Zimmet PZ. Definition, diagnosis and classification of diabetes mellitus and its complications. Part 1: Diagnosis and classification of diabetes mellitus. Provisional report of a WHO consultation. Diabet Med. 1998;15:539–93.

[21] Expert Panel on Detection, Evaluation, and Treatment of High Blood Cholesterol in Adults. Executive summary of the Third Report of The National Cholesterol Education Program (NCEP) Expert Panel on Detection, Evaluation, And High Blood Cholesterol in Adults (Adult Treatment Panel III). JAMA. 2001;285:2486–97.

[22] Balkau B, Charles MA. Comment on the provisional report from the WHO consultation. European Group for the Study of Insulin Resistance (EGIR). Diabet Med. 1999;16:442–3.

[23] Alberti KG, Zimmet P, Shaw J, IDF Epidemiology Task Force Consensus Group. The metabolic syndrome—a new worldwide definition. Lancet. 2005;366:1059–62.

[24] Goodman E, Daniels S, Morrison J, Huang B, Dolan LM. Contrasting prevalence of and demographic disparities in the World Health Organization and National Cholesterol Education Program Adult Treatment Panel III definitions of metabolic syndrome among adolescents. J Pediatr. 2004;145:445–51.

[25] López-Capapé M, Alonso M, Colino E, Mustieles C, Corbatón J, Barrio R. Frequency of the metabolic syndrome in obese Spanish pediatric Population. Eur J Endocrinol. 2006; 155:313–19.

[26] Reinehr T, de Sousa G, Toschke AM, Andler W. Comparison of metabolic syndrome prevalence using eight different definitions: a critical approach. Arch Dis Child. 2007; 92: 1067–72.

[27] Tapia-Ceballos L, López-Siguero JP, Jurado-ortiz A. Prevalence of metabolic syndrome and its componentes in obese children and adolescents. An Pediatr (Barc). 2007 ; 67 : 352–61.

[28] Olza J, Gil-Campos M, Leis R, Bueno G, Aguilera CM, Valle M, et al. Presence of the metabolic syndrome in obese children at prepubertal age. Ann Nutr Metab. 2011; 58:343–50.

[29] Martos-Moreno GA, Gil-Campos M, Bueno G, Bahillo P, Bernal S, Feliu A, et al. Obesity associated metabolic impairment is evident at early ages: Spanish collaborative study. Nutr Hosp. 2014; 30:787–93.

[30] Marti A, Martinez JA. Leptin and body weight regulation. ANALES Sis San Navarra. 1999; 22:353–63.

[31] Moreno LA, Pineda I, Rodríguez G, Fleta J, Giner A, Juste MG, et al. Leptin and metabolic syndrome in obese and non-obese children. Horm Metab Res. 2002; 34:394–9.

[32] Zuo H, Chu NF, Rimm EB, Wang D-J, Liou H-S, Shie S-M. Clustering of cardiovascular disease risk factors among obese schoolchildren: the Taipei Children Heart Study. Am J Clin Nutr. 1998; 67:1141–6

[33] Ferrández A, Baguer L, Labarta JL. Longitudinal study of normal Spanish children from birth to adulthood (anthoprometric, pubertal, radiological and intellectual data. Pediatr Endocr Rev. 2005; 2:423–559.

[34] Task Force on Blood Pressure Control in Children: Report of the Second Task Force on Blood Pressure Control in children – 1987. Pediatrics. 1987; 79: 1–25.

[35] Tresaco B, Bueno G, Pinerda I, Moreno LA, Garagorri JM, Bueno M. Homeostatic model assessment (HOMA) index cut-off values to identify the metabolic syndrome in children. J Physiol Biochem. 2005; 61:381–8.

[36] Pouliot MC, Després JP, Lemieux S, Moorjani S, Bouchard C, Tremblay A, et al. Waist circumference and abdominal sagittal diameter: best simple anthropometric indexes of abdominal visceral adipose tissue accumulation and related cardiovascular risk in men and women. Am J Cardiol. 1994; 73:460–8.

[37] Savva SC, Tornaritis M, Savva ME, Kourides Y, Panagi A, Silikiotou N, et al. Waist circumference and waist-to-height ratio are better predictors of cardiovascular disease risk factors in children than body mass index. Int J Obes. 2000; 24:1453–8.

[38] Cook S, Auinger P, Daniels S. What best predicts medical complications of obesity? BMI, waist circumference pr both. Obes Res. 2003; 11 Suppl:A27–28.

[39] Velásquez-Rodríguez CM, Velásquez-Villa M, Gómez-Ocampo L, Bermúdez-Cardona J. Abdominal obesity and low physical activity are associated with insulin resistance in overweight adolescents: a cross-sectional study. BMC Pediatr. 2014; 14:258.

[40] Reaven G. Role of insulin resistance in human disease. Diabetes. 1988; 37:1595–607.

[41] Arner P. Human fat cell lipolysis: biochemistry, regulation and clinical role. Best Pract Res Clin Endocrinol Metab. 2005; 1:471–82.

[42] Cardona F, Gónzalo-Marín M, Tinahones FJ. Association between postprandial hypertriglyceridemia and insulin resistance in patients with the metabolic syndrome. Endocrinol Nutr. 2006; 53:237–41.

[43] Klop B, Elte JW, Castro-Cabezas M. Dislipidemia in obesity: mechanisms and potential targets. Nutrients. 2013; 5:1218–40.

[44] Zuo H, Shi Z, Yuan B, Dai Y, Wu G, Hussain A. Association between serum leptin concentrations and insulin resistance: a population-based study from China. PLoS ONE. 2013; 8(1): e54615.

[45] Yadav A, Kataria MA, Saini V, Yadav A. Role of leptin and adiponectin in insulin resistance. Clin Chim Acta. 2013; 417:80–84

[46] Falahi E, Rad AHK, Sajjad Roosta S. What is the best biomarker for metabolic syndrome diagnosis?. Diab Met Syndr: Clin Res Rev (2013), http://dx.doi.org/10.1016/j.dsx.2013.06.014 (article in press)

[47] Labruna G, Pasanisi F, Nardelli C, Caso R, Vitale DF, Contaldo F, Sacchetti L. High leptin/adiponectin ratio and serum triglycerides are associated with an "at-risk" phenotype in young severely obese patients. Obesity. 2011; 19: 1492–96.

[48] Donoso MA, Muñoz-Calvo MT, Barrios V, Martínez G, Hawkins F, Argente J. Increased leptin/adiponectin ratio and free leptin index are markers of insulin resistance in obese girls during pubertal development. Horm Res Paediatr. 2013; 80:363–70

[49] Angın Y, Arslan N, Kuralay F. Leptin-to-adiponectin ratio in obese adolescents with 16 nonalcoholic fatty liver disease. Turk J Pediatr. 2014; 56: 259–66

2

Multimodal Lifestyle Intervention: Outlines and Outcomes

Mahmoud M. A. Abulmeaty

Multimodal lifestyle intervention is an essential step in obesity management. This chapter will discuss the structure and components of a proper multimodal lifestyle intervention. The setting for suppling this intervention is preferred to be served by a multidisciplinary team in a secondary care setting, but primary healthcare or even online setting is effective. The results of this type of holistic intervention are much more promising than single-discipline outcome. Success rates of intensive multimodal lifestyle intervention are growing to make it as a potential alternative to bariatric surgery in selected morbidly obese cases. However, this intervention has some limitations such as unpredicted outcomes and high dropout rates. Future studies should augment its curing effects and address the underlying mechanisms.

Keywords: multimodal lifestyle intervention, obesity management, obesity multidisciplinary teams

1. Introduction

Study and management of obesity are hot points in medical research and healthcare services worldwide. This increasing importance of studying and combating obesity came as a result of rapid pandemic prevalence of obesity and being one of the most preventable risk factors of many comorbidities. The traditional management of obesity included many disciplines of healthcare providers through many remedies including dietary manipulations, physical activity (PA) plans, behavioral modification, pharmacotherapy, bariatric surgery, and other complementary therapies [1]. Shift toward trial of complementary methods, such as acupuncture, homeopathy, chiropractic spinal manipulation, and herbal remedies, reflects the limited success rates of the nonsurgical methods for management of obesity. However, single use of a complementary remedy showed small effects with unconvincing evidence in addition to some adverse effects [2]. Low success rates of nonsurgical treatments of obesity and inadequate results may not only result in a management failure but may increase severity of obesity [3]. Even in surgical solutions of obesity, one can find a promising rate of weight loss in short-term basis, but after few years, weight regained especially if not combined with lifestyle modifications such as compliance to dietary and physical activity prescriptions [4]. Accordingly, it can be concluded that single treatment modality is not sufficient for obesity management even with bariatric surgery. The multifactorial nature of obesity as a chronic disease emphasizes this theory. Combined different remedies for weigh loss such as diet plus physical activity achieved a synergistic result rather than using combined protocols in the same remedy such as low-fat diet and low-carbohydrate diet [5].

Teamwork management including different disciplines is increasingly emphasized in management of many chronic diseases. Depth of collaboration among allied disciplines created many levels of multimodal intervention. A multidisciplinary-team approach refers to the cooperation among members from different specialties, but each one stays within his boundaries and works independently or sequentially, each from his or her own disciplinary-specific perspective (i.e., no overlap), in order to improve patient care. The second level is interdisciplinary approach, which harmonizes links between the different disciplines, in a coordinated and integrated fashion toward a common goal for the patient. The third level is transdisciplinary team in which specialists work jointly using a shared conceptual framework that draws together discipline-specific approaches, to address a common problem. Here, the traditional boundaries among different specialties were transcended [6]. Obesity is a good candidate for applying any of these levels for teamwork management because of its multifactorial nature, diversity in response to separate treatment approaches, and predisposition to multiple comorbidities belong to different medical specialties.

2. Multimodal lifestyle intervention for obesity management

From practical point of view, the nonsurgical obesity-related disciplines are much easier to collaborate in a teamwork at any level of multidisciplinary structure. Diet, physical activity, and behavioral modification represent the cornerstone of nonsurgical management of obesity. Combination of these three modalities, which collectively seek to achieve a healthier and less obesogenic lifestyle, is the multimodal lifestyle intervention.

The barriers to a healthful lifestyle are numerous and complex but can be sorted in four levels: intrapersonal, interpersonal, community, and public policy levels. For adolescents, as an example, the main intra/interpersonal barriers were improper perception of the condition, lack of willingness, priority of studying, unsatisfactory weight loss results, and low self-esteem, while lack of family and cultural support, inadequate nutritional education, and scarcity of resources were the common community/public barriers [7]. Perspective of clinical nutrition, as a main medical specialty interested in obesity management, cannot combat these entire barriers resulting in high dropout and failure rates of obesity management. Clinical nutritionist with obesity interest should add some skills about physical activity prescription and behavioral modification to achieve better results. Therefore, integrated efforts of clinical nutritionist, physical activity trainer, and behavioral therapist could overcome much more of these barriers with better commitment and higher success rates of obesity management.

2.1. Which specialties should share the responsibility?

2.1.1. Main medical specialties

The first two components of multimodal lifestyle intervention were clinical nutrition and physical activity. Addition of physical activity augments diet-induced weight loss through many mechanisms. One study examined the total energy expenditure by doubly labeled water and resting metabolic rate by indirect calorimetry in 116 severely obese patients undergoing intervention with diet alone or diet plus physical activity (PA). The results were lower reduction in the daily total energy expenditure (−122 ± 319 vs. −376 ± 305 kcal day^{-1}), elimination of the usual decrease of the activity-induced energy expenditure (83 ± 279 vs. −211 ± 284 kcal day^{-1}), and greater weight loss (13.0 ± 7.0 vs. 8.1 ± 6.3 kg) in diet plus PA group vs. diet alone. Increased PA was associated with greater adherence to low-calorie prescriptions and maintenance of greater weight loss after 6 months [8]. Furthermore, combination of PA modalities such as aerobic training and resistance training adds more to the healthy eating lifestyle than one PA modality. A randomized, parallel-group clinical trial at community-based exercise facilities in two Canadian cities examined 304 adolescents with obesity and revealed that resistance, aerobic, and combined training decreased total percent body fat and waist circumference in adolescents with obesity. Additionally, adherent cases with combined training might cause greater results than aerobic or resistance training alone [9]

Adding a new player to the obesity managing team such as behavioral modification/therapy raises the success rates and gives promising results not only in weight loss but also in body composition. Therefore, it is now accepted that behavioral therapy is an essential component of any adequate obesity managing team. Behavioral management includes many techniques such as goal setting, stimulus control, stress management, problem-solving procedures, self-monitoring, reinforcement techniques, cognitive restructuring, rewarding changes in behavior, social and family support, and relapse anticipation/prevention training [10]. Detailed description of these techniques is out of scoop of this chapter. Another alternative psychological approach for obesity management was reported [11]. It is based on food dependency model of obesity. This model considers obesity as a form of addiction, similar to psychoactive substance abuse, that is, obesity is a combination of the inability to control eating and exercise behaviors to control body fat as a result of an addictive process produced by a vicious circle of distorted thinking and physiological disturbances. According to this model, recommendation for weigh loss included reasonable caloric restriction, gradual decrease of fat quantity in food, physical exercise, strategies for improving self-regulation of eating and exercise, and social/family support [12]. A large number of clinical trials examined the effects of behavioral treatment on weight loss. Most of these trials structured group meetings weekly for the initial 3–6 months of treatment period, biweekly meetings later on up to 12 months, and then become monthly or bimonthly for the later phases of the study (up to 2 years). Group therapy may be more effective than individual treatment as it is less costly and provides a combination of empathy, social support, and healthy competition [13].

Another member of the team could enhance weight loss outcomes, which is adding a pharmacotherapy to previous approaches. Medications try either to modify the internal environment centrally or peripherally or to minimize the obesity-related physiological disturbances as a trial to predispose to a healthier internal environment. Orlistat, phentermine/topiramate, glucagon-like peptide-1 receptor agonists, lorcaserin, dipeptidyl peptidase-4 inhibitors, pramlintide, and dapagliflozin are available medications of variable adjuvant effects, when integrated with the multimodal lifestyle intervention yield more success [14]. In the future, novel therapeutic targets should extend beyond appetite control to include new strategies, such as taste preferences (e.g., Umami), energy expenditure, gut microbiota, bile acid signaling, preservation of β-cell function and hepatic glucose output, and so on.

2.1.2. Other disciplines

Complementary and alternative medicine (CAM) is defined as a group of varied medical and healthcare systems, practices, and products that are not considered to be part of any current Western healthcare system [15]. CAM included a wide range of remedies that were used in obesity management such as herbal supplements, acupuncture, and noninvasive body-contouring devices in addition to homeopathy, yoga therapy, relaxation techniques, massage, and chiropractic medicine. Despite the lack of a strong evidence about efficacy and safety, CAM is widely used especially at private centers and as a folk medicine. The positive results may appear more with mild degrees of obesity [2]. For acupuncture as an example, a meta-analysis published in 2009 [16] investigated the randomized controlled trials (RCTs) for acupuncture compared either with placebo-controlled or with dietary intervention for obesity management and revealed that acupuncture is an effective modality for obesity treatment. However, the amount of evidence is not highly convincing because of the poor methodological quality of trials reviewed. Addition of one or more remedies of CAM to the multimodal lifestyle intervention might produce more success in obesity cure. This evident in a study performed a retrospective analysis of patients attending a 13-week weight loss program consisting of chiropractic/spinal manipulative therapy in addition to nutritional intervention, physical activity, and one-on-one counseling. The results were statistically and clinically significant as regarding changes in weight and BMI. This might provide supporting evidence on the effectiveness of a multimodal approach to weight loss supplemented with chiropractic therapy [17].

2.2. Where? or In which setting?

2.2.1. Obesity multidisciplinary teams (OMDTs)

Construction of multidisciplinary, interdisciplinary, or transdisciplinary centers for obesity management is necessary for augmentation of success rates of lifestyle intervention. The National Institute of Health and Care Excellence (NICE) has recommended that multidisciplinary teams (MDTs) should be used in the treatment of complex obesity. In each hospital, OMDT should consist of a bariatric physician with a specialist interest in obesity as a leader, a registered dietitian, a clinical/counseling psychologist, a specialist nurse, and an access to a physical therapist/exercise physiologist. MDT weight management services should be delivered in the secondary care setting where bariatric physician (such as an endocrinologist or a physician nutrition specialist) can assess etiology, severity of obesity, and its related comorbidities through the medical history and physical examination. The physician will then prescribe appropriate antiobesity drugs or medication for associated comorbidities. Patient should be referred or shifted to other members of OMDT. A dietitian is required to assess the dietary habits of the patient and to tailor an individualized management plan that will aid sustainable weight loss. The role of a psychologist is to identify the psychosocial factors that contributed to the body weight and the factors that maintain the problem and prevent making meaningful lifestyle changes. Then he recommends a plan for how these factors can be managed either by a psychological support within the MDT service or by referring them to an appropriate psychiatric subspecialty. A physical therapist is essential to assess the patient's physical capability and prescribe the appropriate plan of physical activity. The specialist nurse is required to assist with medical assessments, provide advice regarding comorbidity management, and assist in the administration and scoring of dietary or mental questionnaires [18], see **Figure 1**.

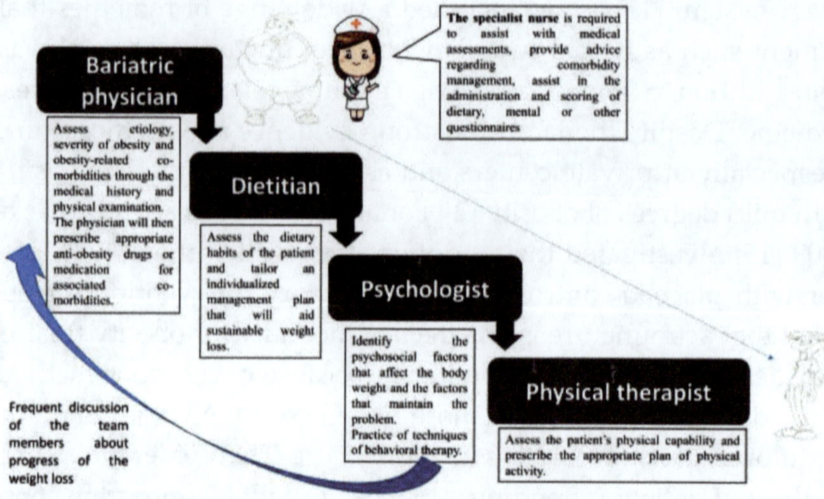

Figure 1. Construction and job specification of the obesity multidisciplinary team.

2.2.2. *Primary healthcare setting*

Primary healthcare (PHC) practitioners are encouraged to screen all adults for obesity and to offer nutritional education and behavioral counseling to cases with obesity. Training of PHC practitioners on implementation of the basic components of multimodal lifestyle intervention especially dietary, physical activity, and behavioral counseling is mandatory. In the year 2006, the National Heart, Lung, and Blood Institute (NHLBI) funded practice-based opportunities for weight reduction (POWER) trials for this purpose [19]. Three clinical trials [20–22] proved that PHC practitioners produced mean weight losses ranged from 3.6 to 9.7 at 6 to 12 months when they provided a brief behavioral counseling to obese patients in their daily practices. A fourth study randomly enrolled overweight 113 women into a dietitian-led intervention, a dietitian-led intervention plus meal replacements, or a PHC intervention with meal replacements. Participants were instructed to attend brief every-other-week visits with their primary care physician or nurse. After 1 year, adherent cases (65%) in PHC group lost weight slightly more than dietitian-led group (4.3% vs. 4.1% of initial weight). However, participants in the dietitian-led plus meal replacements group lost 9.1%, that is, PHC intervention using meal replacements was as effective as the traditional dietitian-led group intervention not using meal replacements [23].

2.2.3. Via telephone or the internet

Multimodal lifestyle intervention is now being delivered by the telephone or Internet (rather than in face-to-face setting). Web-based programs such as Weight Watchers and Nutrisystem allow individual to record their weight, dietary intake, and physical activity online and to receive colorful dietary regimens, tips for physical activity, and behavioral modification, together with graphic displays of weight changes. Even in some programs, a personalized intervention by a lifestyle specialist can be offered. Internet intervention generally produces mean weight losses about one-third of the traditional face-to-face programs and about three times of the self-help controls. These commercial interventions proved their effects via RCTs against self-help controls [13, 19].

3. Outcomes of multimodal lifestyle intervention

Outcomes of the multimodal lifestyle intervention are still inferior to surgical results. However, it is increasingly promising especially if implemented via OMDT. Clinical studies comparing intensive multimodal lifestyle intervention with bariatric surgery provide a convincing evidence about the growing effect of nonsurgical solutions of obesity. A randomized controlled, clinical trial with a 2-year intervention aimed to compare the efficacy of the three levels of obesity intervention, that is, conventional obesity therapy (COT), intensive multimodal obesity management including behavioral therapy (IMOM), and bariatric surgery (BS) as regarding changes in body weight and metabolic parameters in morbidly obese patients. IMOM group resulted in a greater percentage of weight loss than COT patients (−11.3% vs. −1.6%; $P < 0.0044$). Furthermore, 31.4% of patients in the IMOM group became non-morbidly obese within six months of intervention, and at the end of the study, they increased to 44.4%. By comparison with BS group, percentage weight loss grew from 5% for COT group to 38% for IMOM from surgical achievement, that is, percentage of weight loss in IMOM achieved more than one-third of the results of bariatric surgery without complication of surgery. Accordingly, IMOM could be an alternative therapy to patients with obesity, who cannot tolerate bariatric surgery [24].

Look AHEAD study is an interesting 8-year randomized clinical trial. They investigated the effects of intentional weight loss via intensive multimodal lifestyle intervention that included behavioral therapy vs. usual care (education and medication of diabetes), on cardiovascular morbidity and mortality in 5145 overweight/obese adults with type 2 diabetes. Dropout rate was only 12%, and in adherent cases, a clinically significant weight loss (≥5%) at year 8 occurs in 50% of patients with type 2 diabetes [25]. Furthermore, they proved that severely obese participants had similar adherence, percentage of weight loss, and improvement in CVD risk compared with less obese participants, indicating that multimodal lifestyle intervention including behavioral therapy should be considered an effective option for this high-risk category [26].

A recent meta-analysis assessed the impact of lifestyle interventions including a physical activity plan on health outcomes of patients with class II and class III obesity. After the analysis of 56 articles, they concluded that lifestyle interventions including a PA plan can improve weight and various cardiometabolic risk factors in class II and class III obese individuals [27]. By shifting to prospective studies, Karlsen et al. [28] reported that the predictors of weight loss after intensive multimodal lifestyle intervention for one year in morbidly obese patients were excess weight loss at 12 weeks, baseline mental health-related quality of life, occupational status, and age.

Data from pediatric studies are also promising. Morano et al. [29] designed a 6-month multimodal lifestyle intervention for children (ages 10–12 years) with obesity, incorporating school- and family-based components, nutritional education, fun-type physical activities, and exercise training. The results were significant reduction in body mass index z-score, body fat percentage, arm and waist circumferences, and skinfold thickness (for all $P < 0.05$), in addition to improvement of actual and perceived physical abilities, physical activity enjoyment, psychosocial health-related quality of life, and dietary pattern. This indicates the importance of combined dietary-physical activity-behavioral interventions in children with overweight and obesity. Meta-analysis of 64 pediatric and adolescent RCTs (5230 participant) including lifestyle interventions focused on physical activity and sedentary behavior (12 studies), diet only (6 studies), and multimodal interventions concentrated on behavioral modification/therapy (36 studies), and antiobesity drug interventions (metformin, orlistat, and sibutramine) were found in 10 studies. The studies varied greatly in design, outcome measurements, and methodological quality. The authors concluded that combined behavioral lifestyle interventions compared to standard care or self-help can produce a significant and clinically meaningful weight reduction in children and adolescents. However, the limited quality data cannot recommend one treatment program to be superior over another [30].

Efforts should be directed toward explanation and extraction of the underlying mechanisms of proper lifestyle intervention of obesity. As a trial, many studies examined body compositional changes during and after intervention. I have one published article about this issue, where a cohort of adult men with overweightness and obesity underwent to a multicomponent lifestyle intervention including dietary restriction, gradual physical plan, and techniques of behavioral modification for 12 months. In regards to the short-term changes in the body composition, there were a significant loss of fat-free mass (FFM), fat-free mass index (FFMI), and total body water (TBW) in obesity group rather than overweight group. This indicates that patients with obesity lose water and fat-free tissues together with fat loss in the early weeks of multimodal lifestyle intervention for obesity management. On the other hand, long-term body compositional changes after 6 to 12 months showed progressive significant reduction of weight, BMI, waist circumference, percent body fat, fat mass, and fat mass index throughout the study, in addition to preservation of FFM, FFMI, and TBW [31]. Unpublished data revealed also a significant reduction of estimated visceral fat area and improvement of lipid panel. A new meta-analysis of RCTs, which assessed the effect of caloric restriction and exercise training on bone mineral density (BMD), was published [32]. It proved that diet-induced weight reduction led to reduction of BMD at the hip and lumbar spine, while exercise-induced weight loss did not. Furthermore, a running RCT investigating body composition and bone mass changes among children undergoing multimodal lifestyle intervention was started by

Cohen et al. [33]. They designed a RCT for 6- to 8-year-old children with overweightness or obesity, where participants were randomized to a family-centered intervention including nutritional education, physical activity, and behavioral control vs. standard treatment.

Unpredicted outcomes are a common feature of lifestyle intervention for chronic diseases especially for obesity. Karlsen et al.'s study [28] tried to report some predictors of weight loss after intensive multimodal lifestyle intervention in morbidly obese patients (see above). In Abulmeaty [31] study comparison of the basal characteristics adherent with non-responding and dropped out cases revealed that cases with high percent body fat were more prone to dropping out. Furthermore, Suchánek et al. [34] reported that body composition changes in adult females after lifestyle intervention were influenced by the NYD-SP18 gene polymorphism, where overweight/obese female carriers of the NYD-SP18 rs6971091 GG genotype exhibited a more beneficial response to the intensive lifestyle intervention than others.

Another significant limitation of multimodal lifestyle intervention is high rates of dropout. One systemic review searched the literature to find an answer of that question "what are the dropout rates in lifestyle intervention programs for overweight and obese infertile women?" Ten out of studied fifteen articles reported dropout rates. The median dropout rate was 24% (ranged from 0% to 31%). They also concluded that women who drop out lose less weight and have lower spontaneous pregnancy chances than adherents [35]. About 64% is another published rate of dropout from Kuwaiti adult males and females with chronic diseases including diabesity [36]. They also reported the main causes of dropout from dietary intervention, which included unwillingness (48.6%), difficulty adhering to a diet different from that of the family (30.2%), and social meetings (13.7%). The main reasons of exercise dropout were lack of time (39.0%), co-morbid conditions (35.6%), and bad weather conditions (27.8%). The factors interfering with adherence to lifestyle measures were use of cars more than walking (83.8%), traditional fatty food, (79.9%), daily stress (70.7%), high frequency of social meetings (59.6%), high consumption of fast food (54.5%), and the presence of house cleaners (54.1%).

Author details

Mahmoud M. A. Abulmeaty

Address all correspondence to: dr.abulmeaty@gmail.com

1 Clinical Nutrition Program, Department of Community Health Sciences, College of Applied Medical Sciences, King Saud University, Riyadh, KSA

2 Obesity Research and Management Unit, Department of Medical Physiology, Faculty of Medicine, Zagazig University, Zagazig, Egypt

References

[1] Hainer V, Toplak H, Mitrakou A. Treatment modalities of obesity: what fits whom?. Diabetes Care. 2008; 31 Suppl 2: S269–S277. Doi: 10.2337/dc08-s265.

[2] Pittler MH, Ernst E. Complementary therapies for reducing body weight: a systematic review. International Journal of Obesity. 2005; 29: 1030–1038. Doi:10.1038/sj.ijo.0803008

[3] Quilliot D, Roché G, Mohebbi H, Sirvaux MA, Böhme P, Ziegler O. Nonsurgical management of obesity in adults. Presse Médicale. 2010; 39 (9): 930–944. Doi: 10.1016/j.lpm.2010.05.017.

[4] Bradley LE, Forman EM, Kerrigan SG, Goldstein SP, Butryn ML, Thomas JG, Herbert JD, Sarwer DB. Project HELP: a remotely delivered behavioral intervention for weight regain after bariatric surgery. Obesity Surgery. 2016. [Epub ahead of print]. Doi:10.1007/s11695-016-2337-3.

[5] Alexandraki I, Palacio C, Mooradian AD. Relative merits of low-carbohydrate versus low-fat diet in managing obesity. Southern Medical Journal. 2015; 108 (7): 401–416.

[6] Choi BCK, Pak AWP. Multidisciplinarity, interdisciplinarity, and transdisciplinarity in health research, services, education and policy: 3. Discipline, inter-discipline distance, and selection of discipline. Clinical and Investigative Medicine. 2008; 31 (1): E41–E48.

[7] Amiri P, Ghofranipour F, Ahmadi F, Hosseinpanah F, Montazeri A, Jalali-Farahani S, Rastegarpour A. Barriers to a healthy lifestyle among obese adolescents: a qualitative study from Iran. International Journal of Public Health. 2011; 56 (2): 181–189. Doi: 10.1007/s00038-010-0119-6.

[8] DeLany JP, Kelley DE, Hames KC, Jakicic JM, Goodpaster BH. Effect of physical activity on weight loss, energy expenditure, and energy intake during diet induced weight loss. Obesity (Silver Spring). 2014; 22 (2): 363–370. Doi: 10.1002/oby.20525.

[9] Sigal RJ, Alberga AS, Goldfield GS, Prud'homme D, Hadjiyannakis S, Gougeon R, Phillips P, Tulloch H, Malcolm J, Doucette S, Wells GA, Ma J, Kenny GP. Effects of aerobic training, resistance training, or both on percentage body fat and cardiometabolic risk markers in obese adolescents: the healthy eating aerobic and resistance training in youth randomized clinical trial. JAMA Pediatrics. 2014; 168 (11): 1006–1014. Doi: 10.1001/jamapediatrics.2014.1392.

[10] Hainter V, Toplak H, Mitrakou A. Treatment modalities of obesity: what fits whom? Diabetes Care. 31 (Suppl. 2): S269–S277, 2008

[11] Goodrick GK, Foreyt JP. Why treatments for obesity don't last. Journal of American Dietetic Association. 1991; 91: 1243–1247.

[12] Foreyt JP, Goodrick GK. Factors common to successful therapy for the obese patient. Medicine and Science in Sports and Exercise. 1919; 23: 292–297.

[13] Butryn ML, Webb V, Wadden TA. Behavioral treatment of obesity. The Psychiatric Clinics of North America. 2011; 34 (4): 841–859. Doi:10.1016/j.psc.2011.08.006.

[14] Miras AD, le Roux CW. Can medical therapy mimic the clinical efficacy or physiological effects of bariatric surgery? International Journal of Obesity. 2014; 38: 325–333; Doi: 10.1038/ijo.2013.205.

[15] Esteghamati A, Mazaheri T, Rad MV, Noshad S. Complementary and alternative medicine for the treatment of obesity: a critical review. International Journal of Endocrinology and Metabolism. 2015; 13 (2): e19678. Doi: 10.5812/ijem.19678.

[16] Cho SH, Lee JS, Thabane L, Lee J. Acupuncture for obesity: a systematic review and meta-analysis. International Journal of Obesity. 2009; 33: 183–196. Doi: 10.1038/ijo.2008.269.

[17] DeMaria A, DeMaria C, DeMaria R, Alcantara J. A weight loss program in a chiropractic practice: a retrospective analysis. Complementary Therapies in Clinical Practice. 2014; 20: 125–129.

[18] Kmietowicz Z. Multidisciplinary teams are needed throughout UK to manage obesity. BMJ 2013; 346: e8679. Doi: 10.1136/bmj.e8679.

[19] Wadden TA, Volger S, Tsai AG, Sarwer DB, Berkowitz RI, Diewald L, Carvajal R, Moran CH, Vetter M. Managing obesity in primary care practice: an overview and perspective from the POWER-UP study. International Journal of Obesity (London). 2013; 37 (0 1): S3–S11. Doi: 10.1038/ijo.2013.90.

[20] Cohen MD, D'Amico FJ, Merestein JH. Weight reduction in obese hypertensive patients. Family Medicine. 1991; 23: 25–28.

[21] Ockene IS, Hebert JR, Ockene JK, Saperia GM, Stanek E, Nicolosi R, Merriam PA, Hurley TG. Effect of physician-delivered nutrition counseling training and an office-support program on saturated fat intake, weight, and serum lipid measurements in a hyperlipidemic population: Worcester Area Trial for Counseling in Hyperlipidemia (WATCH). Archives of International Medicine. 1999; 159: 725–731.

[22] Martin PD, Rhode PC, Dutton GR, Redmann SM, Ryan DH, Brantley PJ. A primary care weight management intervention for low-income African-American women. Obesity. 2006; 14: 1412–1420. Doi:10.1038/oby.2006.160.

[23] Ashley JM, St Jeor ST, Schrage JP, Perumean-Chaney SE, Gilbertson MC, McCall NL, Bovee V. Weight control in the physician's office. Archives of Internal Medicine. 2001; 161: 1599–1604.

[24] Burguera B, Tur JJ, Escudero AJ, Alos M, Pagán A, Cortés B, González XF, Soriano JB. An intensive lifestyle intervention is an effective treatment of morbid obesity: the TRAMOMTANA study—a two-year randomized controlled clinical trial. International Journal of Endocrinology. 2015; 2015: 194696. Doi: 10.1155/2015/194696.

[25] Wadden TA, Bantle JP, Blackburn Gl, and the Look AHEAD Research Group. Eight-year weight losses with an intensive lifestyle intervention: the look AHEAD study. Obesity (Silver Spring). 2014; 22 (1): 5–13. Doi: 10.1002/oby.20662

[26] Unick JL, Beavers D, Jakicic JM, Kitabchi AE, Knowler WC, Wadden TA, Wing RR; Look AHEAD Research Group. Effectiveness of lifestyle interventions for individuals with severe obesity and type 2 diabetes: results from the look AHEAD trial. Diabetes Care. 2011; 34 (10): 2152–2157. Doi: 10.2337/dc11-0874.

[27] Baillot A, Romain AJ, Boisvert-Vigneault K, Audet M, Baillargeon JP, Dionne IJ, Valiquette L, Abou Chakra CN, Avignon A, Langlois M. Effects of lifestyle interventions that include a physical activity component in class II and III obese individuals: a systematic review and meta-analysis. PLoS One. 2015; 10 (4): e0119017. Doi: 10.1371/journal.pone.0119017.

[28] Karlsen T, Søhagen M, Hjelmesæth J. Predictors of weight loss after an intensive lifestyle intervention program in obese patients: a 1-year prospective cohort study. Health and Quality of Life Outcomes. 2013; 11: 165. Doi: 10.1186/1477-7525-11-165.

[29] Morano M, Rutigliano I, Rago A, Pettoello-Mantovani M, Campanozzi A. A multicomponent, school-initiated obesity intervention to promote healthy lifestyles in children. Nutrition. 2016; 32: 1075–1080.

[30] Oude Luttikhuis H, Baur L, Jansen H, Shrewsbury VA, O'Malley C, Stolk RP, Summerbell CD. Interventions for treating obesity in children. Cochrane Database of Systematic Reviews. 2009, Issue 1: Art. No.: CD001872. Doi: 10.1002/14651858.CD001872.pub2.

[31] Abulmeaty MMA. Multimodal-lifestyle intervention produces reduction of the fat mass rather than body weight loss in men with obesity: a prospective cohort study. Nutrition Clinique et Metabolisme. 2016; 30 (2): 163–171.

[32] Soltani S, Hunter GR, Kazemi A, Shab-Bidar S. The effects of weight loss approaches on bone mineral density in adults: a systemic review and meta-analysis of randomized controlled trials. Osteoporosis International. 2016; 27 (9): 2655–2671. Doi: 10.1007/s00198-016-3617-4.

[33] Cohen TR, Hazell TJ, Vanstone CA, Plourde H , Rodd CJ, Weile HA. A family-centered lifestyle intervention to improve body composition and bone mass in overweight and obese children 6 through 8 years: a randomized controlled trial study protocol. BMC Public Health. 2013; 13: 383.

[34] Suchánek P, Lánská V, Hubáček JA. Body composition changes in adult females after lifestyle intervention are influenced by the NYD-SP18 variant. Central European Journal of Public Health. 2015; 23 (Supplement):S19–S22. Doi: 10.21101/cejph.a4105.

[35] Mutsaerts MAQ, Kuchenbecker WKH, Mol BW, Land JA, Hoek A. Dropout is a problem in lifestyle intervention programs for overweight and obese infertile women: a systematic review. Human Reproduction. 2013; 28 (4): 979–986.

[36] Serour M, Alqhenaei H, Al-Saqabi S, Mustafa A, Ben-Nakhi A. Cultural factors and patients' adherence to lifestyle measures. British Journal of General Practice. 2007; 57: 291–295.

3

Network Analysis of Obesity Expression Data

Ashok Kumar and Kanika Gupta

Abstract

There are numerous genetic and environmental factors associated significantly with obesity, which could be used as potential diagnostic biomarkers. The molecular mechanisms, development, differentiation, and disease gene expression data provide crucial insights as these differentially expressed genes could have major effects on diet-induced obesity and such effect is not seen in animals. Genomics and proteomics are major branches for better understanding the normal function of the tissues and their interactions with the environment i.e. characterizing the tissues in which the newly discovered genes are expressed, helps in understanding the development of tissues, ageing mechanisms, and signalling routes that enable the tissues to function and also direct the similitude, parallelism and other levels of aptness betwixt two or more gene artefacts. It is traditionally known that hypothalamic and brain stem centres are intricate in the mandate of food absorption and energy equilibrium, but statistics on the associated governing elements and their genes was scant until the utmost decagon and have been identified to be strongly expressed in variety of tissues. NPY plays a notable part in anxiety, tension, corpulence, and vitality homeostasis through incitement of NPY-Y1 receptors (Y1Rs) in the mind. NPY1R quality is the protein accomplice of qualities that are utilized as model as a part of mouse and in addition in people. Utilizing diverse bioinformatics instruments, the relative examination of NPY1R at quality and additionally at protein level can be assessed for biomarker of stoutness malady. In this manner, the system science thinks about point to predict the quality of heftiness which could be taken as a biomarker in human by examining with the quality that already has been utilized as marker as a part of model life forms.

Keywords: network biology, text mining, obesity, bioinformatics databases and tools

1. Introduction

Creation of networks and all their known associations [1], enabled valuable insights into human disease and disease therapy. Protein-protein interaction mapping focused on specific human diseases which identified novel interactions among proteins encoded by known disease genes, and have also predicted new disease susceptibility genes. Rapid advances in network biology indicated that cellular networks are governed by universal laws and offer a new conceptual framework that could potentially revolutionize our view of biology and disease pathologies in the twenty-first century [2]. Due to the wide quota of research being conducted on this topic, much has been inscribed in the biomedical literature about the coalition betwixt genes and diseases. Therefore, obtaining disease–gene coalition from script is an evident use case for text mining, and disease–gene coalitions have actually formerly been obtained by postulated co-occurrence-based text-mining structures [3–6]. Text mining is the discovery by computer of new, previously unknown information, by automatically extracting information from different written resources. The purpose of text mining is to process unstructured (textual) information, extract meaningful numeric indices from the text, and, thus, make the information contained in the text accessible to the various data mining (statistical and machine learning) algorithms. As the research on obesity is carried out by large groups in scientific community, this becomes the problem of big data analytics that is, the process of examining large data sets containing a variety of data types to uncover hidden patterns and unknown correlations. Obesity is an abnormal accumulation of body fat, usually 20% or more over an individual's ideal body weight. Excess bodyweight is the sixth most important risk factor contributing to the overall burden of disease worldwide. Genetic factors significantly influence how the body regulates the appetite and the rate at which it turns food into energy (metabolic rate). A lot is known about the genetic aspects of obesity, but much more remains to be discovered. The primary goals are to identify the specific genetic variations and the biologic consequences that are produced, or as commonly put, discovering the genes and pathways involved in producing phenotypic variation and the factors that influence obesity [7]. Thus from the present work we would find markers for obesity in humans which would help in the diagnosis and prognosis of obesity and the same process could find its applications for other diseases.

2. Network biology and text mining approach to find potential human biomarkers in obesity

Network science concerns with biological entanglement by condensing composite structures as elements (nodes) and interactions (edges) betwixt them [8]. In biological structures nodes are metabolites and macromolecules such as proteins, RNA molecules and gene sequences, while the edges are physical, biochemical and functional interactions that can be recognised with a profusion of automation. Creation of networks of genetic disorders and all their known gene associations [1], or of drugs and all their known protein targets [9], enabled worthwhile insights into human disease and disease therapy. Protein-protein interaction mapping efforts focused on specific human diseases (like ataxia [10, 11], autism [12] and breast cancer [13] have identified novel interactions among proteins encoded by known disease genes, and have also predicted new disease susceptibility genes. The common finding among these disease interactomes is the discovery of unexpected relationships between disease genes that initially appeared unrelated [14]. Building and analysing more disease-centric networks is accordingly a critical step towards deeper understanding of underlying disease mechanisms (http://ccsb.dfci.harvard.edu/web/www/ccsb/Research/ networks.html). A key aim of postgenomic biomedical research is to systematically catalogue all molecules and their interactions within a living cell as shown in **Figure 1**. There is a comprehensible necessity to comprehend how these molecules and the interactions betwixt them decide the role of this extremely composite mechanism, both in detachment and when encompassed by different cells. Fast advances in system science determine that cell systems are hegemonize by general laws and offer another calculated structure that could change the perspective of science and infection pathologies in the twenty-first century [2].

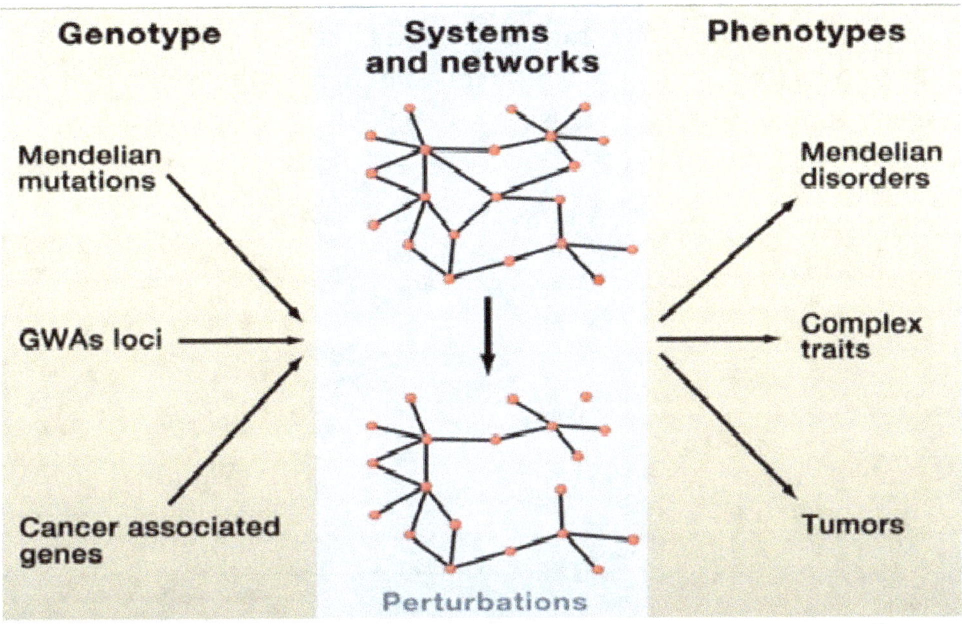

Figure 1. Uproars in Biological Systems and Cellular Networks may stamp genotype-phenotype connections. By communicating with each other, qualities and their items from complex cell systems. The connection between upheavals in system and frameworks properties and phenotypes, for example, Mendelian issue, complex qualities, and tumour, may be as major as that amongst genotypes and phenotypes [8].

Three distinct approaches have been used to capture interactome networks: (1) compilation or curation of hitherto prevailing data accessible in the writing, more often than not removed from one or only a couple sorts of physical or biochemical associations [15]; (2) computational expectations in light of available "orthogonal" data separated from physical or biochemical collaborations, for example, arrangement likenesses, quality request protection, co-nearness and co-nonappearance of qualities in totally sequenced genomes and protein basic data [16]; and (3) orderly, unprejudiced high throughput experimental mapping strategies applied at the scale of whole genomes or proteomes [17]. These approaches, though compatible, differ greatly in the feasible interpretations of the resulting maps. Literature-curated maps extend the benefit of using already accessible information, but are restricted by the intrinsically variable quality of the published data, the absence of orderliness, and the absence of describing of negative data [18, 19]. Computational prediction maps are fast and efficient to implement, and usually include satisfyingly large numbers of nodes and edges, but are necessarily imperfect because they use indirect information [20]. While high-throughput maps attempt to report unbiased, deliberate, and all around controlled information, they were at first all the more difficult to start, albeit late mechanical methodology predict that close achievement can come within a couple of years for profoundly reliable, comprehensive protein-protein connection and quality administrative system maps for human [21]. Content mining is the disclosure by PC of new, beforehand obscure data, by normally acquiring data from various composed courtesy. A key part is the association of the acquired data together to frame new truths or new theories to be viewed as further by a more basic method for examination (http://people.ischool.berkeley.edu/~hearst/text-mining.html). The reason of text mining is to handle unstructured (literary) data, extricate important numeric records from the content, and, in this way, make the data required in the content accessible to the different information mining (factual and machine learning) techniques as shown in **Figure 2**. Data can be acquired to get synopses for the words required in the records or to register outlines for the archives in light of the words contained in them (http://documents.software.dell.com/statistics/textbook/text-mining# overview).

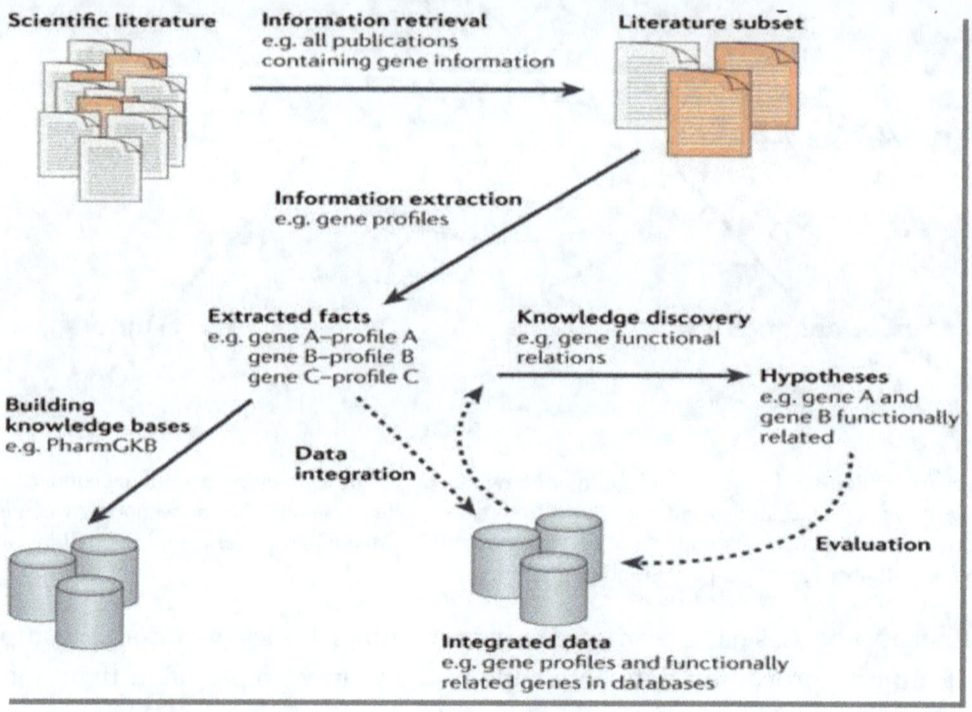

Figure 2. The approach followed by text mining method in general.

The heterogeneous data types are generated by experiments done. To communicate with these scientific discoveries natural language is used which is amenable for direct human interpretations. Natural language is the simple human language, different from programming language, through which human talks to computer. Functional information and annotations can be derived from published text directly or indirectly. Currently databases are only capable of covering a small fraction of biological context information encountered in the literature. For bench scientists, published data is the best source for interpreting high-throughput experiments, but automated text processing methods are required to integrate them into the data analysis workflow. So, the user demands better information access that is beyond just keyword searches. Moreover, due to rapid growth of information, manual extraction of information is a difficult task. So, there is a need of an efficient approach that can retrieve the meaningful information from this vast and unstructured text [22]. Excess bodyweight is the sixth most important risk factor contributing to the overall burden of disease worldwide; 1.1 billion adults and 10% of children are now classified as overweight or obese. The main adverse consequences of being obese are cardiovascular disease, type 2 diabetes, and several cancers as shown in **Figure 3** [23]. The incidence of obesity appears to be levelling in the world and started to be a big concern in the public health that causes social and economic costs of the twenty-first century. The pathogenesis of obesity is complex at all levels of biology as shown in **Figure 4** that is genetics, cell and tissue biology, physiology, and behaviour. The International Diabetes Federation considers central obesity as a primary evidence of metabolic syndrome, with the additional features which include, (1) increased triglyceride levels, (2) increased blood pressure, (3) increased fasting plasma glucose and (4) reduced HDL-cholesterol [24]. In 1997, there was serious buoyancy because, for the first time in 25 years, a new drug for the treatment of obesity had been endorsed by the US Food and Drug Administration (FDA). Then, in April 1996, two more drugs were starting their way through the acceptance procedure [25, 26]. In June 2013, the American Medical Association classified obesity as a disease (http://www.medscape.com/viewarticle/806566).

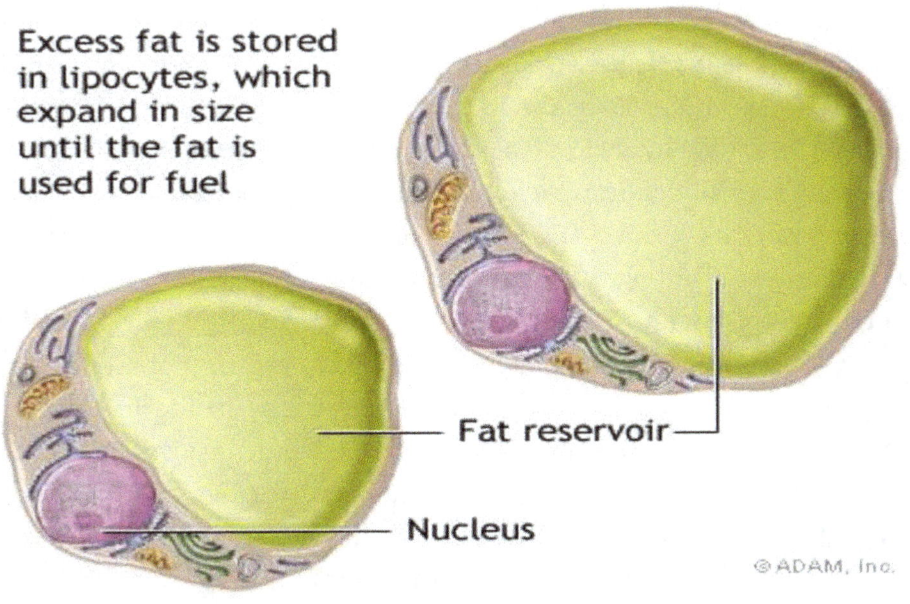

Figure 3. Consequences of obesity.

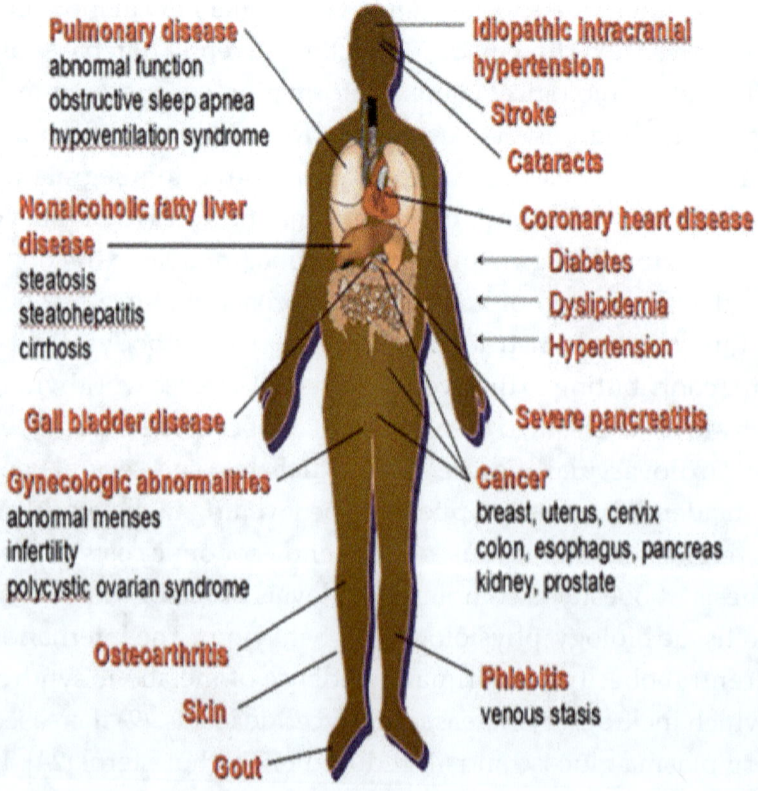

Figure 4. Showing extra calories in fat cells (lipocytes).

A lot is known about the genetic aspects of obesity, but much more remains to be discovered. Medical genetics is fundamentally interested in understanding the relationship between genetic variation and human health and disease. The primary goals are to identify the specific genetic variations and the biologic consequences that are produced, or as commonly put, discovering the genes and pathways involved in producing phenotypic variation, and the factors that influence obesity [7]. Network study on genes and proteins offers functional basics of the complexity of gene and protein, and its interacting partners as shown in **Figure 5**. Obese adults and children are more likely to display elevations in plasma *fabp4* levels [27, 28]. *Pparg* appeared to be a core obesity gene, which interacts with lipid metabolism and inflammation genes [25]. Genetic variants within *FTO* (*fat mass and obesity associated*) have been identified to exhibit the strongest association with obesity in humans [29–32]. The well-known obesity-related *FTO* gene interacts with *APOE* which in turn, is associated with Alzheimer's disease [33] and with *MC4R*, resulting in a higher chance of breast cancer [34]. Gene networks can be constructed by ensembling previously reported interactions in the literature and various databases like STRING, DISEASES, etc. [35]. The network could be visualized and constructed using cytoscape. Cytoscape supported several algorithms for the layout of networks which included spring embedded layout, hierarchical layout, circular layout and attribute based layout [36]. It was generally accepted that hypothalamic and brain stem centres are involved in the regulation of food intake and energy balance but information on the relevant regulatory factors and their genes was scarce until the last decade [37].

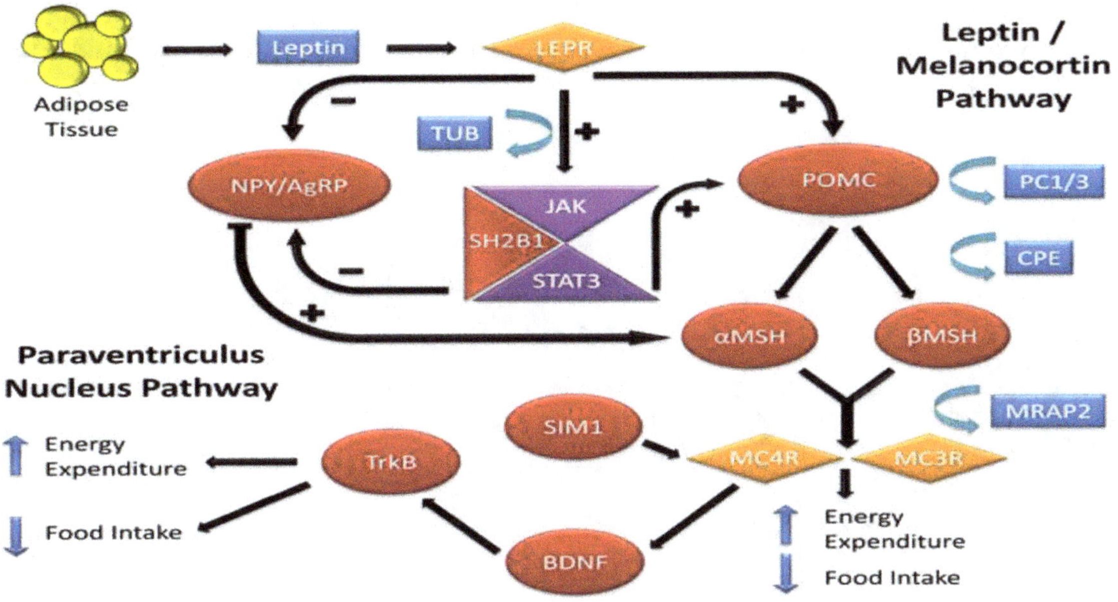

Figure 5. Genes involved in the leptin-melanocortin pathway that have been associated with monogenic obesity through their influence on food intake and energy expenditure.

There are numerous genetic factors, like Melanocortin-4 receptor (MC4R), Proopiomelanocortin (POMC), Single Minded Gene (SIM1), etc., important in obesity, which can be used as biomarkers in humans [38]. In the past literature studies, NPY1R was used as a knockout marker in mouse for obesity but not used as a biomarker in humans [39]. NPY1R (Neuropeptide Y Receptor Y1), have been recognized to actively express in variety of tissues, including trigeminal V ganglion, heart, brain, spleen, lungs, skeletal muscle, kidney and embryo, in embryonic as well as in postnatal Theiler stages as adamanted by RNA in situ and Northern blot [38, 40]. Therefore, interacting patterns of NPY1R were analysed using STRING version 10.0 [41] as shown in **Figure 6**.

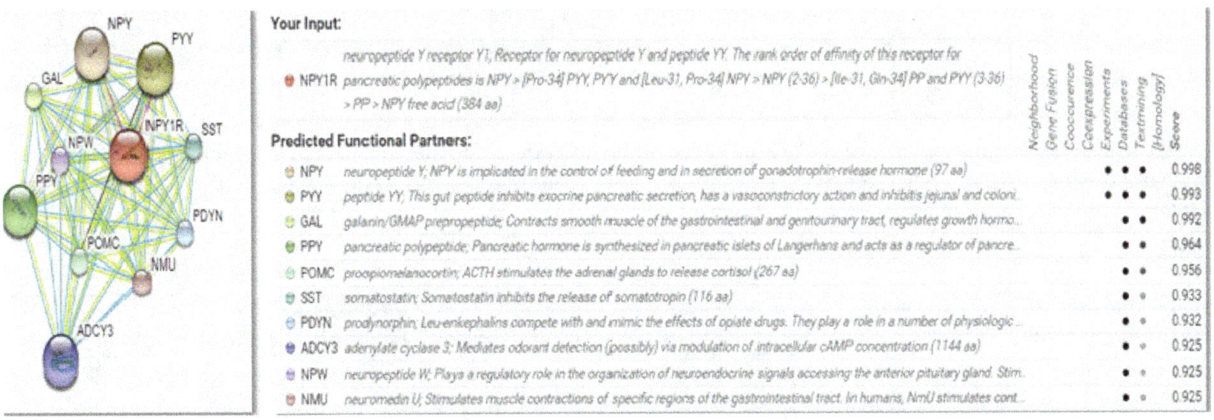

Figure 6. The interacting patterns of NPY1R in *Homo sapiens* obtained from known (curated databases and experimentally determined), predicted (gene-neighbourhood, gene fusions and gene co-occurrence) and other (text mining, protein homology and co-expression) interactions.

As NPY1R was used as an obesity marker in obesity model organisms like mouse and rat, therefore their interactions were also observed using STRING version 10.0 as shown in **Figures 7** and **8**.

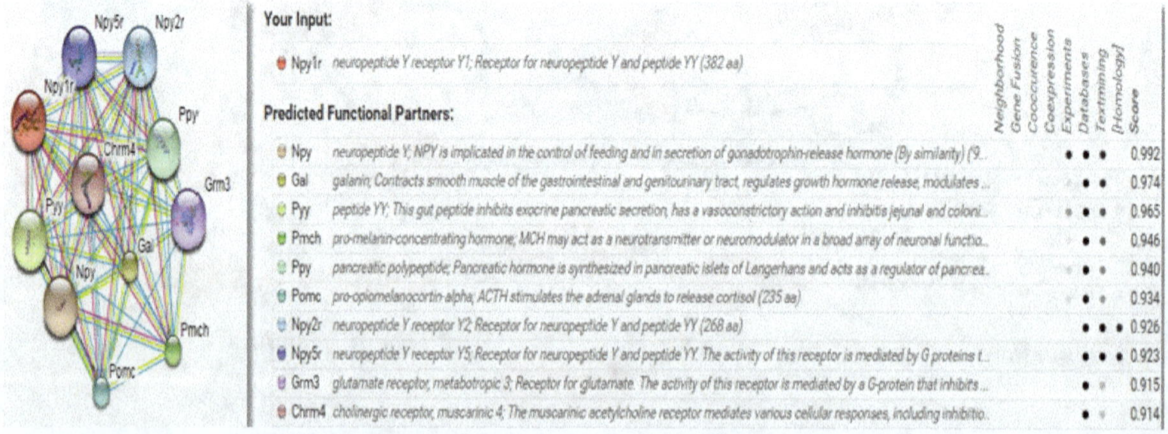

Figure 7. The interacting patterns of NPY1R in *Mus musculus* obtained from known (curated databases and experimentally determined), predicted (gene-neighbourhood, gene fusions and gene co-occurrence) and other (text mining, protein homology and co-expression) interactions.

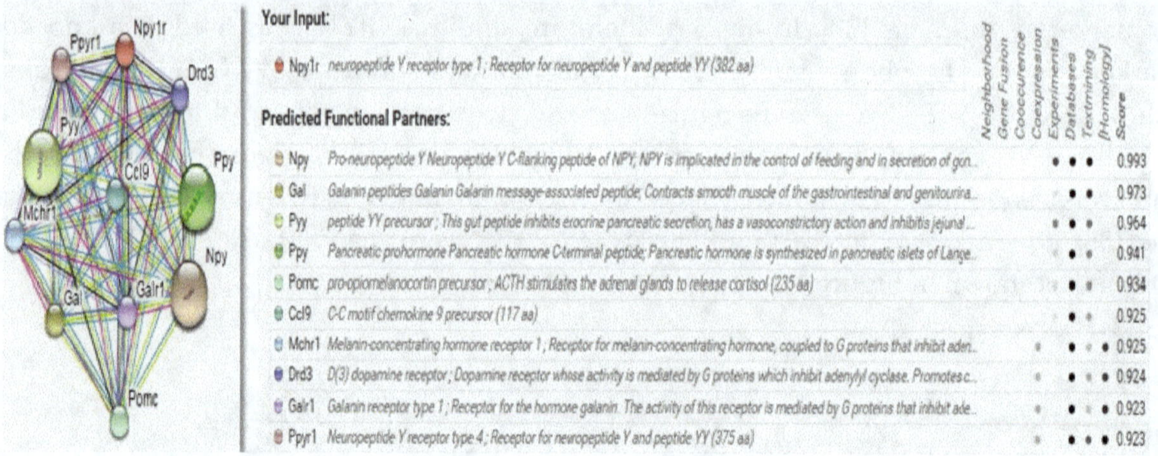

Figure 8. The interacting patterns of NPY1R in *Rattus norvegicus* obtained from known (curated databases and experimentally determined), predicted (gene-neighbourhood, gene fusions and gene co-occurrence) and other (text mining, protein homology and co-expression) interactions.

Homo sapiens		*Mus musculus*		*Rattus norvegicus*	
Functional partners	**Score**	**Functional partners**	**Score**	**Functional partners**	**Score**
NPY	0.998	*Npy*	0.992	*Npy*	0.993
PPY	0.993	*Gal*	0.974	*Gal*	0.973
GAL	0.992	*Pyy*	0.965	*Pyy*	0.964
ppy	0.964	*pmch*	0.946	*ppy*	0.941

Table 1. Lists the top scoring functional partners in *Homo sapiens, Mus musculus* and *Rattus norvegicus*.

After finding the functional partners for NPY1R in human and obesity model organisms that is, mouse and rat, top four high scoring genes were considered and further their functional partners were retrieved from STRING version 10.0 as shown in **Table 1**. The score of the functional partners were mostly on the basis of known experimental and curated databases interactions, other interactions like text mining interactions.

The networks obtained from STRING for all the interactions were merged separately for three organisms using cytoscape version 2.7.0 as shown in **Figures 9–11**.

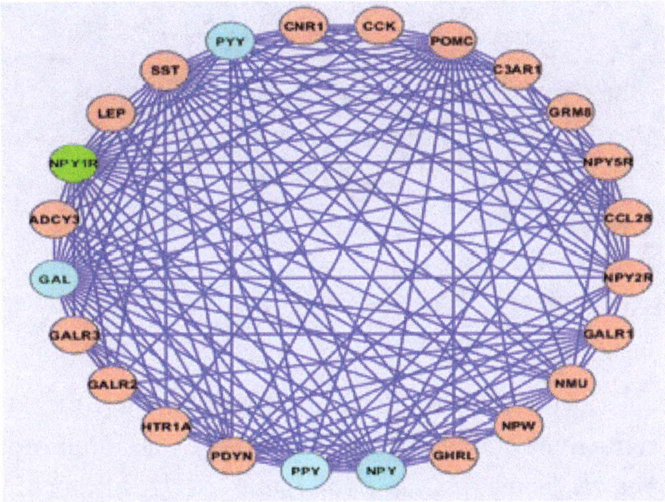

Figure 9. The merged network for *Homo sapiens* interacting functional partners. The green colour node shows the main input NPY1R for which the functional partners were searched. The sea green nodes show the top scoring functional partners of NPY1R.

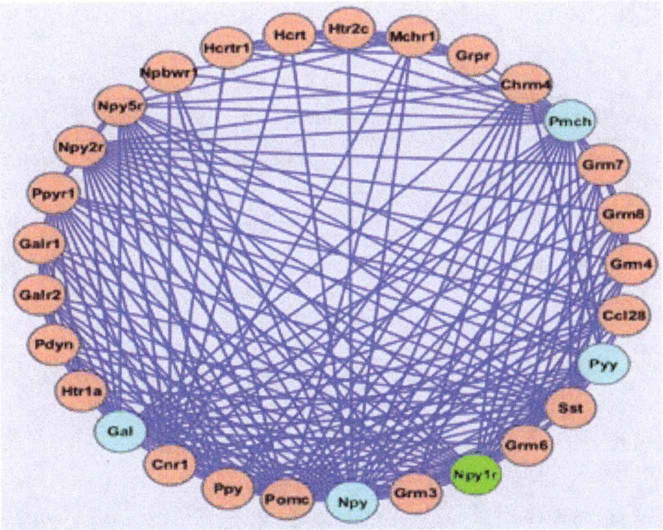

Figure 10. The merged network for *Mus musculus* interacting functional partners. The green colour node shows the main input NPY1R for which the functional partners were searched. The sea green nodes show the top scoring functional partners of NPY1R.

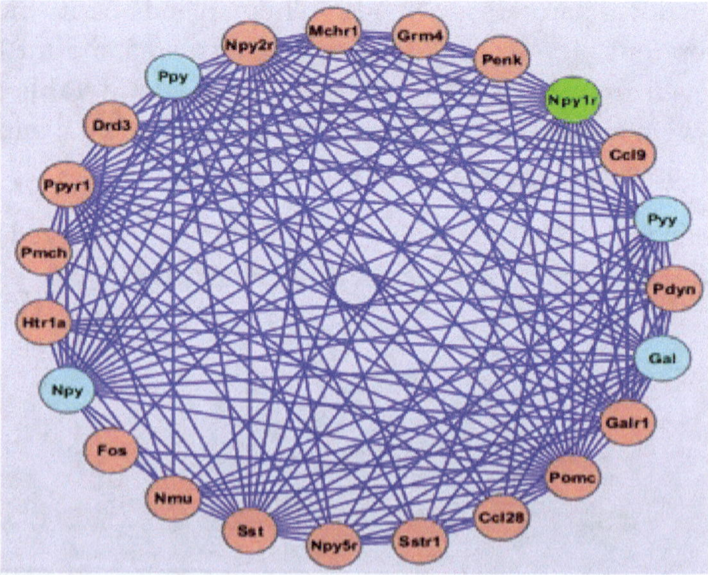

Figure 11. The merged network for *Rattus norvegicus* interacting functional partners. The green colour node shows the main input NPY1R for which the functional partners were searched. The sea green nodes show the top scoring functional partners of NPY1R.

Then these merged networks were manually analysed and it was found that there are 11 genes which were common in the merged networks of the three considered organisms. The common genes were *npy, ppy, pdyn, gal, pomc, npy1r, sst, galr1, npy2r, ccl28* and *npy5r*. Then these common genes were used to find disease-gene associations, in this case, association of common genes with obesity using DISEASES web source [42] that integrates evidence on disease-gene associations from automatic text mining, manually curated literature, cancer mutation data, and genome-wide association studies was found. From DISEASES web source 8 genes out of 11 were found related to obesity, where 7 genes had evidence from text mining and 1 gene had database evidence and no gene was found from experimental results as shown in **Table 2.**

Gene Name	Disease	Evidence	Confidence
NPY	Obesity	Text mining	****
NPY1R	Obesity	Text mining	**
NPY2R	Obesity	Text mining	**
NPY5R	Obesity	Text mining	**
PPY	Obesity	Text mining	****
GAL	Obesity	Text mining	**
CCL28	Obesity	Text mining	**
POMC	Obesity	Database	****

Table 2. List of disease-genes associations acquired from automatic text mining of the biomedical literature and DISEASES web source, where the confidence of each association is signified by stars, where ***** is the highest confidence and * is the lowest.

All the above gathered data was cross checked for networks and its disease associations using KEGG pathway [43, 44] which is a collection of manually drawn pathway maps representing the knowledge on the molecular interaction and reaction networks and Online Mendelian Inheritance in Man (OMIM) [45] which is a comprehensive, authoritative compendium of human genes and genetic phenotypes. Two pathways were found in humans which showed roles in obesity containing the respective genes obtained after disease-gene associations as shown in **Figures 12** and **13**.

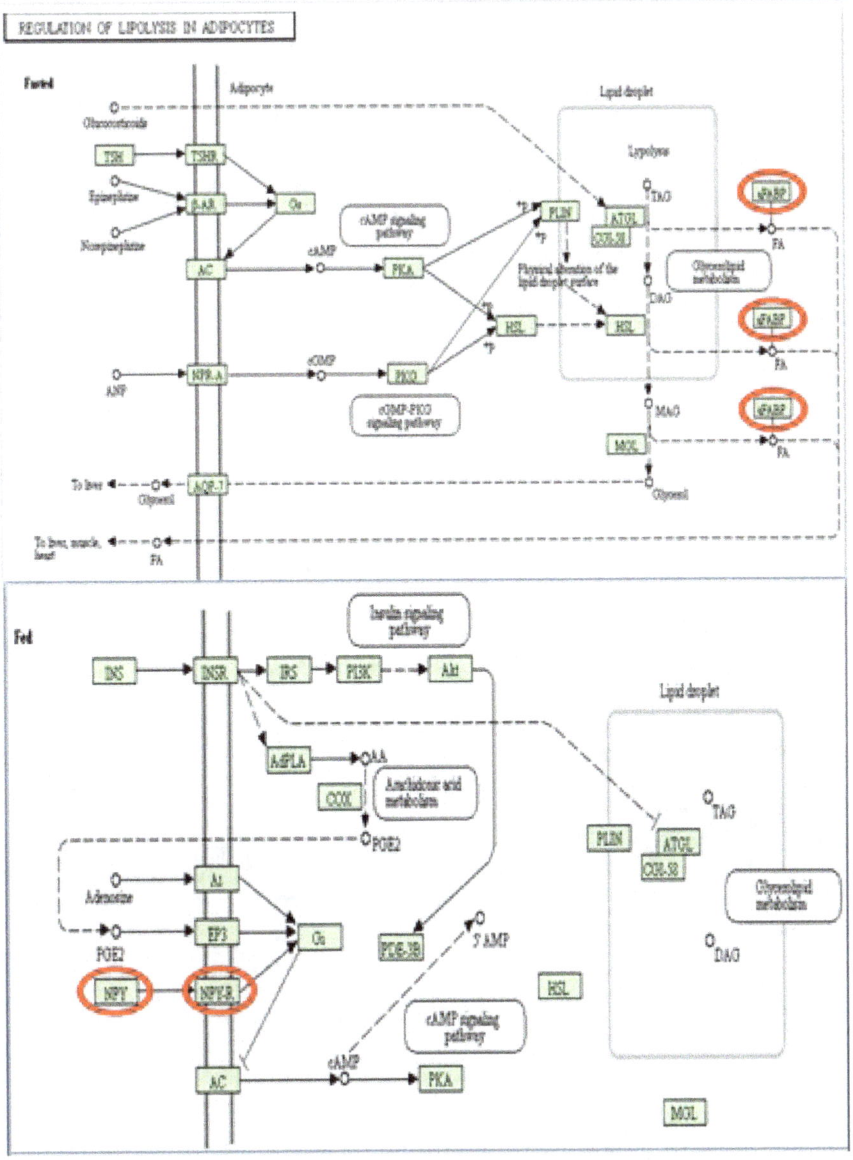

Figure 12. Regulation of lipolysis in adipocytes. This pathway shows the presence of genes *NPYR* and *NPY* in the fed state. This pathway also shows the presence of genes like *FABP* but in the fasting state and is the known marker for obesity [46–60].

Thus, from the above work we could conclude that NPY, NPY1R, NPY2R, NPY5R and POMC which in the past literature studies were used as knockout markers in mouse and rats for obesity but not used as a biomarker in humans could be considered as potential biomarkers for obesity in humans. By finding optimal biomarkers, diagnostic criteria for cardiovascular diseases can be refined in the obese beyond "traditional" risk factors to identify early pathologic processes. Identifying diagnosis and prognosis biomarkers from expression profiling data is of great significance for achieving personalized medicine and designing a therapeutic strategy in complex diseases. A similar methodology can be used to predict other biomarkers for different diseases. For progression and maintenance of life saving diseases, the expression data of biomarkers could be used in future applications.

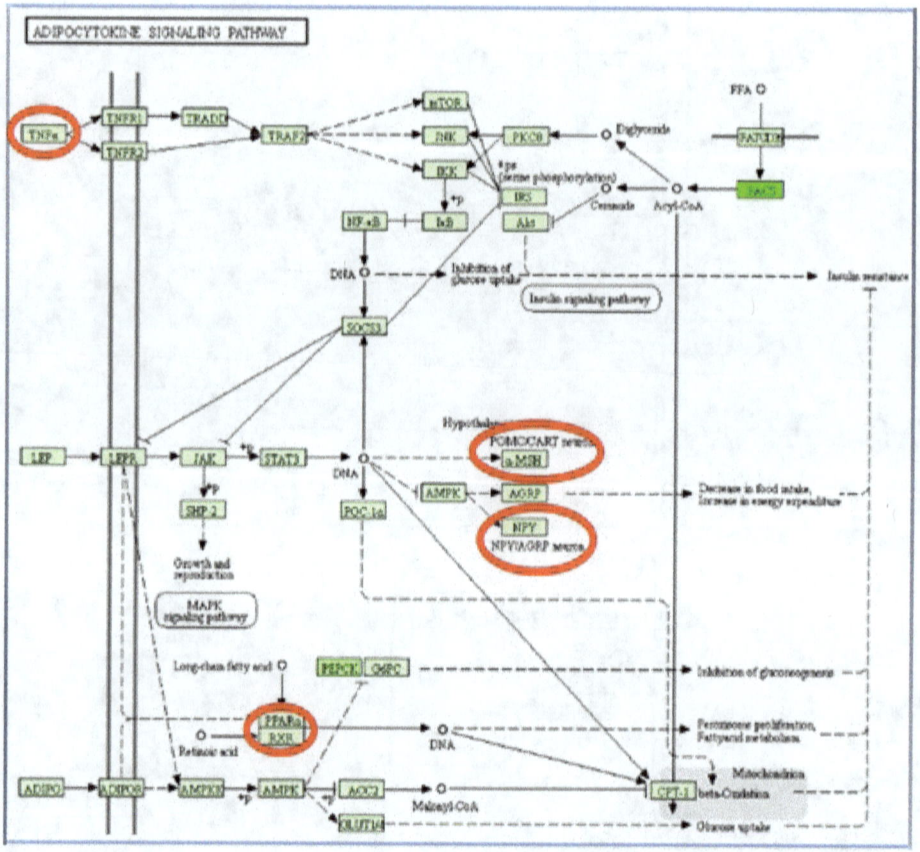

Figure 13. Adipocytokine signalling pathway. This pathway again marks the presence of NPY and POMC in obesity along with already known markers of obesity like PPAR and TNF α [61–74].

Author details

Ashok Kumar* and Kanika Gupta

*Address all correspondence to: ashokkumar@pu.ac.in

Centre For Systems Biology & Bioinformatics, UIEAST, Panjab University, Chandigarh

References

[1] Goh KI, Cusick ME, Valle D, Childs B, Vidal M, Barabasi AL. The human disease network. Proceedings of the National Academy of Sciences of the United States of America. 2007;104(21):8685–8690.

[2] Barabasi AL, Oltvai ZN. Network biology: understanding the cell's functional organization. Nature reviews Genetics. 2004;5(2):101–113.

[3] Alako BT, Veldhoven A, van Baal S, Jelier R, Verhoeven S, Rullmann T, et al. CoPub Mapper: mining MEDLINE based on search term co-publication. BMC bioinformatics. 2005;6:51.

[4] Fleuren WW, Verhoeven S, Frijters R, Heupers B, Polman J, van Schaik R, et al. CoPub update: CoPub 5.0 a text mining system to answer biological questions. Nucleic acids research. 2011;39(Web Server issue):W450–W454.

[5] Tsuruoka Y, Tsujii J, Ananiadou S. FACTA: a text search engine for finding associated biomedical concepts. Bioinformatics. 2008;24(21):2559–2560.

[6] Tsuruoka Y, Miwa M, Hamamoto K, Tsujii J, Ananiadou S. Discovering and visualizing indirect associations between biomedical concepts. Bioinformatics. 2011;27(13):i111–i119.

[7] Drake TA. Genes and pathways contributing to obesity: a systems biology view. Progress in molecular biology and translational science. 2010;94:9–38.

[8] Vidal M, Cusick ME, Barabasi AL. Interactome networks and human disease. Cell. 2011;144(6):986–998.

[9] Yildirim MA, Goh KI, Cusick ME, Barabasi AL, Vidal M. Drug-target network. Nature biotechnology. 2007;25(10):1119–1126.

[10] Lim J, Hao T, Shaw C, Patel AJ, Szabo G, Rual JF, et al. A protein-protein interaction network for human inherited ataxias and disorders of Purkinje cell degeneration. Cell. 2006;125(4):801–814.

[11] Lim J, Crespo-Barreto J, Jafar-Nejad P, Bowman AB, Richman R, Hill DE, et al. Opposing effects of polyglutamine expansion on native protein complexes contribute to SCA1. Nature. 2008;452(7188):713–718.

[12] Sakai Y, Shaw CA, Dawson BC, Dugas DV, Al-Mohtaseb Z, Hill DE, et al. Protein interactome reveals converging molecular pathways among autism disorders. Science translational medicine. 2011;3(86):86ra49.

[13] Pujana MA, Han JD, Starita LM, Stevens KN, Tewari M, Ahn JS, et al. Network modeling links breast cancer susceptibility and centrosome dysfunction. Nature genetics. 2007;39(11):1338–1349.

[14] Kahle JJ, Gulbahce N, Shaw CA, Lim J, Hill DE, Barabasi AL, et al. Comparison of an expanded ataxia interactome with patient medical records reveals a relationship between macular degeneration and ataxia. Human molecular genetics. 2011;20(3):510–527.

[15] Roberts PM. Mining literature for systems biology. Briefings in bioinformatics. 2006;7(4):399–406.

[16] Marcotte E, Date S. Exploiting big biology: integrating large-scale biological data for function inference. Briefings in bioinformatics. 2001;2(4):363–374.

[17] Walhout AJ, Vidal M. Protein interaction maps for model organisms. Nature reviews Molecular cell biology. 2001;2(1):55–62.

[18] Cusick ME, Yu H, Smolyar A, Venkatesan K, Carvunis AR, Simonis N, et al. Literature-curated protein interaction datasets. Nature methods. 2009;6(1):39–46.

[19] Turinsky AL, Razick S, Turner B, Donaldson IM, Wodak SJ. Literature curation of protein interactions: measuring agreement across major public databases. Database: the journal of biological databases and curation. 2010;2010:baq026.

[20] Plewczynski D, Ginalski K. The interactome: predicting the protein-protein interactions in cells. Cellular & molecular biology letters. 2009;14(1):1–22.

[21] Venkatesan K, Rual JF, Vazquez A, Stelzl U, Lemmens I, Hirozane-Kishikawa T, et al. An empirical framework for binary interactome mapping. Nature methods. 2009;6(1): 83–90.

[22] Ananiadou S, Mcnaught J. Text mining for biology and biomedicine. Artech House; 2005. 286. DOI: 978-1580539845.

[23] Haslam DW, James WP. Obesity. Lancet. 2005;366(9492):1197–1209.

[24] Alberti KG, Zimmet P, Shaw J. Metabolic syndrome – a new world-wide definition. A Consensus Statement from the International Diabetes Federation. Diabetic medicine: a journal of the British Diabetic Association. 2006;23(5):469–480.

[25] Bray G. Drug treatment of obesity: don't throw the baby out with the bath water. The American journal of clinical nutrition. 1998;67(1):1–2.

[26] Bray GA, Greenway FL. Current and potential drugs for treatment of obesity. Endocrine reviews. 1999;20(6):805–875.

[27] Reinehr T, Stoffel-Wagner B, Roth CL. Retinol-binding protein 4 and its relation to insulin resistance in obese children before and after weight loss. The journal of clinical endocrinology and metabolism. 2008;93(6):2287–2293.

[28] Yun KE, Kim SM, Choi KM, Park HS. Association between adipocyte fatty acid-binding protein levels and childhood obesity in Korean children. Metabolism: clinical and experimental. 2009;58(6):798–802.

[29] Scuteri A, Sanna S, Chen WM, Uda M, Albai G, Strait J, et al. Genome-wide association scan shows genetic variants in the FTO gene are associated with obesity-related traits. PLoS genetics. 2007;3(7):e115.

[30] Frayling TM, Timpson NJ, Weedon MN, Zeggini E, Freathy RM, Lindgren CM, et al. A common variant in the FTO gene is associated with body mass index and predisposes to childhood and adult obesity. Science. 2007;316(5826):889–894.

[31] Church C, Moir L, McMurray F, Girard C, Banks GT, Teboul L, et al. Overexpression of FTO leads to increased food intake and results in obesity. Nature genetics. 2010;42(12): 1086–1092.

[32] Dina C, Meyre D, Gallina S, Durand E, Korner A, Jacobson P, et al. Variation in FTO contributes to childhood obesity and severe adult obesity. Nature genetics. 2007;39(6): 724–726.

[33] Keller L, Xu W, Wang HX, Winblad B, Fratiglioni L, Graff C. The obesity related gene, FTO, interacts with APOE, and is associated with Alzheimer's disease risk: a prospective cohort study. Journal of Alzheimer's disease: JAD. 2011;23(3):461–469.

[34] da Cunha PA, de Carlos Back LK, Sereia AF, Kubelka C, Ribeiro MC, Fernandes BL, et al. Interaction between obesity-related genes, FTO and MC4R, associated to an increase of breast cancer risk. Molecular biology reports. 2013;40(12):6657–6664.

[35] Bag S, Ramaiah S, Anbarasu A. fabp4 is central to eight obesity associated genes: a functional gene network-based polymorphic study. Journal of theoretical biology. 2015;364:344–354.

[36] Shannon P, Markiel A, Ozier O, Baliga NS, Wang JT, Ramage D, et al. Cytoscape: a software environment for integrated models of biomolecular interaction networks. Genome research. 2003;13(11):2498–2504.

[37] Choquet H, Meyre D. Genetics of Obesity: what have we learned? Current genomics. 2011;12(3):169–179.

[38] Kumar A, Puri R, Gupta K, Pal A. To predict human biomarker for the obesity using mouse homologous expression data at different Theiler stages. ILNS. 2015;45(9):9–17.

[39] Shawky RM, Sadik DI. Genetics of obesity. Egyptian Journal of Medical Human Genetics. 2012;13(1):11–17.

[40] Bertocchi I, Oberto A, Longo A, Mele P, Sabetta M, Bartolomucci A, et al. Regulatory functions of limbic Y1 receptors in body weight and anxiety uncovered by conditional knockout and maternal care. Proceedings of the National Academy of Sciences of the United States of America. 2011;108(48):19395–19400.

[41] Szklarczyk D, Franceschini A, Wyder S, Forslund K, Heller D, Huerta-Cepas J, et al. STRING v10: protein-protein interaction networks, integrated over the tree of life. Nucleic acids research. 2015;43(Database issue):D447–D452.

[42] Pletscher-Frankild S, Palleja A, Tsafou K, Binder JX, Jensen LJ. DISEASES: text mining and data integration of disease-gene associations. Methods. 2015;74:83–89.

[43] Kanehisa M, Sato Y, Kawashima M, Furumichi M, Tanabe M. KEGG as a reference resource for gene and protein annotation. Nucleic acids research. 2016;44(D1):D457–D462.

[44] Kanehisa M, Goto S. KEGG: kyoto encyclopedia of genes and genomes. Nucleic acids research. 2000;28(1):27–30.

[45] Hamosh A, Scott AF, Amberger JS, Bocchini CA, McKusick VA. Online Mendelian Inheritance in Man (OMIM), a knowledgebase of human genes and genetic disorders. Nucleic acids research. 2005;33(Database issue):D514–D517.

[46] Ahmadian M, Wang Y, Sul HS. Lipolysis in adipocytes. The international journal of biochemistry & cell biology. 2010;42(5):555–559.

[47] Ahmadian M, Duncan RE, Sul HS. The skinny on fat: lipolysis and fatty acid utilization in adipocytes. Trends in endocrinology and metabolism: TEM. 2009;20(9):424–428.

[48] Wang S, Soni KG, Semache M, Casavant S, Fortier M, Pan L, et al. Lipolysis and the integrated physiology of lipid energy metabolism. Molecular genetics and metabolism. 2008;95(3):117–126.

[49] Lafontan M. Historical perspectives in fat cell biology: the fat cell as a model for the investigation of hormonal and metabolic pathways. American journal of physiology—Cell physiology. 2012;302(2):C327–C359.

[50] Fruhbeck G, Mendez-Gimenez L, Fernandez-Formoso JA, Fernandez S, Rodriguez A. Regulation of adipocyte lipolysis. Nutrition research reviews. 2014;27(1):63–93.

[51] Proenca AR, Sertie RA, Oliveira AC, Campana AB, Caminhotto RO, Chimin P, et al. New concepts in white adipose tissue physiology. Brazilian journal of medical and biological research = Revista brasileira de pesquisas medicas e biologicas/Sociedade Brasileira de Biofisica [et al.]. 2014;47(3):192–205.

[52] Duncan RE, Ahmadian M, Jaworski K, Sarkadi-Nagy E, Sul HS. Regulation of lipolysis in adipocytes. Annual review of nutrition. 2007;27:79–101.

[53] Lafontan M. Advances in adipose tissue metabolism. International journal of obesity. 2008;32(Suppl 7):S39–S51.

[54] Jaworski K, Sarkadi-Nagy E, Duncan RE, Ahmadian M, Sul HS. Regulation of triglyceride metabolism. IV. Hormonal regulation of lipolysis in adipose tissue. American journal of physiology: gastrointestinal and liver physiology. 2007;293(1):G1–G4.

[55] Thompson D, Karpe F, Lafontan M, Frayn K. Physical activity and exercise in the regulation of human adipose tissue physiology. Physiological reviews. 2012;92(1):157–191.

[56] Lafontan M, Langin D. Lipolysis and lipid mobilization in human adipose tissue. Progress in lipid research. 2009;48(5):275–297.

[57] Arner P, Langin D. Lipolysis in lipid turnover, cancer cachexia, and obesity-induced insulin resistance. Trends in endocrinology and metabolism: TEM. 2014;25(5):255–262.

[58] Brasaemle DL. Thematic review series: adipocyte biology. The perilipin family of structural lipid droplet proteins: stabilization of lipid droplets and control of lipolysis. Journal of lipid research. 2007;48(12):2547–2559.

[59] Lampidonis AD, Rogdakis E, Voutsinas GE, Stravopodis DJ. The resurgence of Hormone-Sensitive Lipase (HSL) in mammalian lipolysis. Gene. 2011;477(1–2):1–11.

[60] Bickel PE, Tansey JT, Welte MA. PAT proteins, an ancient family of lipid droplet proteins that regulate cellular lipid stores. Biochimica et biophysica acta. 2009;1791(6):419–440.

[61] Gual P, Le Marchand-Brustel Y, Tanti JF. Positive and negative regulation of insulin signaling through IRS-1 phosphorylation. Biochimie. 2005;87(1):99–109.

[62] Hardie DG, Scott JW, Pan DA, Hudson ER. Management of cellular energy by the AMP-activated protein kinase system. FEBS letters. 2003;546(1):113–120.

[63] Hurley RL, Anderson KA, Franzone JM, Kemp BE, Means AR, Witters LA. The Ca2+/calmodulin-dependent protein kinase kinases are AMP-activated protein kinase kinases. The journal of biological chemistry. 2005;280(32):29060–29066.

[64] Schwartz MW, Woods SC, Porte D, Jr., Seeley RJ, Baskin DG. Central nervous system control of food intake. Nature. 2000;404(6778):661–671.

[65] Munzberg H, Myers MG, Jr. Molecular and anatomical determinants of central leptin resistance. Nature neuroscience. 2005;8(5):566–570.

[66] Puigserver P, Rhee J, Donovan J, Walkey CJ, Yoon JC, Oriente F, et al. Insulin-regulated hepatic gluconeogenesis through FOXO1-PGC-1alpha interaction. Nature. 2003;423 (6939):550–555.

[67] Yoon JC, Puigserver P, Chen G, Donovan J, Wu Z, Rhee J, et al. Control of hepatic gluconeogenesis through the transcriptional coactivator PGC-1. Nature. 2001;413 (6852):131–138.

[68] Inoue H, Ogawa W, Ozaki M, Haga S, Matsumoto M, Furukawa K, et al. Role of STAT-3 in regulation of hepatic gluconeogenic genes and carbohydrate metabolism in vivo. Nature medicine. 2004;10(2):168–174.

[69] Zhou YT, Shimabukuro M, Wang MY, Lee Y, Higa M, Milburn JL, et al. Role of peroxisome proliferator-activated receptor alpha in disease of pancreatic beta cells. Proceedings of the National Academy of Sciences of the United States of America. 1998;95(15): 8898–8903.

[70] Kelley DE, Mandarino LJ. Fuel selection in human skeletal muscle in insulin resistance: a reexamination. Diabetes. 2000;49(5):677–683.

[71] Yamauchi T, Kamon J, Minokoshi Y, Ito Y, Waki H, Uchida S, et al. Adiponectin stimulates glucose utilization and fatty-acid oxidation by activating AMP-activated protein kinase. Nature medicine. 2002;8(11):1288–1295.

[72] Yamauchi T, Kamon J, Waki H, Terauchi Y, Kubota N, Hara K, et al. The fat-derived hormone adiponectin reverses insulin resistance associated with both lipoatrophy and obesity. Nature medicine. 2001;7(8):941–946.

[73] Minokoshi Y, Alquier T, Furukawa N, Kim YB, Lee A, Xue B, et al. AMP-kinase regulates food intake by responding to hormonal and nutrient signals in the hypothalamus. Nature. 2004;428(6982):569–574.

[74] Weisberg SP, McCann D, Desai M, Rosenbaum M, Leibel RL, Ferrante AW, Jr. Obesity is associated with macrophage accumulation in adipose tissue. The journal of clinical investigation. 2003;112(12):1796–1808.

4

New Potential Beta-3 Adrenergic Agonists with Beta-Phenylethylamine Structure, Synthesized for the Treatment of Dyslipidemia and Obesity

Simona Negreș, Cornel Chiriță,
Andreea Letiția Arsene, Denisa Margină,
Elena Moroșan and Cristina Elena Zbârcea

Abstract

Beta-3 adrenergic receptors have important physiological implications, being expressed in many places in the body, including brown adipose tissue. Of the effects studied in preclinical research on lipid metabolism attributable to stimulation of these receptors, we can mention the increased thermogenesis and metabolic rate in the brown adipose tissue, reduction of body weight in obese diabetic rats, lowering of intra-abdominal and subepithelial fat in nonobese and nondiabetic rats, decrease of triglyceride, and increase of HDL cholesterol levels. Carbohydrate metabolism is also changed by beta-3 adrenergic agonists, the most prevalent effects being blood glucose lowering in diabetic rats, increasing insulin secretion of the pancreas, or increasing glucose tolerance. Metabolic effects of 13 newly synthesized compounds of beta-phenylethylamine structure and reference BRL 37344 were investigated in order to identify a potential affinity for beta-3 adrenergic receptors. The antidiabetic and hypolipemiant effects were investigated on a rat model of alloxan-induced diabetes. The results demonstrated that new beta-phenylethylamine derivatives produced marked biological activity over lipid profile. All compounds have markedly decreased the values of total cholesterol, LDL cholesterol, and triglycerides and also have increased the values of antiatherogenic HDL cholesterol. The effects were significantly more intense than the reference substance BRL 37344.

Keywords: beta-3 adrenergic agonists, antidiabetic, hypolipemiant, glucose-6-phosphate dehydrogenase, glucose-6-phosphatase, hexokinase, beta-phenylethylamine

1. Introduction

The sympathetic nervous system is part of the autonomic nervous system and innervates tissues in almost every organ system. Adrenergic system is important for maintaining the organism homeostasis and mediates the neuronal and hormonal stress response commonly known as the fight-or-flight response.

Central and peripheral adrenergic neurotransmitters are epinephrine and norepinephrine, which act on their specific adrenergic receptors.

Adrenergic receptors types and subtypes		Tissue localization	Dominant effects
α-Adrenergic receptors	α_{1A}	Heart, blood vessels, smooth muscle, liver, lung, vas deferens, prostate, cerebellum, cortex, hippocampus	Contraction of vascular smooth muscle; vasoconstriction of large resistant arterioles in skeletal muscle
	α_{1B}	Heart, kidney, spleen, lung, blood vessels, cortex, brainstem	Promotes cardiac growth and structure
	α_{1D}	Aorta, coronary artery, platelets, prostate, cortex, hippocampus	Vasoconstriction in aorta and coronary artery
	α_{2A}	Sympathetic neurons, platelets, pancreas, locus coeruleus, brainstem, spinal cord	Main inhibitory receptor on sympathetic neurons
	α_{2B}	Liver, kidney, pancreas, blood vessels	Mediates α_2 vasoconstriction
	α_{2c}	Basal ganglia, cortex, cerebellum, hippocampus	Modulates dopamine neurotransmission Inhibits hormone release from adrenal medulla
β-Adrenergic receptors	β_1	Heart, kidney, skeletal muscle, cortex, olfactory nucleus, brain stem	Positive inotropic and chronotropic effects
	β_2	Bronchial and gastrointestinal smooth muscle, blood vessels, heart, lung, skeletal muscle, cortex	Smooth muscle relaxation, skeletal muscle hypertrophy
	β_3	Adipose tissue, gastrointestinal tract, gallbladder, urinary bladder	Lipolysis, thermogenesis, relaxation of the bladder

Tissue localization and dominant effects (after Goodman & Gillman's 2011, modified).

Table 1. Types and subtypes of adrenergic receptors.

Adrenergic receptors were described for the first time by Ahlquist in 1948, who hypothesized the existence of two different types of receptors, α and β, based on the consideration that adrenaline, noradrenaline, and other pharmacological agonists regulate various physiological functions [1]. This differentiation of receptors was confirmed by the finding that there are antagonists, which selectively block α receptors (e.g., phenoxybenzamine or phentolamine) or β receptors (e.g., propranolol). Every type of adrenergic receptors has different subtypes, which are mentioned in **Table 1** [2–4].

1.1. Beta-3 adrenergic receptor discovery and structure

In the early 1980s, Tan S and Curtis-Prior PB proposed the term of beta-3 or beta-hybrid receptor for a new type of beta-adrenergic receptor, based on some studies of four beta-adrenergic agonists on isolated rat adipose cells. They observed that lipolytic potency decreased in the order: isoprenaline (beta-1 and beta-2 agonist) > noradrenaline (beta-1 >>> beta-2 agonist) > salbutamol (beta-2 agonist) > prenalterol (beta-1 agonist). They also studied the effects of some beta-antagonists on lipolysis induced by various agonists. Propranolol (nonselective beta-antagonist) was more potent than betaxolol (selective beta-1 antagonist) or ICI 118551 (selective beta-2 antagonist). All results conducted to the idea that lipolysis in adipose tissue is regulated by other adrenergic receptor than the classical ones, beta-1 and beta-2 [5].

In 1989, Emorine et al. first characterized beta-3 receptor by discovering the gene that encodes it [6]. Before that Arch et al. observed that some nonspecific classical beta-receptor agonists, named BRL 26830A, BRL 33725A, and BRL 35135A, had antiobesity actions on obese and diabetic mice [7].

Further studies have shown that beta-3 receptor is different than beta-1 and beta-2 by some important issues:

- the specific agonists CL 316243 and BRL37344 stimulate only beta-3 receptor [8, 9];
- lack of beta-3 receptor desensitization after agonists activation [10]; and
- the need to use larger quantities of catecholamines to stimulate beta-3 receptors [11].

The structures of beta-1, beta-2, and beta-3 receptors are similar, being all members of G protein-coupled receptors. Beta-3 receptor is a protein which contains 396 amino acids, found in seven transmembrane segments, with three intracellular and three extracellular loops. The amino-terminal region is extracellular, glycosylated, and with variable length. The carboxyl-terminal region is intracellular and it does not possess phosphorylation sites, which are present at beta-1 and beta-2 receptors. Essential for interaction with the ligands are the disulfide bond between the second and the third extracellular loops and also four of the seven transmembrane segments. Other two segments are implicated in G-protein stimulation, with adenylate cyclase and second messenger activation [12].

1.2. Metabolic effects of beta-3 adrenergic receptor stimulation

Some of the most important effects of beta-3 receptor activation are the metabolic ones, especially in the brown adipose tissue. This thermogenic tissue has the role of keeping constant body core temperature of small animals at cold ambient temperatures. Stimulation of beta-3 adrenergic receptors not only activates brown adipose tissue thermogenesis in the short term, but also increases mitochondrial biogenesis and the expression of thermogenin

(UCP1) [13–15]. This protein mediates transport across the internal mitochondrial membrane and interrupts oxidative phosphorylation of the beta oxidation of fatty acids, increasing the use of energy [16]. There have been investigations about the effects of beta-3 adrenergic agonists on thermogenin. The results have shown that beta-3 agonists activated thermogenin, and also other uncoupling proteins, as follows:

- UCP2 that is found in many tissues.
- UCP3 that is found in skeletal muscle and has an important role in basal thermogenesis [17].

The stimulation of thermogenesis by beta-3 adrenergic agonists resulted in a number of experimental studies, which have shown that in animals, these substances lead to weight loss, a selective fat decrease, but without reducing food intake [18].

An *in vitro* study was performed on cells with high levels of beta-3 adrenoreceptors such as the adipocytes of the murine cell line 3T3-F442A. The study demonstrated that insulin and glucocorticoids downregulate beta-3 adrenoreceptor expression through a transcriptional effect. The impairment of beta-3 adrenoceptor gene expression in adipocytes of congenitally obese ob/ob mice could be related to the higher glucocorticoid plasma levels when compared to lean mice [19].

The main studied metabolic actions in preclinical research of beta-3 adrenergic agonists were the reduction of plasma insulin levels, increase glucose tolerance, and reducing body weight in obese diabetic rats. The major implication of beta-3 adrenergic receptor in glucose metabolism and hence in the release of insulin and in obesity has been demonstrated [20, 21].

The development of beta-3 adrenergic agonists was a step forward for the treatment of metabolic diseases by sympathetic activation, because norepinephrine and other relative nonselective derivatives have cardiovascular side effects which limit their use.

1.3. Preclinical studies of beta-3 agonists on carbohydrate and lipid metabolism

Numerous nonclinical studies have shown that administration of beta-3 agonists decreased glucose and lipids plasma concentrations in diabetic mice derived from genetically modified strains (kk, C57BL/KsJ- db/db) or in rats with experimentally induced diabetes [22, 23].

Several mechanisms of action were highlighted and reported:

- improving insulin resistance and increased tissue response to insulin [24],
- increasing insulin secretion in beta cells of the pancreas [25],
- decrease in glucose release from the liver, increase noninsulin-dependent uptake of glucose from white and brown adipose tissue and skeletal muscles [26], and
- increase of glucose tolerance at doses lower than those that stimulate lipolysis in adipose tissue, without affecting the amount of food intake or body weight [27].

The nonclinical research for proving the effects of beta-3 agonists on obesity were conducted on rodent species [28–30] from various strains, both normal and genetically modified to generate predisposition to obesity.

Studies in obese rats treated with the selective beta-3 adrenergic agonists have shown a significant reduction in body weight and reduction of adipose tissue, without food intake being affected by them. It was also demonstrated that an increase of two to three times of the mRNA level and of UCP-type protein, as well as of the guanidine 5'-diphosphate coupled, a relevant index of thermogenesis, in brown and white adipose tissues for the tested rats. In addition, it has been found, after the administration of beta-3 adrenergic agonists, an improvement of glucose tolerance and a decrease of hyperinsulinemia. The researchers suggested two possible mechanisms for defining this aspect, increase of the number of insulin receptors or decrease of glucose transporters in brown and white adipose tissues, which implies an increase in glucose uptake into muscle tissue [31].

Lorente Ferrer et al. investigated the effect of beta-3 receptors agonists on thermogenesis in deep adipose tissue. In general, these agonists increase energy consumption but their effects are quickly counteracted by glucocorticoids. Thus, their potential for long-term treatment of obesity is reduced. Since the metabolic effects of beta-3 receptor agonists (β_3A) overlap only partially with those of oleoyl-estrone (OE) (loss of appetite, weight change, loss of body fat), the possibility of combining them in the energy balance in order to accelerate the decrease of fat deposits was studied. Rats receiving OE or OE + β_3A significantly reduced weight compared with the control group, the maximum reduction corresponding to the group which received the combination [32].

The effect of beta-3 adrenergic receptor agonists was investigated on two strains of rats with different genetic predisposition to obesity: male rats aged 8 weeks Osborne Mendel (OM) strain and S5B/P1 (S5B) strain. Animals were treated with beta-3 adrenergic agonist CL316243 after they have been adapted to either a high fat diet (56% fat-based energy) or low fat (10% fat-based energy), but both equivalent diets in terms of protein content (24% based on protein energy). The animals were fed *ad libitum* and were injected with CL316243 in three doses: 0.1; 0.3; and 3 mg/kg at the beginning of the night. Food intake was measured at 1, 3, and 24 hours after injection. The results showed that CL316243 significantly reduced food intake for all measurements, in both types of rats. Inhibition of food intake was still higher in S5B-type mice. CL316243 significantly decreased serum leptin and serum glucose at both types of rats, especially at S5B. In OM rats, beta-3 adrenergic agonist increased serum insulin levels, while in S5B rats fed with a low-fat diet, the level of serum insulin decreased. In another experiment, CL316243 was administered to rats kept fasting overnight. It was observed after 30 minutes a significant reduction in insulin levels in both types, more pronounced in S5B. The glucose level in OM rats decreased after 30 and 60 minutes, while in rats S5B a decrease was observed only after 30 minutes from the administration. Experiments have shown that beta-3 agonist CL316243 has a much more obvious effect on rat strain resistant to obesity induced by high-fat diet [33].

Another study used a transgenic model of mice, lacking beta-3 adrenergic receptors. CL316243 blocked the activation of adenylate cyclase and lipolysis when it was administered to these mice. A modest growth of fat tissues especially in females was observed. These mice showed an increase in the level of mRNA for beta-1 receptor, but not for receptor beta-2. This showed a functional compensation between the genes for beta-1 and beta-3 receptors. Finally, a sharp increase of insulin levels and lipolysis after administration of CL316243 in normal mice was noted; effects were not found after administration of beta-3 adrenergic agonists in beta-3 receptor-deficient mice [34].

In another model of knockout mice lacking functional beta-3 adrenoreceptors, there were no responses for food intake and insulin secretion in white and brown adipocytes after administration of beta-3 adrenergic agonist CL316243, indicating the implication of beta-3 receptors in these metabolic effects [35].

An increase in insulin levels during "fasted/fed" transition in rats has been demonstrated, associated with a decrease in the mRNA level of beta-3 adrenergic receptor and a decrease of the response in brown and white adipose tissues. It was concluded that there is a close relationship between the food intake, plasma levels of insulin, and beta-3 adrenergic receptors. Downregulation of the beta-3 receptors could be a possible mechanism by which insulin determines lipid storage and prevents lipid mobilization after food intake [36].

In another study, CL316243 was administered in obese diabetic KKAy mice for 2 weeks. The results showed a decrease of serum levels of glucose, insulin, triglyceride, free fatty acid, and tumor necrosis factor-alpha (TNF-alpha) and an increase of adiponectin. The beta-3 adrenergic receptor agonist recovered the mRNA expressions of adiponectin, adiponectin receptors, and beta-3 adrenoreceptor, which were reduced in epididymal white adipose tissue in KKAy mice. Also, CL316243 suppressed the overexpressed mRNA level of TNF-alpha in both epididymal white and brown adipose tissues. It was concluded that the normalization of adiponectin, adiponectin receptors and TNF-alpha could contribute at the amelioration of obesity-induced insulin resistance [28].

In the study conducted on nonobese/nondiabetic Sprague-Dawley rats, the selective beta-3 agonist CL 312243 increased food intake, metabolic rate, and body temperature after 7 days of treatment. The author also showed a decrease in intra-abdominal and subepithelial fat, a hepatic glucose level independent of variations in body weight, an increase in interscapular fat, and in total glucose, which stimulates the production of insulin. According to the results, only white and brown adipose tissues have been affected. A more important role of adipose tissue in glucose uptake underlining the potential role of beta-3 adrenergic agonist drugs for the treatment of obesity and insulin-resistant diabetes was suggested [8].

By a critical analysis of the published data in nonclinical research, it was concluded that beta-3 adrenergic receptor activation in the experiment-induced diabetes and obesity [37, 38] determines an increase of glucose tolerance and lipolysis activation in adipose tissue [22]. It seems that the effects are dose dependent and the selectivity of actions for glucose metabolism occurs at lower doses than those used for influencing lipid metabolism.

Comparing the effects of beta-3 agonists in rats and humans, Arch and Wilson stated that these compounds, with remarkable effects on rodents, have not convinced in clinical studies because of limited efficacy or serious side effects. The explanations mentioned by the authors included low pharmacokinetic properties and a low biotransformation to active compounds. A possible more important distinction between rats and humans is the different structure of beta-3 receptors, leading to lower efficacy of compounds in humans than in rats. In addition, it seems that the number of beta-3 receptors is lower than beta-1 and beta-2 receptors in the tissues that mediate thermogenesis in humans [39]. This is one of the reasons why the clinical studies conducted on beta-3 selective agonists had some contradictory results.

Mirabegron, a currently approved drug for the treatment of overactive bladder, was recently studied in humans for its effects on brown adipose tissue. This drug has several advantages over other members of its class, including a higher bioavailability and a higher *in vitro* affinity for the human beta-3 adrenoreceptor. Mirabegron was orally administered in the dose of 200 mg to 12 healthy male subjects with detectable brown adipose tissue. The results showed that all treated subjects had a higher brown adipose tissue metabolic activity, measured with ^{18}F-fluorodeoxyglucose (^{18}F-FDG) using positron emission tomography (PET) combined with computed tomography (CT). These are promising results for a possible future use of beta3 agonists for metabolic disease [40].

Based on all these preclinical and clinical considerations new chemical entities with beta-phenylethylamine nucleus, substituted in various positions on the nucleus or side chain, with potential action on diabetes and/or obesity were synthesized [41, 42]. Chemists led synthesis in order to obtain derivatives with increased beta-3 receptor selectivity. The compounds were conventionally named A1-βPhEA–A13-βPhEA (**Figure 1**).

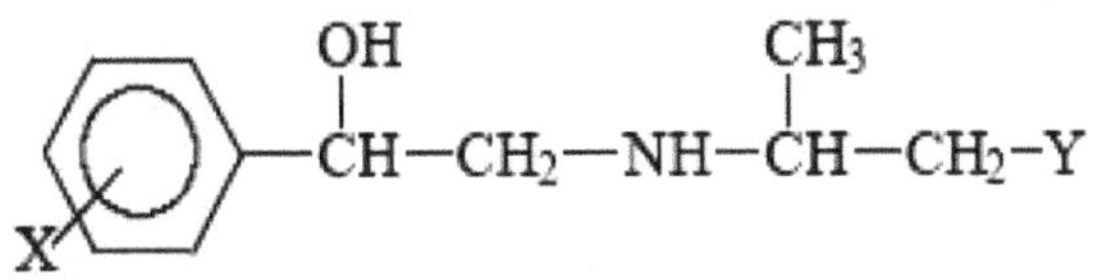

- X = H, alkoxy, halogen, dihalogen
- Y = 4-carbopropoxy-phenoxy, 4-carbomethoxymethylene-phenoxy, 4-carbomethoxyethylene-phenoxy

Figure 1. General structure of the newly synthesized compounds. X = H, alkoxy, halogen, dihalogen; Y = 4-carbopropoxy-phenoxy, 4-carbomethoxymethylene-phenoxy, 4-carbomethoxyethylene-phenoxy.

2. Objectives

The purpose of this study was to test the effects of the newly synthesized compounds over lipid profile and body weight of rats to which alloxanic diabetes was induced, being a known fact that this metabolic disorder induces alterations in plasma lipids.

Alloxan was chosen for induction of type II diabetes mellitus because its pancreatic toxicity was demonstrated in nonclinical trials using isolated islet cell or entire perfused rat pancreas and afterwards by directly administering the substance to rodent or nonrodent animals. In the first stage, alloxan stimulates on short-term insulin secretion, which is followed by total suppression of the response of the islet cells to glucose, regardless of its concentration [43].

Alloxan is readily absorbed by beta pancreatic cell, a process that contributes to diabetogenic action. Its absorption also takes place in liver although hepatocytes are more resilient to its action compared to beta cells, therefore more protected against its toxicity [44].

2.1. Mechanism of alloxan toxicity

The mechanism of toxic action resides in formation of reactive species of oxygen [45], the alloxan exhibiting increased affinity to substrates containing thiolic groups (reduced glutathione, cysteine, proteins with sulfide groups, enzymes) [46]. The product of alloxan reduction, the dialuric acid, is reoxidized to alloxan, the redox cycle thus formed being responsible for releasing superoxide radicals—see **Figure 2** [47].

$$AH_2 + O_2 \rightarrow AH\bullet + O_2{\bullet^-} + H^+$$

$$AH\bullet + O_2 \rightarrow A + O_2{\bullet^-} + H^+$$

$$AH_2 + O_2{\bullet^-} + H^+ \rightarrow AH\bullet + H_2O_2$$

$$AH\bullet + O_2{\bullet^-} + H^+ \rightarrow A + H_2O_2$$

$$H_2O_2 + e^- \rightarrow OH\bullet + OH^-$$

$$Fe^{2+} + H_2O_2 \rightarrow Fe^{3+} + OH\bullet + OH^-$$

$$\text{Net: } O_2{\bullet^-} + H_2O_2 \rightarrow O_2 + OH\bullet + OH^-$$

Figure 2. Mechanism of diabetes induction by administration of alloxan [47]. A, Alloxan; AH·, alloxan radical; AH_2, dialuric acid; $O_2{\cdot^-}$, superoxide radical; OH·, hydroxyl radical.

An optimal protection against cytotoxic action of alloxan and dialuric acid is offered by an association between superoxide-dismutase (SOD) and catalase (CAT), in order to completely prevent the redox cycle and consecutively the formation of any reactive oxygen species [48].

Glucose confers complete protection against toxic effects of alloxan both *in vivo* and *in vitro*, by blocking glucokinase inhibition by it and also contributing to maintaining the antioxidant protection mechanism of the beta cells [49].

One of the targets for the reactive oxygen species is the DNA of the pancreatic islet cells. The DNA fragmentation occurs in beta cells exposed to alloxan [49, 50].

The DNA alteration stimulates poly-ADP-ribose, enzyme which contributes to affected DNA repair. In several trials it was stated that glucose administration contributes to counteracting the alloxan cytotoxicity. Such ability is the result not only of glucokinase protection but also of interaction with glucose carrier GLUT2 resulting in reduced alloxan absorption [51].

3. Materials and methods

Diabetes was induced to white Wistar male rats by intraperitoneal administration of extemporaneously prepared alloxan (Sigma-Aldrich) solution, in the dose of 130 mg/kg weight [52]. After 48 hours, glycemia was determined using ACCU-CHEK Active device (Roche Diagnostics GmbH, D-68298 Mannheim, Germany). The blood was harvested from tail veins by vein puncture. The determination was used for the selection of diabetic animals, thus presenting a glycemia over 200 mg/dL.

From the total rat collectivity, a percentage of 66.34% became diabetic with the remaining 33.66% becoming hyperglycemic. Fifteen groups of diabetic animals were designated for experimental research (eight animals/group), being treated as follows:

- diabetic control group (D Control)—distilled water, 1 mL/100 g weight p.o.;
- reference group—BRL 37344, 50 mg/kg weight, p.o.;
- A1-βPhEA—20 mg/kg weight, p.o.;
- A2-βPhEA—50 mg/kg weight, p.o.; and
- A3-βPhEA through A13-βPhEA, 100 mg/kg weight, p.o.

At the same time, a nondiabetic control group was designated (ND control), treated with distilled water, 1 mL/100 g weight p.o. Administration of tested and reference substances (BRL 37344) continued for 14 days, once daily.

The doses chosen for investigating the metabolic effects of the newly synthesized derivatives were established following previous determinations of acute toxicity which allowed to set the LD_{50} [53, 54].

At the end of the experiment, the animals were sacrificed and biochemical and enzymatic determinations were performed: glycemia, glucose-6-phosphate dehydrogenase (transforming glucose by pentose-phosphate pathway), glucose–6–phosphatase (catalyzes the hydrolysis of glucose–6–phosphate to glucose and inorganic phosphate), hexokinase (catalyzes the phosphorylation of glucose), total cholesterol, LDL cholesterol, HDL cholesterol, and triglycerides.

4. Results and discussion

The model of alloxan-induced diabetes has produced alterations in the activity of the three enzymes [55–57] involved in glucose metabolism homeostasis (**Figure 3**).

Moreover, the lipid profile was altered by the administration of the pancreatic toxic, registering statistically significant increases in total cholesterol, LDL cholesterol, and triglycerides, together with decreases in HDL cholesterol (**Figure 4**).

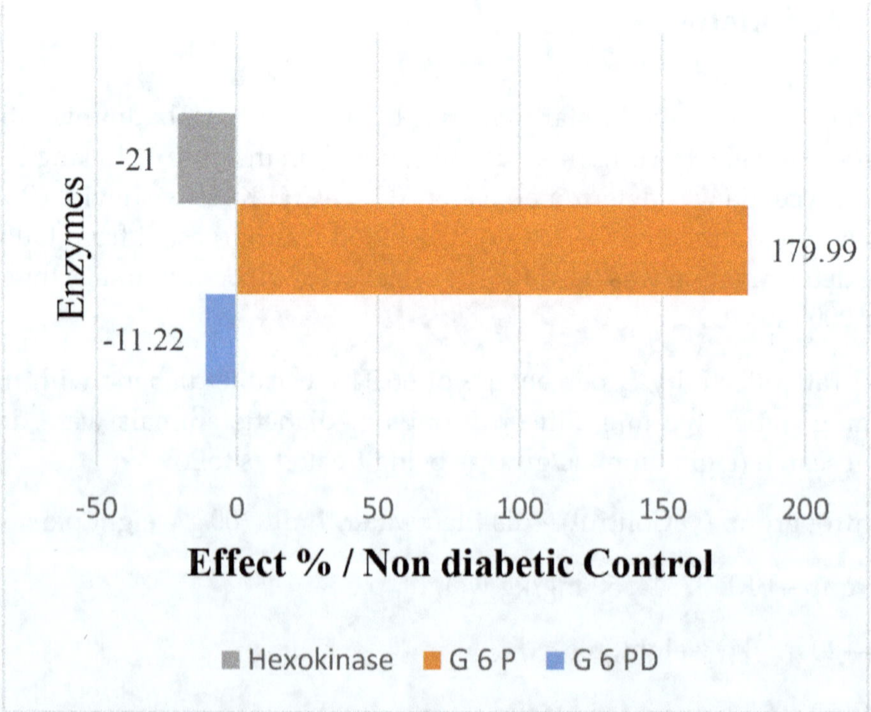

Figure 3. Variations of the activity of the enzymes involved in glucose metabolism in diabetic animals compared to nondiabetic animals.

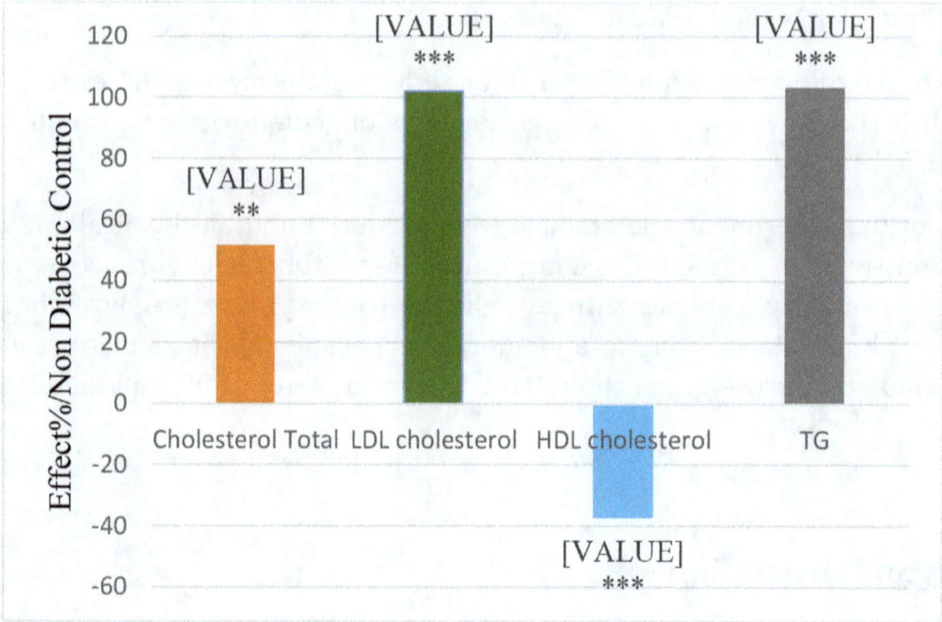

Figure 4. Variation of plasma lipids in diabetic animals compared to nondiabetic animals ** $p<0.01$; *** $p<0.001$.

To what concern the effect of new compounds with possible affinity for beta-3 adrenergic receptors, seven of those (A1-βPhEA, 20 mg/kg weight; A3-βPhEA, 100 mg/kg weight; A4-βPhEA, 100 mg/kg weight; A6-βPhEA, 100 mg/kg weight; A8-βPhEA, 100 mg/kg weight; A9-

βPhEA, 100 mg/kg weight; A13-βPhEA, 100 mg/kg weight) have markedly reduced the values of total cholesterol (**Table 2, Figure 5**).

Group	M ± SE	ANOVA	Dunnett posttest/ND control	ANOVA	Dunnett posttest/D control
Nondiabetic control	78.22 ± 9.553	0.0002***		<0.0001***	**
Diabetic control	119.3 ± 11.89		**		
BRL 37344 50 mg/kg	77.65 ± 2.196		ns		*
A1-βPhEA 20 mg/kg	62.03 ± 5.005		ns		***
A2-βPhEA 50 mg/kg	74.83 ± 13.10		ns		*
A3-βPhEA 100 mg/kg	70.42 ± 9.716		ns		**
A4-βPhEA 100 mg/kg	69.27 ± 6.423		ns		**
A5-βPhEA 100 mg/kg	113.0 ± 11.41		ns		ns
A6-βPhEA 100 mg/kg	61.00 ± 4.749		ns		***
A7-βPhEA 100 mg/kg	75.05 ± 5.286		ns		*
A8-βPhEA 100 mg/kg	72.31 ± 6.148		ns		**
A9-βPhEA 100 mg/kg	69.25 ± 6.542		ns		**
A10-βPhEA 100 mg/kg	77.73 ± 7.884		ns		*
A11-βPhEA 100 mg/kg	66.60 ± 3.331		ns		*
A12-βPhEA 100 mg/kg	75.32 ± 5.966		ns		*
A13-βPhEA 100 mg/kg	62.15 ± 6.673		ns		**

Table 2. The effect of new derivatives of beta-phenylethylamine on total cholesterol in rats with alloxan-induced diabetes * p<0.05; ** p<0.01; *** p<0.001.

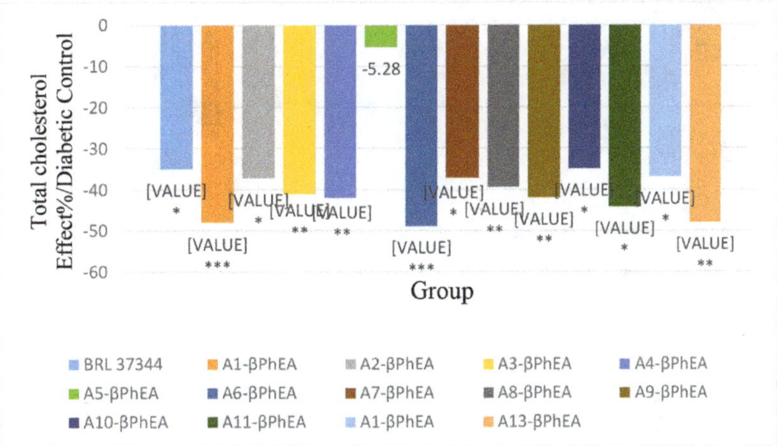

Figure 5. Alterations of total cholesterol in diabetic animals treated with reference substance (BRL 37344) or newly synthesized derivatives of beta-phenyl ethylamine compared to diabetic control group * p<0.05; ** p<0.01; *** p<0.001.

The majority of the tested compounds (**Table 3**) have markedly reduced the values of LDL cholesterol (**Figure 6**), the effect probably due to increased plasma clearance for this lipid fraction as total cholesterol serum concentration decreased. Smaller reductions, still statistically significant (**Table 3**) in values of LDL cholesterol, and comparable to those of the beta-3adrenergic agonist, BRL 37344, were produced by the compounds: A7-βPhEA, A10-βPhEA, A12-βPhEA, and A13-βPhEA (**Figure 6**).

Group	M ± SE	ANOVA	Dunnett posttest/ND control	ANOVA	Dunnett posttest/D control
Nondiabetic control	51.07 ± 3.610	<0.0001***		<0.0001***	***
Diabetic Control	103.2 ± 7.899		***		
BRL 37344 50 mg/kg	78.71 ± 4.940		ns		**
A1-βPhEA 20 mg/kg	56.87 ± 1.887		ns		***
A2-βPhEA 50 mg/kg	57.47 ± 2.831		ns		***
A3-βPhEA 100 mg/kg	50.91 ± 1.205		ns		***
A4-βPhEA 100 mg/kg	57.08 ± 2.302		ns		***
A5-βPhEA 100 mg/kg	56.26 ± 2.134		ns		***
A6-βPhEA 100 mg/kg	56.88 ± 2.496		ns		***
A7-βPhEA 100 mg/kg	75.91 ± 6.447		**		***
A8-βPhEA 100 mg/kg	54.62 ± 2.458		ns		***
A9-βPhEA 100 mg/kg	53.70 ± 2.128		ns		***
A10-βPhEA 100 mg/kg	76.00 ± 7.567		**		***
A11-βPhEA 100 mg/kg	57.52 ± 3.112		ns		***
A12-βPhEA 100 mg/kg	66.77 ± 7.334		ns		***
A13-βPhEA 100 mg/kg	50.21 ± 1.188		ns		***

Table 3. The effect of new derivatives of beta-phenylethylamine on LDL cholesterol values in alloxan-induced diabetic rats ** p<0.01; *** p<0.001.

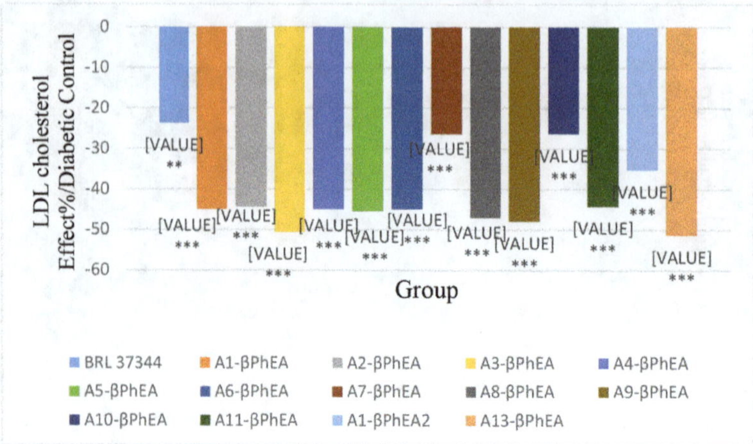

Figure 6. Alterations of LDL cholesterol values in diabetic animals treated with reference substance (BRL 37344) or new derivatives of beta-phenylethylamine compared to diabetic control group ** p<0.01; *** p<0.001.

The results for lowered total cholesterol and LDL cholesterol are in line with other literature data showing that several beta-3adrenergic agonists have induced similar effects in mice with apolipoprotein E deficiency and in wild C57BL/6J strain animals. For such substances an increase in apolipoprotein A1 and PPARα and PPARγ receptors (peroxisome proliferator-activated receptor) expression in liver was demonstrated [58].

Other trials showed that, due to effects on lipid metabolism but also to glycemia reduction, the β_3 adrenergic agonist BRL 37344 has induced a reduction in the process of formation of atherosclerotic plaque in ApoE(-/-) mice [59].

A pivotal role in slowing down the process of atherosclerosis stands with HDL cholesterol, which is a small size alpha-lipoprotein, formed in liver or shed from chylomicrons dismemberment. These lipoproteins have a cholesterol-rich core with type 1 and 2 apolipoproteins at the surface, ensuring the reverse transport of cholesterol, from tissues to liver. The trial conducted by Shi et al. demonstrated the increases in mARN and apoA1 expression.

Group	M ± SE	ANOVA	Dunnett posttest/ND control	ANOVA	Dunnett posttest/D control
Nondiabetic control	46.36 ± 2.930	<0.0001***		<0.0001***	***
Diabetic control	29.34 ± 3.478		***		
BRL 37344 50 mg/kg	34.82 ± 3.216		ns		ns
A1-βPhEA 20 mg/kg	48.09 ± 3.621		ns		***
A2-βPhEA 50 mg/kg	42.96 ± 2.102		ns		*
A3-βPhEA 100 mg/kg	46.24 ± 4.104		ns		***
A4-βPhEA 100 mg/kg	53.35 ± 4.875		ns		***
A5-βPhEA 100 mg/kg	49.79 ± 2.926		ns		***
A6-βPhEA 100 mg/kg	46.07 ± 3.679		ns		***
A7-βPhEA 100 mg/kg	52.18 ± 3.653		ns		***
A8-βPhEA 100 mg/kg	51.04 ± 1.662		ns		***
A9-βPhEA 100 mg/kg	47.81 ± 4.664		ns		***
A10-βPhEA 100 mg/kg	45.66 ± 4.880		ns		***
A11-βPhEA 100 mg/kg	38.04 ± 2.596		ns		ns
A12-βPhEA 100 mg/kg	38.46 ± 2.095		ns		ns
A13-βPhEA 100 mg/kg	41.94 ± 1.330		ns		*

Table 4. The effect of new derivatives of beta-phenyl ethylamine on HDL cholesterol in rats with alloxan-induced diabetes * $p<0.05$; *** $p<0.001$.

The results of the experimental research have shown that all tested compounds have induced statistically significant increases in HDL cholesterol, compared to diabetic control group (**Table 4**). A smaller effect of increase of the values for this lipid fraction was produced by the compounds A11-βPhEA and A12-βPhEA, still being similar to the one for beta$_3$ adrenergic agonist BRL 37344 (**Figure 7**).

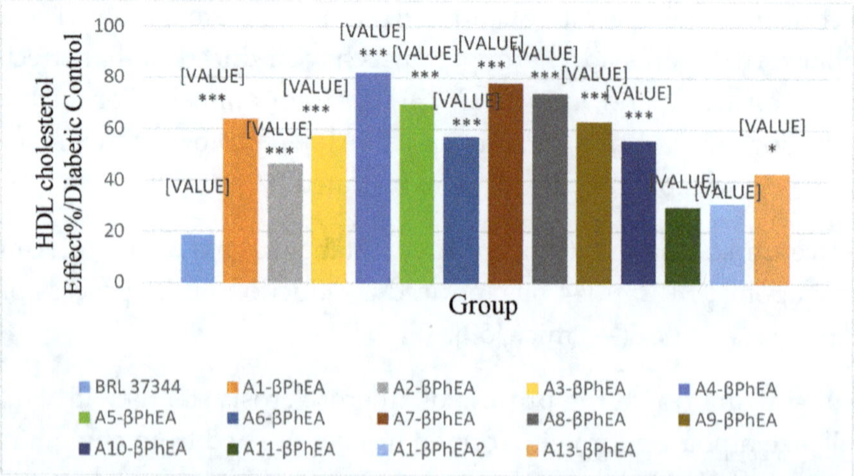

Figure 7. Alteration of HDL cholesterol in diabetic animals treated with reference substance (BRL 37344) or with derivatives of beta-phenylethylamine compared to diabetic control group * $p<0.05$; *** $p<0.001$.

Group	M ± SE	ANOVA	Dunnett posttest/ND control	ANOVA	Dunnett posttest/D control
Nondiabetic control	81.74 ± 2.261	0.0002***		<0.0001***	***
Diabetic control	166.3 ± 6.793		***		
BRL 37344 50 mg/kg	77.13 ± 3.639		ns		***
A1-βPhEA 20 mg/kg	91.25 ± 4.573		ns		***
A2-βPhEA 50 mg/kg	88.01 ± 4.158		ns		***
A3-βPhEA 100 mg/kg	90.23 ± 4.643		ns		***
A4-βPhEA 100 mg/kg	67.38 ± 8.630		ns		***
A5-βPhEA 100 mg/kg	66.32 ± 5.682		ns		***
A6-βPhEA 100 mg/kg	66.58 ± 9.860		ns		***
A7-βPhEA 100 mg/kg	80.60 ± 3.113		ns		***
A8-βPhEA 100 mg/kg	84.24 ± 2.831		ns		***
A9-βPhEA 100 mg/kg	87.80 ± 4.384		ns		***
A10-βPhEA 100 mg/kg	86.21 ± 2.935		ns		***
A11-βPhEA 100 mg/kg	87.86 ± 5.032		ns		***
A12-βPhEA 100 mg/kg	84.35 ± 3.656		ns		***
A13-βPhEA 100 mg/kg	91.25 ± 6.193		ns		***

Table 5. The effect of new derivatives of beta-phenyl ethylamine on serum TG in rats with alloxan-induced diabetes *** $p<0.001$.

In Wistar rats alloxan has induced a high increase, statistically significant, of serum triglycerides (TG) (**Table 5**). Compared to diabetic control group, all the tested compounds have reduced the values of serum triglycerides with high statistical significance. These effects could be due to increased expression [58] of PPARα (liver, kidney, muscle, adipose tissue) and PPAR γ receptors (subtypes 1, 2, 3 in adipose tissue) resulting in increased expression of the gene for lipoprotein lipase.

4.1. Effects on body weight

During the research, animals had free access to standard food and water. The body weight was determined initially, at 48 hours after alloxan administration and then in day 5, 10, and 14 of the experiment. For nondiabetic control group the same determination were performed as in the case of diabetic groups. The food was dispensed daily in same amounts and body weight was determined before the next feeding.

Throughout this determination it was apparent that alloxan-induced diabetes produces, in 48 hours from administration, a statistically nonsignificant reduction (**Figure 8**) of body weight in treated animals (203.4 ± 0.7004 vs. 205.9 ± 0.7078).

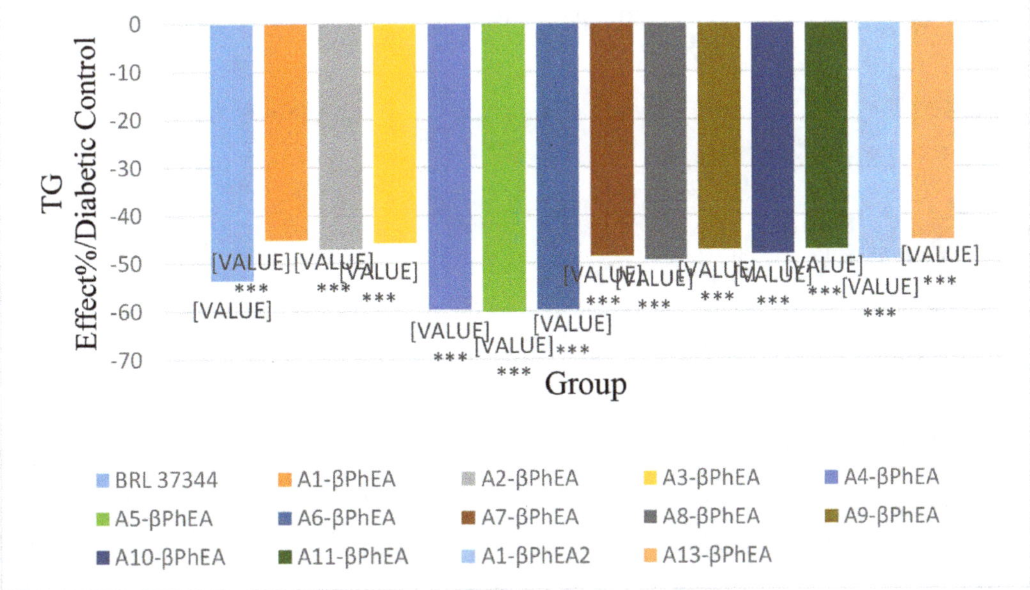

Figure 8. Body weight of animals initially and at 48 hours after alloxan administration *** p<0.001.

The research results showed that, for diabetic control group, animal body weight increases after alloxan administration, reaching a significant higher value in day 14 of the experiment (p = 0.0097**). For the groups treated with reference substance, the body weight varied statistically nonsignificantly in all moments of determination (**Table 6**). The amount of consumed food increased for the diabetic control group, while for the treated groups, it remained constant. In the determinations of day 14, for nondiabetic control group it was registered an increase of 1.07% in body weight against the initial measurement, while for the diabetic control group the increase reached 5.65%. The variation in body weight at the end of the experiment against initial and compared to diabetic control group was calculated using the formulas:

Group	Parameter	Body weight basal	Body weight 48 h after alloxan	Body weight Day 5	Body weight Day 10	Body weight Day 14
ND control	M ± SE	203.8 ± 3.301	200.2 ± 4.176	204.3 ± 2.894	205.5 ± 2.766	206.0 ± 2.733
	ANOVA/48 h	0.7341 ns				
D control	M ± SE	203.2 ± 3.429	197.0 ± 3.967	206.5 ± 2.363	209.7 ± 2.305	214.7 ± 1.382**
	ANOVA/48 h after A	0.0097**				
BRL 37344	M ± SE	204.3 ± 2.963	198.7 ± 3.920	203.8 ± 2.868	202.7 ± 2.246	201.5 ± 2.513
	ANOVA/48 h after A	0.6778 ns				
A1-βPhEA	M ± SE	202.5 ± 2.872	197.2 ± 3.640	201.7 ± 2.836	200.8 ± 3.114	199.8 ± 3.092
	ANOVA/48 h after A	0.7823 ns				
A2-βPhEA	M ± SE	200.2 ± 3.781	195.5 ± 4.123	198.5 ± 3.667	198.7 ± 3.556	199.0 ± 3.540
	ANOVA/48 h after A	0.9238 ns				
A3-βPhEA	M ± SE	208.0 ± 2.206	201.8 ± 3.936	206.0 ± 2.145	205.5 ± 2.247	205.0 ± 2.556
	ANOVA/48 h after A	0.6202 ns				
A4-βPhEA	M ± SE	204.8 ± 2.701	199.5 ± 3.805	202.8 ± 2.651	203.2 ± 2.151	202.0 ± 3.088
	ANOVA/48 h after A	0.4047 ns				
A5-βPhEA	M ± SE	207.2 ± 2.868	201.1 ± 4.083	206.0 ± 3.044	204.7 ± 2.552	206.7 ± 3.232
	ANOVA/48 h after A	0.6717 ns				
A6-βPhEA	M ± SE	205.0 ± 2.966	199.1 ± 3.973	203.2 ± 2.868	202.5 ± 2.754	202.0 ± 2.781
	ANOVA/48 h after A	0.7505 ns				
A7 -βPhEA	M ± SE	206.7 ± 2.552	201.1 ± 3.989	204.8 ± 2.358	204.2 ± 2.167	203.7 ± 2.290
	ANOVA/48 h after A	0.7213 ns				
A8-βPhEA	M ± SE	204.8 ± 1.990	201.7 ± 3.802	203.5 ± 1.586	202.7 ± 1.926	203.7 ± 2.290
	ANOVA/48 h after A	0.9261 ns				
A9 -βPhEA	M ± SE	208.2 ± 1.249	202.1 ± 3.667	205.5 ± 0.7638	204.7 ± 1.022	203.8 ± 1.558
	ANOVA/48 h after A	0.3638 ns				
A10-βPhEA	M ± SE	206.3 ± 2.741	200.8 ± 4.036	205.0 ± 2.477	204.8 ± 2.587	204.0 ± 2.671
	ANOVA/48 h after A	0.7431 ns				
A11-βPhEA	M ± SE	208.0 ± 3.066	202.2 ± 4.401	206.2 ± 2.738	205.8 ± 2.713	205.7 ± 2.813
	ANOVA/48 h after A	0.7922 ns				
A12-βPhEA	M ± SE	207.3 ± 2.894	201.7 ± 4.234	205.7 ± 2.565	205.3 ± 2.603	204.5 ± 2.320
	ANOVA/48 h after A	0.7561 ns				
A13-βPhEA	M ± SE	209.3 ± 2.591	203.0 ± 4.244	206.7 ± 2.028	206.7 ± 2.390	205.0 ± 2.266
	ANOVA/48 h after A	0.6257 ns				

ns, nonsignificant; A, alloxan.

Table 6. The effect of new derivatives of beta-phenylethylamine on body weight in rats with alloxan-induced diabetes ** $p<0.01$.

$$\text{Effect }\%\frac{\text{BW}}{\text{basal}}=\frac{\text{BW basal}(\text{g})-\text{BW day14}(\text{g})}{\text{BW basal}(\text{g})}\times 100 \tag{1}$$

$$\begin{aligned}&\textit{Effect \% BWSubstance / Diabetic control } = \textit{Effect \% BW}\\&\textit{Diabetic control } + \textit{ Effect \% BW Substance}\end{aligned} \tag{2}$$

Taking into account that body weight increased for the animals in diabetic control group and that for all tested substances it has decreased against initial, the effect of the tested substances was determined compared to diabetic control group (**Figure 9**). It was therefore noted that newly synthesized derivatives of beta-phenyl ethylamine and the reference substance BRL 37344 had produced decreases in body weight between 5.89 and 7.76%, compared to diabetic control animals after 14 days of treatment.

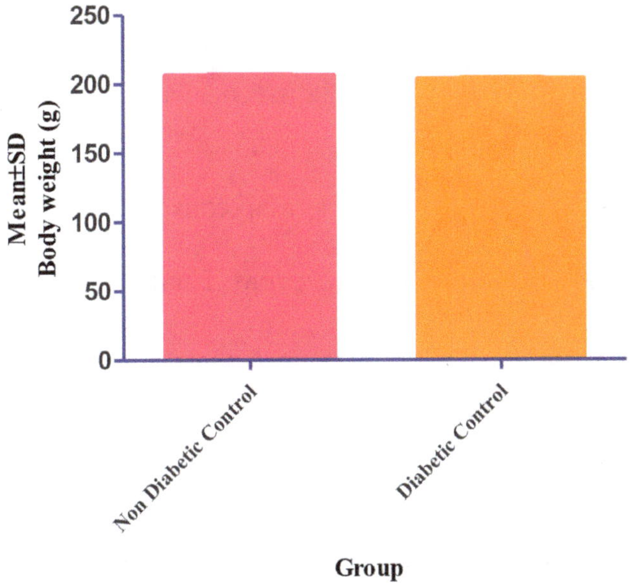

Figure 9. Variation of body weight for animals treated with reference substance and tested substances compared to diabetic control group at day 14 determination.

5. Conclusions

The results of this experimental research have demonstrated that newly synthesized derivatives of beta-phenylethylamine produce marked biological activity over lipid profile which is altered in diabetes induced by alloxan administration in rats.

All tested compounds have markedly decreased the values of total cholesterol, LDL cholesterol, and triglycerides, the effect being more intense than with reference substance BRL 37344. They also have increased the values of antiatherogenic HDL cholesterol, significantly more than the reference substance. Overall, the activity on body weight was of reduction even if the food consumption of the animals was not altered. These experimental data suggest that the tested new chemical entities have high therapeutical potential in the treatment of dislipidemias and/or obesity.

Acknowledgements

The authors acknowledge the contribution of INDCF Bucharest scientific collective who performed the chemical synthesis for the tested compounds and with whom have collaborated previously in two Romanian national research projects: CEEX 51/2005 şi PC NR. 1750/2008.

Author details

Simona Negreş, Cornel Chiriţă*, Andreea Letiţia Arsene, Denisa Margină, Elena Moroşan and Cristina Elena Zbârcea

*Address all correspondence to: chirita.cornel@gmail.com

University of Medicine and Pharmacy "Carol Davila", Faculty of Pharmacy, Bucharest, Romania

References

[1] Ahlquist RP. A study of the adrenotropic receptors. The American Journal of Physiology, 1948; 153(3):586–600. PMID 18882199

[2] Westfall TC, Westfall DP. Neurotransmission: The autonomic and somatic motor nervous systems. Chap. 8, in: Goodman and Gilman`s The Pharmacological Basis of Therapeutics. 12th Ed., McGraw-Hill; 2011. pp. 203–204.

[3] Graham RM, Perez DM, Hwa J, Piascik MT. α_1-Adrenergic receptor subtypes. Molecular structure, function, and signaling. Circulation Research, 1996; 78:737–749. DOI: 10.1161/01.RES.78.5.737

[4] Sawa M, Harada H. Recent developments in the design of orally bioavailable β3-adrenergic receptor agonists. Current Medicinal Chemistry, 2006; 13(1):25–37. DOI: 10.2174/ 092986706775198006

[5] Tan S, Curtis-Prior PB. Characterization of the beta-adrenoreceptor of the adipose cell of the rat. International Journal of Obesity, 1983; 7(5):409–414. PMID: 6139348

[6] Emorine LJ, Marullo S, Briend-Sutren MM, Patey G, Tate K, Delavier-Klutchko C, Strosberg AD. Molecular characterization of the human beta 3-adrenergic receptor. Science, 1989; 245(4922):1118–1121. DOI: 10.1126/science.2570461

[7] Arch JR, Ainsworth AT, Cawthorne MA, Piercy V, Sennitt MV, Thody VE, Wilson C, Wilson S. Atypical beta-adrenoceptor on brown adipocytes as target for anti-obesity drugs. Nature, 1984; 309(5964):163–165. PMID: 6325935

[8] de Souza CJ, Hirshman MF, Horton ES. CL-316,243, a beta3-specific adrenoceptor agonist, enhances insulin-stimulated glucose disposal in nonobese rats. Diabetes, 1997; 46(8):1257–1263. PMID: 9231648

[9] Martin CA, Naline E, Manara L, Advenier C. Effects of two beta 3-adrenoceptor agonists, SR 58611A and BRL 37344, and of salbutamol on cholinergic and NANC neural contraction in guinea-pig main bronchi in vitro. British Journal of Pharmacology, 1993; 110(4):1311–1316. PMC2175861

[10] Carpéné C, Galitzky J, Collon P, Esclapez F, Dauzats M, Lafontan M. Desensitization of beta-1 and beta-2, but not beta-3, adrenoceptor-mediated lipolytic responses of adipocytes after long-term norepinephrine infusion. Journal of Pharmacology and Experimental Therapeutics, 1993; 265(1):237–247. PMID: 8097243

[11] Galitzky J, Reverte M, Portillo M, Carpéné C, Lafontan M, Berlan M. Coexistence of beta 1-, beta 2-, and beta 3-adrenoceptors in dog fat cells and their differential activation by catecholamines. American Journal of Physiology, 1993; 264:E403–E412. PMID: 8096365

[12] Coman OA, Păunescu H, Ghiță I, Coman L, Bădărău A, Fulga I. Beta 3 adrenergic receptors: Molecular, histological, functional and pharmacological approaches. Romanian Journal of Morphology and Embryology, 2009; 50(2):169–179. PMID: 19434307

[13] Betz MJ, Enerbäck S. Human brown adipose tissue: What we have learned so far. Diabetes, 2015; 64:2352–2360. DOI: 10.2337/db15-0146

[14] Fisher MH, Amend AM, Bach TJ, Barker JM,Brady EJ, Candelore MR, Carroll D, Cascieri MA,Chiu SH, Deng L, Forrest MJ, Hegarty-Friscino B, Guan XM, Hom GJ, Hutchins JE, Kelly LJ, Mathvink RJ, Metzger JM, Miller RR, Ok HO, Parmee ER, Saperstein R, Strader CD, Stearns RA, Macintyre DE. A selective human beta3 adrenergic receptor agonist increases metabolic rate in rhesus monkeys. Journal of Clinical Investigation, 1998; 101(11):2387–2393. DOI: 10.1172/JCI2496

[15] Klaus S, Seivert A, Boeuf S. Effect of beta 3 adrenergic agonist C1316,243 on functional differentiation of with and brown adipocytes in primary cell culture. Biochimica and Biophysica Acta, 2001; 1539:85–92. PMID: 11389970

[16] Ursino MG, Vasinaa V, Raschia E, Cremab F, De Pontia F. The beta 3- adrenoceptor as a therapeutic target: Current perspectives. Pharmacological Research, 2009; 59:221–234. DOI: 10.1016/j.phrs.2009.01.002

[17] Nedergaard J, Cannon B. The "novel" "uncoupling" proteins UCP2 and UCP3: What do they really do? Pros and cons for suggested functions. Experimental Physiology, 2003; 88(1):65–84. PMID: 12525856

[18] Sleigh SH, Barton CL. Repurposing strategies for therapeutics. Pharmaceutical Medicine, 2010; 24(3):151–159. DOI: 10.1007/BF03256811

[19] Langin D, Tavernier G, Lafontan M. Regulation of beta 3-adrenoreceptor expression in white fat cells. Fundamental and Clinical Pharmacology, 1995; 9(2):97–106. PMID: 7628838

[20] Oana F, Takeda H, Matsuzawa A, Akahane S, Isaji M, Akahane M. Adiponectin receptor 2 expression in liver and insulin resistance in db/db mice given a beta 3 adrenoreceptor agonist. European Journal of Pharmacology, 2005; 518:71–76. DOI:10.1016/j.ejphar.2005.06.004

[21] Bhadada SV, Patel BM, Mehta AA, Goyal RK. β(3) Receptors: Role in cardiometabolic disorders. Therapeutic Advances in Endocrinology and Metabolism, 2011; 2(2):65–79. DOI: 10.1177/2042018810390259

[22] Kenji O, Matsui H, Yasuhiro O, Ryotaro T, Kenichiro M, Hajime I, Akiko I, Tomofumi M, Michitaka T, Yoko K. The polymorfism of the beta 3 adrenergic receptor gene is associated with reduced low-density lipoprotein particle size. Metabolism, 2003; 52(3): 356–361. DOI: 10.1053/meta.2003.50056

[23] Oana F, Takeda H, Matsuzawa A, Akahane S, Hayashi M, Tamura T, Uehara M, Isaji M, Akahane M. KTO-7924, a Beta3-adrenergic receptor agonist, reduces hyperglycemia and protects beta-cells in the islets of Langerhans of db/db mice. Endocrine Research. 2010; 35(4):174–182. DOI: 10.3109/07435800.2010.507733

[24] Ghorbani M, Shafiee Ardestani M, Gigloo SH, Cohan RA, Inanlou DN, Ghorbani P. Antidiabetic effect of CL 316,243 (a β3-adrenergic agonist) by down regulation of tumour necrosis factor (TNF-α) expression. PLoS One. 2012;7(10):e45874. DOI: 10.1371/journal.pone.0045874

[25] Pang Z, Wu N, Zhang X, Avallone R, Croci T, Dressler H, Palejwala V, Ferrara P, Tocci M, Polites G. GPR40 is partially required for insulin secretion following activation of beta 3-adrenergic receptors. Molecular and Cellular Endocrinology, 2010; 325:18–25. DOI: 10.1016/j.mce.2010.04.014

[26] Watts VL, Sepulveda FM, Cingolani OH, Ho AS, Niu X, Kim R, Miller KL, Vandegaer K, Bedja D, Gabrielson KL, Rameau G, O`Rourke B, Kass DA, Barouch LA. Anti-hypertrophic and anti-oxidant effect of beta3-adrenergic stimulation in myocytes requires differential neuronal NOS phosphorylation. Journal of Molecular and Cellular Cardiology, 2013; 62:8–17. DOI: 10.1016/j.yjmcc.2013.04.025

[27] Sen A, Nichani VN. Exploring beta 3 adrenoreceptors for potential clinical applications. International Journal of Pharmaceutical Sciences Review and Research, 2010; 5(3):55–58.

[28] Fu L, Isobe K, Zeng Q, Suzukawa K, Takekoshi K, Kawakami Y. The effects of beta(3)-adrenoceptor agonist CL-316,243 on adiponectin, adiponectin receptors and tumor necrosis factor-alpha expressions in adipose tissues of obese diabetic KKAy mice. European Journal of Pharmacology, 2008; 584(1):202–206. DOI: 10.1016/j.ejphar.2008.01.028

[29] Kanzler SA, Januario AC, Paschoalini MA. Involvement of ß –adrenergic receptors in the control of food intake 3 in rats. Brazilian Journal of Medical and Biological Research, 2011; 44 (11):1141–1147.

[30] Kim-Motoyama H, Yasuda K, Yamaguchi T, Yamada N, Katakura T, Shuldiner AR, Akanuma Y, Ohashi Y, Yazaki Y, Kadowaki T. A mutation of the beta 3-adrenergic receptor is associated with visceral obesity but decreased serumtriglyceride. Diabetologia, 1997; 40(4):469–472. PMID: 9112025

[31] Umekawa T, Yoshida T, Sakane N, Saito M, Kumamoto K, Kondo M. Anti-obesity and anti-diabetic effects of CL316,243, a highly specific beta 3-adrenoceptor agonist, in Otsuka Long-Evans Tokushima fatty rats: Induction of uncoupling protein and activation of glucose transporter 4 in white fat. European Journal of Endocrinology, 1997; 136:429–437. PMID: 9150705

[32] Ferrer-Lorente R, Cabot C, Fernandez Lopez LA, Alemanz M. Combined effects of oleoyl-estrone and beta 3 adrenergic agonist (CL316,243) on lipid stores of diet induced overweight male Wistar rats. Life Sciences, 2005; 77:2051–2058. DOI: 10.1016/j.lfs.2005.04.008

[33] White LC, Ishihara Y, Dotson LT, Hughes DA, Bray GA, York DA. Effect of beta 3 agonist on food intake in two strains of rats that differ in susceptibility to obesity. Physiology & Behavior, 2004; 82:489–496. DOI: 10.1016/j.physbeh.2004.04.059

[34] Susulic VS, Frederich RC, Lawitts J, et al. Targeted disruption of the beta 3-adrenergic receptor gene. J Biol Chem., 1995; 270:29483. PMID: 7493988

[35] Grujic D, Susulic VS, Harper ME, et al. Beta3-adrenergic receptors on white and brown adipocytes mediate beta3-selective agonist-induced effects on energy expenditure, insulin secretion, and food intake. A study using transgenic and gene knockout mice. Journal of Biological Chemistry, 1997; 272:17686. PMID: 9211919

[36] Hadri KE, Charon C, Pairault J, Hauguel-De MS, Quignard B, Feve B. Down-regulation of beta3-adrenergic receptor expression in rat adipose tissue during the fasted/fed transition: Evidence for a role of insulin. Biochemical Journal, 1997; 323:359. PMID: 9163324

[37] Mund RA, Frishman WH. Brown adipose tissue thermogenesis: β3-adrenoreceptors as a potential target for the treatment of obesity in humans. Cardiology in Review, 2013; 21(6):265–269. DOI: 10.1097/CRD.0b013e31829cabff

[38] Sacks H, Symonds ME. Anatomical locations of human brown adipose tissue: Functional relevance and implications in obesity and type 2 diabetes. Diabetes, 2013; 62(6): 1783–1790. DOI: 10.2337/db12-1430

[39] Arch JR, Wilson S. Prospects for beta 3-adrenoceptor agonists in the treatment of obesity and diabetes. International Journal of Obesity and Related Metabolic Disorders, 1996; 20(3):191–199. PMID: 8653138

[40] Cypess AM, Weiner LS, Roberts-Toler C, Elia EF, Kessler SH, Kahn PA, English J, Chatman K, Trauger SA, Doria A, Kolodny GM. Activation of human brown adipose tissue by a β3-adrenergic receptor agonist. Cell Metabolism, 2015; 21(1):33–38. DOI: 10.1016/j.cmet.2014.12.009

[41] Guţă R, Ilie C, Putina G, Nănău-Andreescu D, Negreş S, Caproiu MT. Potential antidiabetic/antiobesity compounds from the beta-3-adrenergic receptors agonists class. Revista de Chimie 2007; 58(10):937–940.

[42] Guţă R, Putina G, Andreescu D, Ghiţă C, Ilie C, Căproiu MT, Negreş S, Chiriţă C. Potential antidiabetes/antiobesity compounds from the beta-3-adrenergic receptors agonists class (II). Revista de Chimie 2012; 63(6): 565–570.

[43] Kliber A, Szkudelski T, Chichlowska J. Alloxan stimulation and subsequent inhibition of insulin release from in situ perfused rat pancreas. Journal of Physiology and Pharmacology, 1996; 47:321–328. PMID: 8807559

[44] Tiedge M, Lortz S, Drinkgern J, Lenzen S. Relation between antioxidant enzyme gene expression and antioxidative defense status of insulin-producing cells. Diabetes, 1997; 46:1733–1742. PMID: 9356019

[45] Heikkila RE, Winston B, Cohen G. Alloxan-induced diabetes-evidence for hydroxyl radical as a cytotoxic intermediate. Biochemical Pharmacology, 1976; 25:1085–1092.

[46] Lenzen S, Munday R. Thiol-group reactivity, lipophilicity, and stability of alloxan, its reduction products and its N-methyl derivatives and a comparison with ninhydrin. Biochemical Pharmacology, 1991; 42:1385–1391. PMID: 1930261

[47] Munday R. Generation of superoxide radical, hydrogen peroxide and hydroxyl radical during the autoxidation of N,N,N',N'-tetramethyl-pphenylenediamine. Chemico-Biological Interactions, 1988; 65:133–143. PMID: 2835187

[48] Lenzen S. Oxidative stress: The vulnerable beta-cell. Biochemical Society Transactions, 2008; 36(Pt 3):343-347. DOI: 10.1042/BST0360343

[49] Sakurai K, Ogiso T. Effect of ferritin on ëDNA strand breaks in the reaction system of alloxan plus NADPH-cytochrome P450 reductase: Ferritin's role in diabetogenic action of alloxan. Biological and Pharmaceutical Bulletin, 1995; 18:262–266. PMID: 7742795

[50] Takasu N, Komiya I, Asawa T. STZ and alloxan induced H_2O_2 generation and DNA fragmentation in pancreatic islets. Diabetes, 1991; 40:1141–1145. PMID: 1834504

[51] Jorns A, Munday R, Tiedge M, Lenzen S. Comparative toxicity of alloxan, N-alkylalloxans and ninhydrin to isolated pancreatic islets in vitro. Journal of Endocrinology, 1997; 155:283–293. PMID: 9415063

[52] Negreş S, Chiriţă C, Moroşan E, Arsene AL. Experimental pharmacological model of diabetes induction with alloxan in rat. Farmacia, 2013; 61(2):313–323.

[53] Negreş S, Chiriţă C, Zbârcea CE, Cristea AN, Moroşan E, Mihele D, Putina G. Experimental pharmacological researches regarding acute toxicity and the efffect on baseline glycaemia of some newly synthetized beta 3 adrenergic receptors agonists. Farmacia, 2007; 6: 662–670.

[54] Negreș S, Dinu M, Ancuceanu RV, Olaru OT, Ghica MV, Șeremet OC, Zbârcea CE, Velescu BȘ, Ștefănescu E, Chiriță C. Correlations in silico/in vitro/in vivo regarding determinating acute toxicity in non-clinical experimental trial, according to bioethic regulations enforced by European union. Farmacia, 2015; 63(6):877–885.

[55] Ansari MA, Gupta BL, Baquer NZ. Changes in insulin receptor, hexokinase and NADPH producing enzymes in Choroid plexus during experimental diabetes. Journal of Biosciences, 1993; 18(3):337–343.

[56] Bugdayci G, Altan N, Sancak B, Bukan N, Kosova F. The effect of the sulfonylurea glyburide on glutathione-S-transferase and glucose-6-phosphate dehydrogenase in streptozotocin-induced diabetic rat liver. Acta Diabetologica, 2006; 43(4):131–134. DOI: 10.1007/s00592-006-0228-0

[57] Ramesh B, Pugalendi KV. Antihyperglycemic effect of umbelliferone in streptozotocin-diabetic rats. Journal of Medicinal Food, 2006; 9(4):562–566. DOI: 10.1089/jmf.2006.9.562

[58] Shi ST, Li YF, Guo YQ, Wang ZH. Effect of beta-3 adrenoceptor stimulation on the levels of ApoA-I, PPARα, and PPARγ in apolipoprotein E-deficient mice. Journal of Cardiovascular Pharmacology, 2014; 64(5):407–411. DOI: 10.1097/FJC.0000000000000133

[59] Wang ZH, Li YF, Guo YQ. β3-Adrenoceptor activation attenuates atherosclerotic plaque formation in ApoE(-/-) mice through lowering blood lipids and glucose. Acta Pharmacologica Sinca, 2013; 34(9):1156–1163. DOI: 10.1038/aps.2013.70

5

Epidemiology of Abdominal Obesity

Maria Teresa Anselmo Olinto,

Heloísa Theodoro and Raquel Canuto

Abdominal obesity (AO) is associated with endothelial dysfunction, inflammation, insulin resistance, diabetes mellitus, hypercholesterolemia, metabolic syndrome, and cancer. AO is a multifactorial disorder arising from genetic, environmental, socioeconomic, and behavioral factors. Thus, in this chapter, we devote ourselves to the exercise of trying to explain the epidemiology of AO in adults. We showed the increasing prevalence of AO around the world, and a gender difference in this determination was observed. Among women, the population group who is the most affected by AO, a higher prevalence of AO is observed in individuals living in low- or middle-income countries (LMIC), who are older, multiparous, and in the menopausal transition, and who belong to the poorest strata and have lower educational level. While among men, the risk of AO is positively associated with socioeconomic status, particularly in LMIC. Regarding behavioral factors (eating frequency, sleep duration, physical activity, and smoking), gender differences are difficult to be detected due to the lack of studies investigating their association with AO according to sex. However, the current evidence suggests that men benefit more from consuming a greater number of meals a day and women are more affected by the harmful effects of physical inactivity. We argued AO, despite biological conditions associated with behavior factors, should be examined as an important issue of gender inequality in health, possibly mediated by socioeconomic and behavioral differences between men and women.

Keywords: abdominal obesity, waist circumference, epidemiology, gender, income

1. Introduction

Obesity is a worldwide epidemic. Beyond the fat mass per se, the pattern of fat distribution has a profound influence on cardiometabolic risk. Visceral abdominal fat (VAF) is metabolically active and pro-inflammatory and presents a higher cardiometabolic risk association and calcification of the coronary arteries than the body mass index (BMI) and has more impact on health than subcutaneous fat, presenting a risk factor for increased incidence of metabolic syndrome [1, 2].

Abdominal obesity (AO) is directly associated with increased VAF, and it is also associated with endothelial dysfunction, inflammation, insulin resistance, diabetes mellitus, hypercholesterolemia, metabolic syndrome [MetS], and cancer [1, 3].

There are several methods available to measure AO. Waist circumference (WC) provides an indicator of central adiposity that is the most practical and easiest method used in large-scale epidemiological studies [4]. It is a good predictor of cardiometabolic morbidity and mortality, and it has also a positive association with visceral abdominal fat. However, WC does not allow us to differentiate between visceral fat and subcutaneous fat; methods such as absorptiometry by dual energy X-ray (DEXA), impedance, or densitometry can be used to handle this differentiation [5–7].

WC measurement requires correct and standardized procedures, which depend mainly on training and adequate equipment. A standardized technique requires that the person being measured removes bulky or tight garments, as well as shoes with heels, empties their bladder then stands in the upright position, with arms loosely positioned to the side. The tape is passed around the body and positioned mid-way between the iliac crest and costal margin of the lower rib, ensuring that it

Population	Organization (References)	Recommended waist circumference threshold for abdominal obesity	
		Men	**Women**
Europid	IDF	≥94 cm	≥80 cm
Caucasian	WHO	≥94 cm [increased risk]≥102 cm [still higher risk]	≥80 cm [increased risk]≥88 cm [still higher risk]
United States	AHA/NHLBI [ATP III]	≥102 cm	≥88 cm
Canada	Health Canada	≥102 cm	≥88 cm
European	European cardiovascular societies	≥102 cm	≥88 cm
Asian [including Japanese]	IDF	≥90 cm	≥80 cm
Asian	WHO	≥90 cm	≥80 cm
Japanese	Japanese obesity society	≥85 cm	≥90 cm
China	Cooperative task force	≥85 cm	≥80 cm
Middle East, Mediterranean	IDF	≥94 cm	≥80 cm
Sub-Saharan African	IDF	≥94 cm	≥80 cm
Ethnic Central and South American	IDF	≥90 cm	≥80 cm

Table 1. Waist circumference cutoffs recommended for the diagnosis of abdominal obesity according to ethnicity and gender [9].

is horizontally oriented and untwisted. The subject is asked to look ahead and breathe out; the measurement is taken at the end of expiration; then, the procedure is repeated [7, 8].

In addition, the definition of cutoffs should consider the characteristics of the study population. In 2009, a method to standardize the diagnosis of metabolic syndrome was established, upon discussions held by the International Diabetes Federation (IDF) and the American Heart Association/National Heart, Lung, and Blood Institute. In this context, it was suggested that ethnicity and gender should be considered for the diagnosis of AO [9] (**Table 1**).

AO is a multifactorial disorder arising from genetic, environmental, socioeconomic, and behavioral factors. These factors differ in their respective contributions to the AO epidemic. In this chapter, we devote ourselves to the exercise of trying to explain the epidemiology of AO. First, we describe the worldwide prevalence of AO. Then, the possible biological and socioeconomic factors that are associated with AO are demonstrated, according to the sex/gender differences. Finally, we describe the role of important behavioral factors determining AO.

2. Prevalence of abdominal obesity

Populations worldwide have faced a growing "epidemics" of AO. Overweight and obesity across low- and middle-income countries (LMIC) have reached levels found in higher-income countries (HIC). Despite its high prevalence, there are differences among regions and countries, and these need to be taken into account for us to understand the etiology of AO.

To better elucidate this picture, **Table 2** depicts the prevalence of AO according to gender in selected high and LMIC. LMIC showed the highest prevalence of AO, compared with HIC; in several studies, an increasing trend of AO in the past 10 years [10, 16, 17] has been observed. For example, in the study called China Health and Nutrition Survey (1993–2009), with 52,621 Chinese adults, the prevalence of AO increased from 8.5 to 27.8% among men and from 27.8 to 45.9% among women [17]. Similarly, in the USA, data from the National Health and Nutrition Examination Survey [NHANES] from 1999 to 2010 identified an increase over time, and the difference between genders was 20% higher for females [10].

Regarding gender, both in LMIC and in HIC, it was observed that women had a higher prevalence of AO than men. Also, recent studies show a higher prevalence of AO in women than men, in all ages. There is a proportional increase in the accumulation of fat in the abdominal region as people get older, but a stabilization or even a small decrease in the prevalence of AO in men after 60 years of age could be perceived [12, 18, 20]. In Brazil, in a study involving data from 3117 subjects, the prevalence of AO was found to be 26 and 73%, respectively, in women aged 24–34 years and 55–65 years. In men, the prevalence of AO was found to be 16.9% (24–34 years) and 27.2% (55–65 years) [20].

But why do women have a higher prevalence of AO than men? On one hand, sex hormones strongly influence body fat distribution and adipocyte differentiation between females and males, showing a physiological difference in the AO determination between sexes. However, in part AO is due to a social construction, since socioeconomic, cultural, and behavioral characteristics play an important role in its causal chain.

Author	Country (year)	Prevalence (%)	Men (%)	Women (%)
High-income countries				
Beltrán-Sánchez et al. [10]	USA (2009–2010)[1]	56.0	46.4	65.4
Gutiérrez-Fisac et al. [11]	Spain (2008–2010)[2]	36.0	32.0	39.0
Riediger and Clara [12]	Canada (2007–2009)[1]	35.0	29.1	40.0
Schienkiewitz et al. [13]	Germany (1997–1999)[1]	33.9	29.7	38.0
Sardinha et al. [14]	Portugal (2008–2009)[2]	–	19.3	37.9
Low-/middle-income countries				
Barquera et al. [15]	Mexico (2010–2012)[3]	74.0	64.5	82.8
Misra and Shivastava [16]	South Asians (2011–2012)[4]	68.9	17.6–62.2	23.7–74.8
Xi et al. [17]	China (2009)[3]	37.4	27.8	45.9
Linhares et al. [18]	Brazil (2010)[1]	30.0	19.5	37.5
Chukwuonye et al. [19]	Nigeria (2013)[1]	21.8	3.2	39.2

Cutoffs of WC for AO = [1]≥102 cm (males) and ≥88 cm (females); [2]>102 cm (males) and >88 cm (females); [3]>90 cm (males) and >80 cm (females); [4]≥90 cm (males) and ≥80 cm (females).

Table 2. Prevalence of AO according to gender in selected high- and low-middle-income countries.

To better understand this topic, it is important to elucidate the differences between sex (biology) and gender (the social). According to Annandale and Hunt [21], this distinction was essential to make it clear that gender inequalities in health were, in the most part, socially produced, rather than biologically given. Olinto [22] also called attention to the operationalization of the gender category in epidemiological studies. Sex only means the genetic, anatomical, and physiological characterization of human beings. However, gender roles are socially constructed and usually framed as an extension of biologically determined social functions. The pioneering feminist Simone de Beauvoir said in her famous quote: "One is not born, but rather becomes, a woman." Though the positions of women and men are not simply parallel, the principle is also true for men: One is not born masculine, but has to become a man [23]. Thus, gender is related to differences in patterns of employment, education, family, and household structure, leisure and consumption at the societal level, and in the everyday experience of individual men and women [21]. In this sense, we describe the possible biological and social factors associated with AO according to gender differences.

3. Physiological differences between the sexes and the characteristics of reproductive life in women

Among the physiological factors related to sex differences, there is a hormonal issue: Sex hormones strongly influence body fat distribution and adipocyte differentiation. Estrogens and testosterone differentially affect the physiology of adipocytes. Visceral fat is higher in men than in premenopausal women. In men, visceral fat accrual generally increases with the amount of total body fat, whereas in women, visceral fat accumulation is less a function of total adiposity. Women had less visceral fat despite having a higher total body fat, BMI, and subcutaneous fat [24–27].

As women reach menopause, depot differences in adipocyte size are attenuated due to the express increase in omental cell size. The propensity of postmenopausal women toward visceral fat accumulation and presence of larger adipocytes suggests that the decline of estrogen may stimulate adipocyte hypertrophy in this depot. In men, adipocytes of the visceral and abdominal subcutaneous fat compartments have similar sizes across the range of adiposity values [24, 28].

In men, a meta-analysis found that those with low concentrations of total testosterone (TT), sex hormone-binding globulin (SHBG), and free testosterone (FT) were more likely to develop metabolic syndrome compared to those having high sex hormone concentrations. The revealed associations were independent of age and lifestyle factors. Associations with TT were strongest for prevalent AO [OR (odds ratio) per quartile decrease = 1.58] (95% CI 1.51–1.66). Low FT concentrations were associated with incident AO [HR (hazard ratio) = 1.13] (95% CI 0.98–1.29), although the latter was not statistically significant [29].

Studies show that the prevention of AO should be focused on lifestyle. However, there are different hormonal factors between the sexes that must be considered, especially for women, whose menopausal transition goes through hormonal changes that favor the redistribution of body fat, being more susceptible to abdominal fat accumulation. Moreover, the life expectancy of women generally exceeds that of men, with a significant increase in the number of women experiencing the menopausal transition phase, which makes this an increasingly relevant issue in terms of public health.

Menarche and menopause set the beginning and the end of women's reproductive life and are important risk factors for chronic diseases, including obesity and cardiovascular disease. Early menarche, before the age of 12, has been associated with a higher prevalence of AO [30–33]. Both early menarche and early menopause can be considered as increased risk factors for cardiovascular disease.

The association between early menarche and obesity is still controversial in the literature. However, some longitudinal studies demonstrated that childhood obesity is the trigger to early pubertal development because of increased exposure to reproductive steroids [estradiol level] [30, 32, 34–36]. Furthermore, many genetic variants associated with the timing of menarche are in or near genes associated with childhood and adulthood obesity, so this fact should be considered [32].

Reproductive life characteristics are directly associated with AO. For example, a cross-sectional study with a sample of 617 women from southern Brazil observed that women with a history of three or more pregnancies and menarche at the age of 11 or earlier had a 25% higher prevalence of AO compared to nulliparous or primiparous women with menarche at 14 years or older [31]. Studies show that the number of parturitions leads to a tendency of decreased hip circumference and increased WC [37–39].

Pregnancy was associated with visceral adiposity gains and central obesity in the study with 122 premenopausal women monitored for 5 years. Throughout the monitoring period, nulliparous women had a 14% increase in the visceral adipose tissue, while those with at least one parturition increased by 40%. Parturition was associated with increased WC. It is suggested that after pregnancy, there is a preference for fat accumulation in the visceral adipose tissue [40]. Similarly, in a sample of 170 American women aged 18–76 years, it has been found that the intra-abdominal fat tissue increased as the number of parturitions increased, regardless of age, body fat percentage, physical activity, and smoking [41].

Changes in the distribution of body fat and AO as a consequence of pregnancy require further investigation. As a modifiable risk factor, weight gain during the pre- and postpartum periods can provide a critical window for performing interventions to prevent substantial weight gain and the development of obesity in women [42].

Epidemiological studies are consistent in the sense that characteristics of reproductive life may have a strong influence on body fat buildup in women during the menopausal transition. The transition from the reproductive phase to the nonreproductive phase is characterized by endocrine changes due to the decline of ovarian activity, biological changes due to decreased fertility, and consequent clinical changes due to menstrual cycle changes, as well as a variety of symptoms [43].

The change in metabolism that accompanies menopausal transition occurs at the expense of a reduction in lipoprotein lipase, responsible, along with estrogen, for regulating fat accumulation and distribution in tissues [44]. Testosterone seems to be a factor influencing the accumulation of visceral adipose tissue, and it seems to be related to the state of hyperandrogenism in women. The accumulation of visceral fat was higher in women after menopause compared to premenopausal women [45].

Several studies have shown a high prevalence of AO in postmenopausal women, ranging from 50 to 85% [31, 46–49]. A systematic review by Mendes et al. [49] found a high prevalence of AO in the menopausal transition, mainly in studies performed in clinics. Among these, the highest prevalence rates were reported in a study based on the Northeast region of Brazil, with 76.6% of premenopausal women and 85.2% of postmenopausal women. The lowest prevalence was found among Asian women, who had prevalence of 16.4% among premenopausal women and of 29.1% among postmenopausal women, suggesting that ethnicity is an outlier factor as far as the accumulation of fat in the abdominal region is concerned, once Western women have a higher prevalence than Eastern women.

The relationship involving women's experience in their reproductive period, their individual characteristics, such as age of menarche and number of parturition, hormonal changes during the menopausal transition, and the accumulation of fat in the abdominal region deserves more attention from health professionals.

4. Socioeconomic status and gender

Gender, as a social construct, plays an important role in the association between socioeconomic characteristics and AO. Socioeconomic status (SES) is a complex and multidimensional construct, in which individuals are classified by being compared to other individuals, based on material and nonmaterial attributes [50]. SES influences the individual access to goods and services regarding nutrition, physical activity, and other healthy practices and environmental conditions, which influence the relationship between socioeconomic position and AO.

Studies have used different SES indicators; nonetheless, we focus primarily on individual characteristics, such as income, education and occupation, and economic development of countries, because they may have greater importance regarding interpretations of linkages between SES and AO which emphasize behavior.

Classic studies showed the direction of association between SES and obesity varied by population and economic status of countries. In developed countries, individuals with lower socioeconomic status were more likely to be obese than those in the higher socioeconomic group. However, in some LMIC the prevalence of obesity has increased among low SES groups, mainly among women. However, Is the association between SES and obesity similar to the association between SES and AO?

Most of these global analyses did not evaluate AO as outcome. This paper aims to show findings on the association between SES and WC in HIC and LMIC. In HIC, a recent study analyzed 50 years of socioeconomic inequities in WC among US-born black and white Americans, using data from the National Health Examination Surveys (NHES) I-III (1959–1970), National Health and Nutrition Examination Surveys (NHANES) I-III [1971–1994], and NHANES 1999–2008. WC increased in socioeconomic strata among both black and white Americans. Regarding income, white people in the 20th [low] income percentile have greater mean WC compared with people in the 80th [high] income percentile [51]. In the same direction, a cross-sectional study carried out with 12,883 individuals representing the Spanish population found that the frequency of obesity and AO decreased as the educational level increased [11]. In addition, a prospective study in the United Kingdom with 8312 subjects and three follow-ups over ten years showed that a lower adult occupational position predicted adverse changes in WC [52]. Finally, 56,556 participants from seven population-based German cohort studies (CARLA, SHIP, KORA, DEGS, EPIC-Heidelberg, EPIC-Potsdam, PopGen) were analyzed by meta-analysis. Men and women in the low education group had a 0.1% point greater annual increase in WC than participants in the high education group. Women with low income had a 0.1% point higher annual increase in WC than women with high income [53].

On the other hand, in LMIC, associations of risk factors with AO differ between men and women. The Thai National Health Examination Survey investigated this association in 64,480 adults. Compared with primary education, the odds of obesity [range I] were higher in men with university education. For women, the association was inverse, the odds of obesity ranges I and II were higher in those with primary education [54]. In Northeast China, a representative sample of 25,196 adults was evaluated. Analysis stratified by gender showed that men with a higher educational level, white-collar job, or cadre job were part of the high risk group, and women with a higher level of education or higher family income were in the low risk group [55]. Finally, in Brazil, a cross-sectional study with 1,720 Brazilian adults found results that point to the same direction. The WC was 4.67 cm higher in women who live in low education neighborhoods compared to the residents of high education areas. In the same group, the chance of AO was 2.05 times higher [56].

Thus, the findings suggest that the association between SES and AO is similar to the association with overall obesity. Separate studies of individual nations showed that high status people tend to have a smaller WC than others, in HIC, and this association is the same for women, in LMIC. On the other hand, among men from LMIC, the association between SES and AO is positive. First, this reversal in the relationship of SES and AO across levels of economic development highlights the importance of the national socioeconomic context of AO. Second, the high prevalence of AO among low SES women, in LMIC, shows an important health inequality. In some LMIC countries, low SES groups may now have sufficient access to cheap, calorie-dense, and processed food, as a consequence of the globalization of the fast food industry and agriculture.

5. Behavioral characteristics

We explored the role of eating frequency, sleep duration, physical activity, and smoking on AO. We also draw a parallel between gender differences and these associations.

5.1. Eating frequency

Since the 1960s, studies have suggested an inverse association between the consumption of a greater number of meals per day and body weight maintenance [57]. Since then, the media, health professionals, and guidelines for health and weight management have followed this recommendation [58]. However, studies that have attempted to determine the effects of eating frequency on weight and body composition have reached different conclusions, and some scientists have called attention to the lack of solid evidence to justify such recommendation.

Thus, several review studies have been recently conducted in order to determine whether there is association between eating frequency and body weight and body composition [59–62]. However, a few studies that investigated AO or WC or waist-to-hip ratio as outcome were retrieved in these reviews [63].

A negative association between eating frequency was found in several observational studies [64–68]. Most of them found that having three or fewer meals/day is associated with excessive abdominal fat, when compared with having more than three meals/day; however, this association can only be seen among men [64–67]. In general, increased eating frequency has been postulated to increase metabolism [69], appetite control, and food intake and to improve glucose and insulin control [70–72]. However, this association only among men could be due to the fact that men who have a high eating frequency also have a healthier lifestyle, including the practice of physical activity and healthier eating habits, which results in reduced body fat and WC [73].

On the other hand, a recent cross-sectional study used data from the NHANES 2003–2012 and found that eating frequency was positively associated with central obesity in men and women.

Compared with the lowest eating frequency (≤3 times/d), the odds for AO in the highest category (≥5 times/d) were OR 1.42 (95% CI 1.15;1.75) in men and OR 1.29 (95% CI 1.05;1.59) in women [74]. This finding seems plausible, given the observed positive association between eating frequency and energy intake [67, 75, 76]. In addition, the authors called attention to the apparent inverse relation between eating frequency and adiposity measures, such as an artifact that in part can be attributed to the underreporting of eating frequency concomitant with the underreporting of energy intake by obese or overweight subjects [74].

Regarding experimental evidence, a meta-analysis study published in 2015 evaluated experimental research on meal frequency with respect to changes in fat mass and lean mass, and its results suggest a small potential benefit of increased feeding frequencies for fat mass and body fat percentage. In studies retrieved in this meta-analysis, only the Arciero's study measured the outcome as abdominal fat. This randomized trial investigated the effects of consuming traditional (15% of total energy) versus higher [35% of total energy] protein intakes as three or six meals/day on abdominal fat. Six meals per day in a high-protein condition were superior to three meals per day with a high-protein or traditional protein intake [15%] for decreasing abdominal fat in the absence of significant differences in total energy intake or expenditure. However, the study design did not rule out the possibility of an interaction between the two [eating frequency and protein intake] playing a role in mediating these responses [63].

Although observational studies suggest that men may benefit from a potential protective effect of a high eating frequency, women may not experience this protective effect. However, there is no sufficient evidence to establish a clear and strong association between eating frequency and AO, and it is necessary to conduct more observational and experimental studies.

5.2. Sleep duration

Over the past several decades, the prevalence of chronic sleep deprivation has grown to epidemic proportions. According to the National Sleep Foundation, by 1998 only 38% of American adults were obtaining 8 h of sleep and that number had fallen to 28% by 2009 [77]. Evidence has grown over the past decades supporting the role of sleep duration as a notable risk factor for overall obesity [78, 79]. More recently, studies have suggested that measures of central adiposity, such as WC, are also associated [80].

Heorell-Haglöw's [80] cross-sectional study investigated the association between sleep duration and WC in 6,461 Swiss women. The study showed a U-shaped association: Both short sleeping (<5 h) and long sleeping (≥10 h) women had greater means of WC compared to normal sleepers (7–8 h) in younger women (<50 years old). Other cross-sectional study involving men and women found a similar U-shaped association, considering short sleepers (<7 h) and long sleepers (>8 h) [81]. However, several studies found that only short sleep, and not long sleep duration, is a risk factor for central obesity [82–84].

A few longitudinal studies have investigated the association between sleep duration and AO. A prospective study with a 10-year follow-up in women confirmed the U-shaped association found in some cross-sectional studies. Among younger women (aged <40 years), both habitual short (<6 h) and long sleep durations (≥9 h) were risk factors for central obesity. In addition, decreased sleep duration from normal to short duration during the follow-up was a risk factor for increased WC [85]. Another prospective cohort investigated the association of short sleep duration (≤5 h) among women in the first year postpartum with adiposity status at 3 years postpartum. The authors demonstrated that postpartum sleep of ≤5 h/day was associated with a higher WC at 3 years postpartum, compared to sleeping >5 h [86].

In order to assess the magnitude and consistency of the relation of insufficient sleep and WC, a meta-analysis of cross-sectional studies was conducted in 2014. The analyses included 21 studies (total of 56,259 participants); the results confirmed a significant negative relation between sleep duration and WC, and longer sleep duration was not investigated [86]. However, What is short sleep and long sleep? Grandner et al. summarized the laboratory findings and epidemiological studies that investigated the consequences of acute reductions in sleep time, and they proposed to describe short sleep duration as <6 h/day [87]. However, there is no robust definition of long sleep duration, although several studies have defined long sleepers as those who have a habitual sleep duration of more than 8 h.

Finally, clinical trials that measured AO as an outcome are sparse, probably because it is difficult to maintain individuals on sleep deprivation for a long period of time. In a randomized study of adults, sleep curtailment was shown to undermine dietary efforts to reduce adiposity, after 14 days of moderate caloric restriction with 8.5- or 5.5-h nighttime sleep opportunity. It reduced the fraction of weight loss by 55% and increased the loss of fat-free body mass by 60% [88]. The hormonal regulation that occurs during sleep and its multiple peripheral effects depend on sleep duration and quality, indicating that sleep deprivation has deleterious health effects. In a randomized study, acute sleep deprivation in adults has been associated with changes in thermoregulation and, consequently, reductions in total energy expenditure in humans. Sleep-deprived individuals may also increase their total caloric intake due to the impact of sleep deprivation on peripheral regulators of satiety. Studies have associated sleep deprivation with lower leptin and higher ghrelin levels, with consequent increases in appetite and weight gain [89–92].

Furthermore, reduced sleep duration is known to have consequences on individuals' social routines and lifestyles, particularly regarding dietary habits and level of physical activity. In this sense, short sleep duration is associated with irregular eating habits, such as a dominance of snacks over meals, increased intake of fat and sweets, increased energy intake and, on the other hand, reduced intake of fruits and vegetables, and lower physical activity level [93–95]. These findings can be explained in part by a disinhibited eating behavior [tendency toward overeating and eating opportunistically], which is associated with less healthy food choices, thus contributing to weight gain. Because short sleep duration inevitably results in more time and opportunities for eating, short-duration sleepers who also have a high disinhibition eating behavior trait will eat more and gain more weight than short-duration sleepers who have a low disinhibition eating behavior trait [96].

After more than three decades of studies about the metabolic consequences of changes in the patterns of sleep duration, we can conclude that there is sufficient evidence to support that short sleep duration plays an important role in the AO etiology in adults. However, the association between long sleep and AO lacks more solid evidence, and explanations about its causal chain are weak. Nonetheless, disrupted eating patterns, such as having a dominance of snacks over meals, a higher intake of fat and sweets, and a lower intake of fruits and vegetables, are associated with both short and long sleep duration [95].

5.3. Physical activity

Strong evidence shows that physical inactivity increases the risk of many adverse health conditions, including coronary heart disease and type 2 diabetes mellitus, and it also shortens life expectancy [97]. The therapeutic role of physical activity in cardiovascular and metabolic disease involves multiple mechanisms, and one of these pathways appears to be via its effect on abdominal fat [98]. Physical activity has a role in the prevention, treatment, and control of AO. However, this chapter has focused on the epidemiology of AO, and thus we have decided to describe the predictor role of physical activity on the occurrence of AO.

Several prospective studies have evaluated the association between physical activity and AO. In the European Prospective Investigation into Cancer and Nutrition [EPIC] prospective cohort study, 84,511 men and 203,987 women were followed for 5.1 years. Physical activity predicted a lower WC in men and in women, regardless of baseline body weight, baseline WC, and other confounding factors [99]. A nationally representative population-based cohort study, The Australian Diabetes, Obesity and Lifestyle Study [AusDiab] found similar results. It followed 2,191 men and 2,650 women for 5 years. Men and women with AO showed the odds of reducing physical levels from baseline to follow-up for 1.40 (95% CI 1.10;1.79) and 1.44 (95% CI 1.16;1.80), respectively, compared to those with a normal WC [100].

In the same direction, long-term longitudinal studies (follow-up ≥ 20 years) have shown that youth physical activity had an effect on AO through the maintenance of physical activity in adulthood [101, 102]. A longitudinal study data by Finns on the cardiovascular risk in young people followed 1319 men and women for 21 years. Structural equation analysis indicated that the prevalence of AO in adulthood was directly affected by adult physical activity and indirectly via youth physical activity. Obesity was significantly reduced from youth to adulthood. The model accounted for 19% of AO in men and 13% in women [103]. Another long-term longitudinal study has showed sex differences in the association between physical activity and AO. The Coronary Artery Risk Development in Young Adults study (CARDIA), a 20-year follow-up prospective longitudinal study with 3,554 men and women, showed that maintaining high levels of activity was associated with smaller gains in WC compared with low activity levels. Men maintaining high activity gained 3.1 fewer centimeters in WC, and women maintaining higher activity gained 3.8 fewer centimeters [104].

Studies only among women showed similar results. In a prospective cohort with 233 middle-aged women, after a 20-month follow-up, changes in physical activity remained as an independent predictor of abdominal fat change after adjusting for changes in total body fat and total energy intake. Compared with women who maintained or decreased physical activity, women who increased physical activity had approximately half the risk [RR (relative risk) = 0.52 95% CI: 0.27;0.98] of gaining abdominal fat [105]. In Southern Brazil, a case-control study investigated the association between the practice of physical activities in adolescence and AO in adulthood among women who were shift workers. Women who participated in five or more physical activities in adolescence were 50% less likely to have AO than women who participated in one activity or no physical activities (OR = 0.50 95% CI: 0.27;0.93) [106].

Finally, evidence from clinical trials can help us understand how physical activity reduces body fat, preferentially from the abdominal area. In the past decade, several systematic reviews have summarized results from randomized controlled and nonrandomized controlled trials [107–109]. They support moderate physical activity as an effective intervention for reducing abdominal fat in overweight or obese subjects. Also increasing physical activity expressed as energy expended per week was positively related to reductions in total adiposity in a dose-response manner. The gender influence presents controversial results due to low numbers for comparison among those reviews. However, the most recent review showed a stronger relationship between physical activity and visceral fat in women than in men. However, it is difficult to compare differences in the amount of visceral fat reduction by aerobic exercise between men and women, as women generally store a greater total fat mass relative to body weight than men. Also, energy cost of exercise interventions and energy expenditure associated with sedentary behavior may differ considerably between genders [109].

Furthermore, the interplay between physical activity and AO may differ by gender. Although the practice of physical activity may be more beneficial for women than men, it has been shown that inactive women with a large WC had a greater risk of cardiovascular heart diseases (CHD) than inactive men with a large WC [98, 110]. In this sense, Kin and Han [98] examined the interaction between physical activity and AO in relation to the Framingham Risk Score in 2,112 adults, using data from the 2007 Korean National Health and Nutrition Examination Survey (NHANES IV). The findings suggested that the risk of CHD associated with physical inactivity and AO was much stronger in women than in men. Inactive men with a large WC had an OR for CHD risk of 2.91 (95% CI 1.63;5.22), compared with physically active men with a normal WC, while inactive women with a large WC had an OR of 6.37 (95% CI 3.44;11.80), compared with active women with a normal WC [98]. Thus, at the same time that women could have greater benefits from the practice of physical activity compared with men, they also have more deleterious effects from physical inactivity.

5.4. Smoking

Smoking is one of the major causes of preventable death in developed countries and presents a complex interaction with abdominal and general obesity. People with both conditions are at high risk of cardiovascular disease and have a substantially reduced life expectancy. Unfortunately, for many smokers, the fear of weight gain is a considerable barrier to cessation. Thus, understanding the role of smoking in the occurrence of AO is a very important issue.

Smokers have a lower body weight and BMI than nonsmokers. Nevertheless, the association between smoking and WC is inverse. Large cross-sectional studies have supported the hypothesis that current smokers tend to have a larger WC than nonsmokers, suggesting that smoking may increase central fat accumulation [111–113]; prospective studies showed that the number of cigarettes plays an important role in this association [111, 114, 115]. A cross-sectional study with a nationally representative sample of 9047 Scotland adults found that in women who were current smokers, the mean WC was higher compared with nonsmokers [111]. In the same way, a prospective study of five consecutive birth cohorts of Finnish twins ($n = 4{,}296$) analyzed the effect of adolescent smoking on AO in early adulthood. Smoking at least 10 cigarettes a day when aged 16–18 years increased the risk of adult AO in 34%, regardless of current smoking status [114]. A cohort of 79,236 white, non-Hispanic healthy adults estimated the effects of behaviors on a 10-year change in odds ratios for WC gain. Women who continued smoking up to a pack a day experienced a small protection against WC gain, but this effect could not be confirmed for women smoking more than a pack a day.

In addition, studies of smokers have shown a dose-response association between total smoking amount during a lifetime and AO. A cross-sectional study with 6,123 Caucasians from Switzerland found that compared with light-smoking men, the odds ratio for AO was 1.28 (95% CI 0.78–2;10) for moderate smokers and 1.94 (95% CI 1.15;3.27) for heavy smokers and 1.07 (95% CI 0.72–1.58) and 2.15 (95% CI 1.26;3.64) in women who were moderate and heavy smokers, respectively [115]. A prospective study in South Korea, with 283 subjects, found results that point to the same direction. WC and VAF area showed a J- or U-shaped association with total smoking during lifetime. And, after restricting the analyses to past/current smokers, they found positive dose-response associations between smoking pack-years and AO [116].

Recently, epigenetic studies have shown that genetic factors may have an important role in this association. A genetic variant in chromosome 15 CHRNA5-CHRNA3-CHRNB4 gene region (rs16969968) was associated with smoking quantity. It was also associated with a lower BMI and a greater WC. In this sense, a Mendelian randomization of the meta-analyses of 29 studies comprising almost 150,000 participants using this genetic variant as a proxy for smoking heaviness was conducted. The results suggested that for every copy of the minor allele associated with cigarette consumption (i.e., increasing cigarette per day consumption by approximately one cigarette), WC will be increased by 0.14%, if BMI were to remain constant. These findings strengthen the hypothesis that a preferential redistribution toward central adiposity is associated with higher cigarette consumption.

The physiological mechanism linking smoking and AO was not fully elucidated, but cortisol and sex hormones could play a possible role in greater WC among smokers. Smokers have higher fasting plasma cortisol concentrations than nonsmokers, and VAF is influenced by the cortisol concentration. In addition, an imbalance between male and female sex hormones [estrogens/androgen in women] and a decrease in testosterone, in men, are observed in smokers [117]. At the same time, unhealthy behavior was also observed in subjects who smoked. Some researchers have pointed to the existence of dangerous behaviors that included smoking, lower physical activity, and unhealthy eating habits in adults, and these behaviors were usual among low SES subjects [106, 118].

Unfortunately, smoking cessation also has deleterious effects on the body composition. Several studies have reported an increase in weight after smoking cessation [119, 120]. A prospective study Inter99 (1-year follow-up) investigated changes in WC after smoking cessation. Smoking cessation resulted in substantial increase in weight and central fat. Women quitters gained more weight and had a higher increase in WC than men [121]. Kahn's cohort study showed that quitting smoking was associated with approximately doubling the likelihood of WC gain compared with those who were current smokers or those who never smoked [122]. However, the increase in WC may be explained by the increase in weight; consequently, future studies are needed to elucidate this issue.

The role of smoking in increased overall obesity is well documented in the literature, while its relationship with AO has received less attention. However, current evidence suggests a causal relationship between smoking and fat distribution. Smoking increases the risk of AO and, among smokers, the number of cigarettes smoked per day was also positively associated with AO. We still need further evidence in order to understand the real impact of smoking cessation in the body composition. Thus, smoking should be avoided in order to prevent AO; current smokers should be informed that they are more prone to central fat accumulation and to the inherent additional health risks; the increase in unhealthy central fat after smoking cessation needs attention, mainly among women, who pay more attention to body shape and could avoid smoking cessation.

6. Conclusion

In this report, we have showed how demographic, socioeconomic, and behavioral characteristics influence the occurrence of AO in adults. **Figure 1** depicts the mainly associated factors of AO in men and in women. Among women, the population group who is the most affected by AO, a higher prevalence is observed in individuals living in LMIC, who are older, multiparous, and in the menopausal transition, belong to the poorest strata, and have lower educational level, while, among men, the risk of AO is positively associated with social position, particularly in LMIC. The characteristics of women's reproductive life are highlighted in the

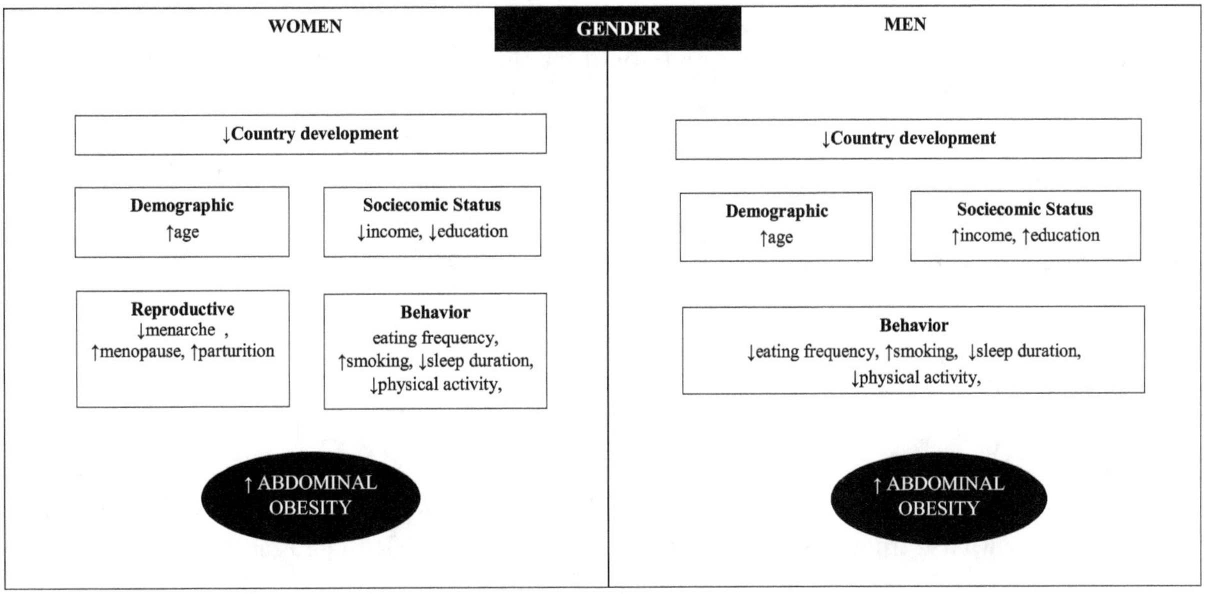

Figure 1. Causal pathway of abdominal obesity according to gender.

figure, such as menarche, menopause, and parturition, because these risk factors only affect women. Regarding behavioral factors [eating frequency, sleep duration, physical activity, and smoking], gender differences are difficult to be detected due to the lack of studies investigating their association with AO according to sex. However, the current evidence suggests that men benefit more from consuming a greater number of meals a day and women are more affected by the harmful effects of physical inactivity.

Finally, this chapter showed the increasing prevalence of AO around the world, mainly in LMIC, and explored the associated factors. We also argued AO, despite biological conditions associated with behavior factors, should be examined as an important issue of gender inequality in health, possibly mediated by socioeconomic and behavioral differences between men and women.

Acknowledgements

This chapter publication was supported by University of Vale do Rios dos Sinos. M.T.A. Olinto received research productivity grants from The Brazilian National Council for Scientific and Technological Development (grants 307257/2013-4)

Author details

Maria Teresa Anselmo Olinto[1,2]*, Heloísa Theodoro[1,3] and Raquel Canuto[4]

*Address all correspondence to: mtolinto@gmail.com

1 University of Vale do Rio dos Sinos, São Leopoldo, Brazil

2 Department of Nutrition, Federal University of Health Science of Porto Alegre, Porto Alegre, Brazil

3 Department of Nutrition, University of Caxias do Sul, Caxias do Sul, Brazil

4 Department of Nutrition, Federal University of Rio Grande do Sul, Porto Alegre, Brazil

References

[1] Shah RV, Murthy VL, Abbasi AS, Blankstein R, Kwong RY, Goldfine AB, et al. Visceral adiposity and the risk of metabolic syndrome across body mass index: the MESA study. JACC Cardiovasc Imaging. 2014;7(12):1221–1235. doi:10.1016/j.jcmg.2014.07.017

[2] Carmienke S, Freitag MH, Pischon T, Schlattmann P, Fankhaenel T, Goebel H, et al. General and abdominal obesity parameters and their combination in relation to

mortality: a systematic review and meta-regression analysis. Eur J Clin Nutr. 2013; 67 (6):573–585. doi:10.1038/ejcn.2013.61

[3] Martins IS, Marino SP. The potential of central obesity antropometric indicators as diagnostic tools. Rev Saúde Pública. 2003;37(6):760–767.

[4] Olinto MTA, Nácul LC, Dias-da-Costa JS, Gigante DP, Menezes AMB, Macedo S. Intervention levels for abdominal obesity: prevalence and associated factors. Cad Saúde Pública. 2006;22(6):1207–1215. doi:10.1590/S0102-311X2006000600010

[5] Lee K, Lee S, Kim YJ, Kim YJ. Waist circumference, dual-energy X-ray absortiometrically measured abdominal adiposity, and computed tomographically derived intra-abdominal fat area on detecting metabolic risk factors in obese women. Nutrition. 2008;24:625–631. doi:10.1016/j.nut.2008.03.004

[6] Lean ME, Han TS, Deurenberg P. Predicting body composition by densitometry from simple anthropometric measurements. Am J Clin Nutr. 1996;63:4–14.

[7] Menezes TN, Rocha FL, Belém PLO, Pedraza DF. Abdominal obesity: a critical review of the measurement techniques and cutoff points of anthropometric indicators adopted in Brazil. Ciência & Saúde Coletiva. 2014;19(6):1741–1754. doi:10.1590/1413-81232014196.15012013

[8] World Health Organization (WHO). Waist Circumference and Waist-Hip Ratio: Report of a WHO Expert Consultation, Geneva, 8–11 December 2008. Geneva: WHO; 2011.

[9] Alberti KG, Eckel RH, Grundy SM, Zimmet PZ, Cleeman JI, Donato KA, et al. Harmonizing the metabolic syndrome: a joint interim statement of the International Diabetes Federation task force on Epidemiology and Prevention; National Heart, Lung, and Blood Institute; American Heart Association; World Heart Federation; International Atherosclerosis Society; and International Association for the Study of Obesity. Circulation. 2009;120:1640–1645. doi:10.1161/CIRCULATIONAHA.109.192644

[10] Beltrán-Sánchez H, Harhay MO, Harhay MM, McElligott S. Prevalence and trends of metabolic syndrome in the adult US population, 1999–2010. J Am Coll Cardiol. 2013;62 (8):697–703. doi:10.1016/j.jacc.2013.05.064

[11] Gutiérrez-Fisac JL, Guallar-Castillón P, León-Muñoz LM, Graciani A, Banegas JR, Rodríguez-Artalejo F. Prevalence of general and abdominal obesity in the adult population of Spain, 2008–2010: the ENRICA study. Obes Rev. 2012;13(4):388–392. doi:10.1111/j.1467-789X.2011.00964

[12] Riediger ND, Clara I. Prevalence of metabolic syndrome in the Canadian adult population. CMAJ. 2011;183(15):E1127–E1134. doi:10.1503/cmaj.110070

[13] Schienkiewitz A, Mensink GBM, Scheidt-Nave C. Comorbidity of overweight and obesity in a nationally representative sample of German adults aged 18–79 years. BMC Public Health. 2012;12:658. doi:10.1186/1471-2458-12-658

[14] Sardinha LB, Santos DA, Silva AM, Coelho-e-Silva MJ, Raimundo AM, Moreira H, et al. Prevalence of overweight, obesity, and abdominal obesity in a representative sample of Portuguese adults. PLoS One. 2012;7(10):1–8. doi:10.1371/journal.pone.0047883

[15] Barquera S, Campos-Nonato I, Hernández-Barrera L, Pedroza A, Rivera-Dommarco JA. Prevalence of obesity in Mexican adults, 2000–2012. Salud Pública Méx. 2013;55(2):S151–S160

[16] Misra A, Shivastava U. Obesity and dyslipidemia in South Asians. Nutrients. 2013;5:2708–2733. doi:10.3390/nu5072708

[17] Xi B, Liang Y, He T. Secular trends in the prevalence of general and abdominal obesity among Chinese adults, 1993–2009. Obes Rev. 2012;13(3):287–296. doi:10.1111/j.1467-789X.2011.00944

[18] Linhares RS, Horta BL, Gigante DP, Dias-da-Costa JS, Olinto MTA. Distribution of general and abdominal obesity in adults in a city in southern Brazil. Cad Saúde Pública. 2012;28(3):438–447. doi:10.1590/S0102-311X2012000300004

[19] Chukwuonye II, Chuku A, Onyeonoro UU, Okpechi IG, Madukwe OO, Umeizudike TI, et al. Prevalence of abdominal obesity in Abia State, Nigeria: results of a population-based house-to-house survey. Diabetes Metab Syndr Obes Targets Ther. 2013;6:285–291. doi:10.2147/DMSO.S43545

[20] Alves RFS, Faerstein E. Educational inequality in the occurrence of abdominal obesity: Pró-Saúde Study. Rev Saúde Pública. 2015;49(65):1–8. doi:10.1590/0102-311X00077415

[21] Annandale E, Hunt K. Gender Inequalities in Health. Buckingham: Open University Press; 2000.

[22] Olinto MTA. Using the concepts of gender and/or sex in epidemiology: an example in the hierarchical approach conceptual framework. Rev Bras Epidemiol. 1998;1:161–169. doi:10.1590/S1415-790X1998000200006

[23] Connell R. Gender In World Perspective, Second ed. Cambridge: Polity Press; 2009.

[24] Pradhan AD. Sex differences in the metabolic syndrome: implications for cardiovascular health in women. Clin Chem. 2014;60(1):44–52. doi:10.1373/clinchem.2013.202549

[25] Kvist H, Chowdhury B, Grangård U, Tylén U, Sjöström L. Total and visceral adipose-tissue volumes derived from measurements with computed tomography in adult men and women: predictive equations. Am J Clin Nutr. 1988;48:1351–1361.

[26] Lemieux S, Prud'homme D, Bouchard C, Tremblay A, Despres JP. Sex differences in the relation of visceral adipose tissue accumulation to total body fatness. Am J Clin Nutr. 1993;58:463–467.

[27] Kuk JL, Lee S, Heymsfield SB, Ross R. Waist circumference and abdominal adipose tissue distribution: influence of age and sex. Am J Clin Nutr. 2005;81:1330–1334.

[28] Lovejoy JC, Champagne CM, de Jonge L, Xie H, Smith SR. Increased visceral fat and decreased energy expenditure during the menopausal transition. Int J Obes (Lond). 2008;32:949–958. doi:10.1038/ijo.2008.25

[29] Brand JS, Rovers MM, Yeap BB, Schneider HJ, Tuomainen T, Haring R. Testosterone, sex hormone-binding globulin and the metabolic syndrome in men: an individual participant data meta-analysis of observational studies. PLoS One. 2014;9(7):1–12. doi:10.1371/journal.pone.0100409

[30] Glueck CJ, Wang P, Woo JG, Morrison JA, Khoury PR, Daniels SR. Adolescent and young adult female determinants of visceral adipose tissue at ages 26–28 years. J Pediatr. 2015;166(4):936–946. doi:10.1016/j.jpeds.2014.12.030

[31] Theodoro H, Rodrigues AD, Mendes KG, Liane RH, Paniz VM, Olinto MT. Reproductive characteristics and obesity in middle-aged women seen at an outpatient clinic in southern Brazil. Menopause. 2012;19:1022–1028. doi:10.1097/gme.0b013e3182503834

[32] Trikudanathan S, Pedley A, Massaro JM, Hoffmann U, Seely EW, Murabito JM, et al. Association of female reproductive factors with body composition: the Framingham Heart Study. J Clin Endocrinol Metab. 2013;98(1):236–244. doi:10.1210/jc.2012-1785

[33] Tzeng CR, Chang YC, Wang CW, Chen CH, Hsu MI. Cluster analysis of cardiovascular and metabolic risk factors in women of reproductive age. Fertil Steril. 2014;101(5):1404–1410. doi:10.1016/j.fertnstert.2014.01.023

[34] Feibelmann TCM, Silva AP, Resende DCS, Rsende AEMR, Scatena LM, Borges MF. Puberty in a sample of Brazilian schoolgirls: timing and anthropometric characteristics. Arch Endocrinol Metab. 2015;59(2):105–111. doi:10.1590/2359-3997000000021

[35] Mueller MT, Pereira MA, Demerath EW, Dreyfus JG, MacLehose RF, Carr JJ. Earlier menarche is associated with non-alcoholic fatty liver disease and abdominal ectopic fat in midlife, independent of young-adult BMI: the CARDIA study. Obesity. 2015;23(2):468–474. doi:10.1002/oby.20950

[36] Zhai L, Liu J, Zhao J, Liu J, Bai Y, Jia L, et al. Association of obesity with onset of puberty and sex hormones in Chinese girls: a 4-year longitudinal study. PLoS One. 2015;10(8): e0134656. doi:10.1371/journal.pone.0134656

[37] Lassek MD, Gaulin SJ. Changes in body fat distribution in relation to parity in American women: a covert form of maternal depletion. Am J Phys Anthropol. 2006;131:295–302. doi:10.1002/ajpa.20394

[38] Stevens J, Katz EG, Huxley RR. Associations between gender, age and waist circumference. Eur J Clin Nutr. 2010;64:6–15. doi:10.1038/ejcn.2009.101

[39] Albarwani SA, Bayoumi RA, Jaju D, Al-Yahyaee SAS, Al-Hadabi S, Lopez-Alvarenga JC, et al. Differing definition-based prevalence of metabolic syndrome in the women of Oman family study: a function of multiparity. Metab Syndr Relat disord. 2008;6(3):197–202. doi:10.1089/met.2008.0009

[40] Gunderson EP, Sternfeld B, Wellons MF, Whitmer RA, Chiang V, Quesenberry JRCP, et al. Childbearing may increase visceral adipose tissue independent of overall increase in body fat. Obesity. 2008;16:1078–1084. doi:10.1038/oby.2008.40

[41] Blaudeau TE, Hunter GR, Sirikul B. Intra-abdominal adipose tissue deposition and parity. Int J Obes. 2006;30:1119–1124. doi:10.1038/sj.ijo.0803252

[42] Gunderson EP. Childbearing and obesity in women: weight before, during and after pregnancy. Obstet Gynecol Clin N Am. 2009;36:317–332.

[43] World Health Organization. Research on the Menopause in the 1990. Reports of a WHO Scientific Group. Geneva: WHO; 1996.

[44] Lovejoy JC. Weight gain in women at midlife: the influence of menopause. Obes Manag.2009;10:52–56. doi:10.1089/obe.2009.0203

[45] Phillips GB, Jing T, Heymsfield SB. Does insulin resistance, visceral adiposity, or a sex hormone alteration underlie the metabolic syndrome? Studies in women. Metabolism. 2008;57(6):838–844. doi:10.1016/j.metabol.2008

[46] Donato GB, Fuchs SC, Oppermann K, Bastos C, Spritzer PM. Association between menopause status and central adiposity measured at different cutoffs of waist circumference and waist-to-hip ratio. Menopause. 2006;13(2):280–285. doi:10.1097/01.gme.0000177907.32634.ae

[47] Orsatti FL, Nahas EA, Nahas-Neto J, Maestá N, Padoani NP, Orsatti CL. Anthropometric measures: predictors of non-transmissible chronic diseases in postmenopausal women in the Southeast region of Brazil. Rev Bras Ginecol Obstet. 2008;30(4):182–189. doi:10.1590/S0100-72032008000400005

[48] Kim HM, Park J, Ryu SY, Kim J. The effect of menopause on the metabolic syndrome among Korean women. Diabete Care. 2007;30(3):701–706. doi:10.2337/dc06-1400

[49] Mendes KG, Theodoro H, Rodrigues AD, Olinto MTA. Prevalence of metabolic syndrome and its components in the menopausal transition: a systematic review. Cad Saúde Pública. 2012;28(8):1423–1437. doi:10.1590/S0102-311X2012000800002

[50] Krieger N, Williams DR, Moss NE. Measuring social class in US public health research: concepts, methodologies, and guidelines. Annu Rev Public Health. 1997;18:341–378. doi:10.1146/annurev.publhealth.18.1.341

[51] Krieger N, Kosheleva A, Waterman PD, Chen JT, Beckfield J, Kiang MV. 50-year trends in US socioeconomic inequalities in health: US-born Black and White Americans, 1959–2008. Int J Epidemiol. 2014;43(4):1294–1313. doi:10.1093/ije/dyu047

[52] Elovainio M, Ferrie JE, Singh-Manoux A, Shipley M, Batty GD, Head J, et al. Socioeconomic differences in cardiometabolic factors: social causation or health-related selection? Evidence from the Whitehall II Cohort Study, 1991–2004. Am J Epidemiol. 2011;174 (7):779–789. doi:10.1093/aje/kwr149

[53] Herzog B, Lacruz ME, Haerting J, Hartwig S, Tiller D, Medenwald D, et al. Socioeconomic status and anthropometric changes-A meta-analytic approach from seven German cohorts. Obesity (Silver Spring, MD). 2016;24(3):710–718. doi:10.1002/oby.21366

[54] Aekplakorn W, Inthawong R, Kessomboon P, Sangthong R, Chariyalertsak S, Putwatana P, et al. Prevalence and trends of obesity and association with socioeconomic status in Thai adults: National Health Examination Surveys, 1991–2009. J Obes. 2014;2014:410259. doi:10.1155/2014/410259

[55] Wang H, Wang J, Liu MM, Wang D, Liu YQ, Zhao Y, et al. Epidemiology of general obesity, abdominal obesity and related risk factors in urban adults from 33 communities

of Northeast China: the CHPSNE study. BMC Public Health. 2012;12:967. doi:10.1186/1471-2458-12-967

[56] Boing AF, Subramanian SV. The influence of area-level education on body mass index, waist circumference and obesity according to gender. Int J Public Health. 2015;60(6):727–736. doi:10.1007/s00038-015-0721-8

[57] Fabry P, Hejl Z, Fodor J, Braun T, Zvolankova K. The frequency of meals. Its relation to overweight, hypercholesterolaemia, and decreased glucose-tolerance. Lancet. 1964;2 (7360):614–615.

[58] Seagle HM, Strain GW, Makris A, Reeves RS. Position of the American Dietetic Association: weight management. J Am Diet Assoc. 2009;109(2):330–346.

[59] Jon Schoenfeld B, Albert Aragon A, Krieger JW. Effects of meal frequency on weight loss and body composition: a meta-analysis. Nutr Rev. 2015;73(2):69–82. doi:10.1093/nutrit/nuu017

[60] Kulovitz MG, Kravitz LR, Mermier C, Gibson AL, Conn CA, Kolkmeyer D, et al. Potential role of meal frequency as a strategy for weight loss and health in overweight or obese adults. Nutrition. 2014;30(4):386–392. doi:10.1016/j.nut.2013.08.009

[61] La Bounty PM, Campbell BI, Wilson J, Galvan E, Berardi J, Kleiner SM, et al. International society of sports nutrition position stand: meal frequency. J Int Soc Sports Nutr. 2011;8:4. doi:10.1186/1550-2783-8-4

[62] Bellisle F, McDevitt R, Prentice AM. Meal frequency and energy balance. Br J Nutr. 1997;77(Suppl 1):S57–S70. doi:10.1079/BJN19970104

[63] Arciero PJ, Ormsbee MJ, Gentile CL, Nindl BC, Brestoff JR, Ruby M. Increased protein intake and meal frequency reduces abdominal fat during energy balance and energy deficit. Obesity (Silver Spring, MD). 2013;21(7):1357–1366. doi:10.1002/oby.20296

[64] Holmback I, Ericson U, Gullberg B, Wirfalt E. A high eating frequency is associated with an overall healthy lifestyle in middle-aged men and women and reduced likelihood of general and central obesity in men. Br J Nutr. 2010;104(7):1065–1073. doi:10.1017/S0007114510001753

[65] Oliveira LP, Assis AM, Silva Mda C, Santana ML, Santos NS, Pinheiro SM, et al. Factors associated with overweight and abdominal fat in adults in Salvador, Bahia State, Brazil Cadernos de Saude Publica. 2009;25(3):570–582. doi:10.1590/S0102-311X2009000300012

[66] Peixoto Mdo R, Benicio MH, Jardim PC. The relationship between body mass index and lifestyle in a Brazilian adult population: a cross-sectional survey. Cadernos de Saude Publica. 2007;23(11):2694–2740. doi:10.1590/S0102-311X2007001100017

[67] Ruidavets JB, Bongard V, Bataille V, Gourdy P, Ferrieres J. Eating frequency and body fatness in middle-aged men. International journal of obesity and related metabolic disorder. J Int Assoc Study Obes. 2002;26(11):1476–1483. doi:10.1038/sj.ijo.0802143

[68] Smith KJ, Blizzard L, McNaughton SA, Gall SL, Dwyer T, Venn AJ. Daily eating frequency and cardiometabolic risk factors in young Australian adults: cross-sectional analyses. Br J Nutr. 2012;108(6):1086–1094. doi:10.1017/S0007114511006398

[69] Jenkins DJ, Wolever TM, Vuksan V, Brighenti F, Cunnane SC, Rao AV, et al. Nibbling versus gorging: metabolic advantages of increased meal frequency. N Engl J Med. 1989;321(14):929–934. doi:10.1056/NEJM198910053211403

[70] Leidy HJ, Campbell WW. The effect of eating frequency on appetite control and food intake: brief synopsis of controlled feeding studies. J Nutr. 2011;141(1):154–157. doi:10.3945/jn.109.114389

[71] Farshchi HR, Taylor MA, Macdonald IA. Beneficial metabolic effects of regular meal frequency on dietary thermogenesis, insulin sensitivity, and fasting lipid profiles in healthy obese women. Am J Clin Nutr. 2005;81(1):16–24.

[72] Schwarz NA, Rigby BR, La Bounty P, Shelmadine B, Bowden RG. A review of weight control strategies and their effects on the regulation of hormonal balance. J Nutr Metab. 2011;2011:15. doi:10.1155/2011/237932

[73] Canuto R, Garcez A, Kac G, Lira P, Olinto MT. Eating frequency and weight and body composition: a systematic review of observational studies. (In press).

[74] Murakami K, Livingstone MB. Eating frequency is positively associated with overweight and central obesity in US adults. J Nutr. 2015;145(12):2715–2724. doi:10.3945/jn.115.219808

[75] Bertéus Forslund BH, Torgerson JS, Sjostrom L, Lindroos AK. Snacking frequency in relation to energy intake and food choices in obese men and women compared to a reference population. Int J Obes. 2005;29(6):711–719. doi:10.1038/sj.ijo.0802950

[76] Mills JP, Perry CD, Reicks M. Eating frequency is associated with energy intake but not obesity in midlife women. Obesity (Silver Spring, MD). 2011;19(3):552–559. doi:10.1038/oby.2010.265

[77] Foundation NS. Sleep in America Poll. Washington, DC: National Sleep Foundation; 2009.

[78] Patel SR, Hu FB. Short sleep duration and weight gain: a systematic review. Obesity (Silver Spring, MD). 2008;16(3):643–653. doi:10.1038/oby.2007

[79] Knutson KL, Spiegel K, Penev P, Van Cauter E. The metabolic consequences of sleep deprivation. Sleep Med Rev. 2007;11(3):163–178. doi:10.1016/j.smrv.2007.01.002

[80] Theorell-Haglow J, Berglund L, Janson C, Lindberg E. Sleep duration and central obesity in women – differences between short sleepers and long sleepers. Sleep Med. 2012;13(8):1079–1085. doi:10.1016/j.sleep.2012.06.013

[81] Hall MH, Muldoon MF, Jennings JR, Buysse DJ, Flory JD, Manuck SB. Self-reported sleep duration is associated with the metabolic syndrome in midlife adults. Sleep. 2008;31(5):635–643.

[82] Moraes W, Poyares D, Zalcman I, de Mello MT, Bittencourt LR, Santos-Silva R, et al. Association between body mass index and sleep duration assessed by objective methods in a representative sample of the adult population. Sleep Med. 2013;14(4):312–318. doi:10.1016/j.sleep.2012.11.010

[83] Rontoyanni VG, Baic S, Cooper AR. Association between nocturnal sleep duration, body fatness, and dietary intake in Greek women. Nutrition. 2007;23(11–12):773–777. doi:10.1016/j.nut.2007.07.005

[84] Ko GT, Chan JC, Chan AW, Wong PT, Hui SS, Tong SD, et al. Association between sleeping hours, working hours and obesity in Hong Kong Chinese: the 'better health for better Hong Kong' health promotion campaign. Int J Obes. 2007;31(2):254–260. doi:10.1038/sj.ijo.0803389

[85] Theorell-Haglow J, Berglund L, Berne C, Lindberg E. Both habitual short sleepers and long sleepers are at greater risk of obesity: a population-based 10-year follow-up in women. Sleep Med. 2014;15(10):1204–1211. doi:10.1016/j.sleep.2014.02.014

[86] Taveras EM, Rifas-Shiman SL, Rich-Edwards JW, Gunderson EP, Stuebe AM, Mantzoros CS. Association of maternal short sleep duration with adiposity and cardiometabolic status at 3 years postpartum. Obesity (Silver Spring, MD). 2011;19(1):171–178. doi:10.1038/oby.2010.117

[87] Grandner MA, Hale L, Moore M, Patel NP. Mortality associated with short sleep duration: the evidence, the possible mechanisms, and the future. Sleep Med Rev. 2010;14 (3):191–203. doi: 10.1016/j.smrv.2009.07.006

[88] Nedeltcheva AV, Kilkus JM, Imperial J, Schoeller DA, Penev PD. Insufficient sleep undermines dietary efforts to reduce adiposity. Ann Intern Med. 2010;153(7):435–441. doi:10.7326/0003-4819-153-7-201010050-00006

[89] Ogawa Y, Kanbayashi T, Saito Y, Takahashi Y, Kitajima T, Takahashi K, et al. Total sleep deprivation elevates blood pressure through arterial baroreflex resetting: a study with microneurographic technique. Sleep. 2003;26(8):986–989.

[90] Gangwisch JE, Heymsfield SB, Boden-Albala B, Buijs RM, Kreier F, Pickering TG, et al. Short sleep duration as a risk factor for hypertension: analyses of the first National Health and Nutrition Examination Survey. Hypertension. 2006;47(5):833–839. doi:10.1161/01.HYP.0000217362.34748.e0

[91] Meier-Ewert HK, Ridker PM, Rifai N, Regan MM, Price NJ, Dinges DF, et al. Effect of sleep loss on C-reactive protein, an inflammatory marker of cardiovascular risk. J Am Coll Cardiol. 2004;43(4):678–683. doi:10.1016/j.jacc.2003.07.050

[92] Stamatakis KA, Punjabi NM. Effects of sleep fragmentation on glucose metabolism in normal subjects. Chest. 2010;137(1):95–101. doi:10.1378/chest.09-0791

[93] Ohida T, Kamal AM, Uchiyama M, Kim K, Takemura S, Sone T, et al. The influence of lifestyle and health status factors on sleep loss among the Japanese general population. Sleep. 2001;24(3):333–338.

[94] Canuto R, Pattussi MP, Macagnan JB, Henn RL, Olinto MT. Sleep deprivation and obesity in shift workers in southern Brazil. Public Health Nutr. 2014;17(11):2619–2623. doi:10.1017/S1368980013002838

[95] Kim J, Jo I. Age-dependent association between sleep duration and hypertension in the adult Korean population. Am J Hypertens. 2010;23(12):1286–1291. doi:10.1038/ajh.2010.166

[96] Chaput JP, Despres JP, Bouchard C, Tremblay A. The association between short sleep duration and weight gain is dependent on disinhibited eating behavior in adults. Sleep. 2011;34(10):1291–1297. doi:10.5665/SLEEP.1264

[97] Lim SS, Vos T, Flaxman AD, Danaei G, Shibuya K, Adair-Rohani H, et al. A comparative risk assessment of burden of disease and injury attributable to 67 risk factors and risk factor clusters in 21 regions, 1990–2010: a systematic analysis for the Global Burden of Disease Study. The Lancet. 2010;380(9859):2224–2260. doi:10.1016/S0140-6736(12)61766-8

[98] Kim J, Han HR. Physical activity, abdominal obesity and the risk of coronary heart disease: a Korean national sample study. Public Health. 2012;126(5):410–416. doi:10.1016/j.puhe.2012.01.034

[99] Ekelund U, Besson H, Luan J, May AM, Sharp SJ, Brage S, et al. Physical activity and gain in abdominal adiposity and body weight: prospective cohort study in 288,498 men and women. Am J Clin Nutr. 2011;93(4):826–835. doi:10.3945/ajcn.110.006593

[100] Lakerveld J, Dunstan D, Bot S, Salmon J, Dekker J, Nijpels G, et al. Abdominal obesity, TV-viewing time and prospective declines in physical activity. Prev Med. 2011;53(4–5):299–302. doi:10.1016/j.ypmed.2011.07.012

[101] Mustelin L, Silventoinen K, Pietilainen K, Rissanen A, Kaprio J. Physical activity reduces the influence of genetic effects on BMI and waist circumference: a study in young adult twins. Int J Obes. 2008;33(1):29–36. doi:10.1038/ijo.2008.258

[102] Waller K, Kaprio J, Kujala UM. Associations between long-term physical activity, waist circumference and weight gain: a 30-year longitudinal twin study. Int J Obes. 2008;32(2):353–361. doi:10.1038/sj.ijo.0803692

[103] Yang X, Telama R, Leskinen E, Mansikkaniemi K, Viikari J, Raitakari OT. Testing a model of physical activity and obesity tracking from youth to adulthood: the cardiovascular risk in young Finns study. Int J Obes. 2007;31(3):521–527. doi:10.1038/sj.ijo.0803459

[104] Hankinson AL, Daviglus ML, Bouchard C, Carnethon M, Lewis CE, Schreiner PJ, et al. Maintaining a high physical activity level over 20 years and weight gain. JAMA. 2010;304(23):2603–2610. doi:10.1001/jama.2010.1843

[105] Davidson LE, Tucker L, Peterson T. Physical activity changes predict abdominal fat change in midlife women. J Phys Act Health. 2010;7(3):316–322. doi:10.1123/jpah.7.3.316

[106] Garcez AS, Olinto MT, Canuto R, Olinto BA, Pattussi MP, Paniz VM. Physical activity in adolescence and abdominal obesity in adulthood: a case-control study among women shift workers. Women Health. 2015;55(4):419–431. doi:10.1080/03630242.2015.1022686

[107] Ross R, Janssen I. Physical activity, total and regional obesity: dose-response considerations. Med Sci Sports Exerc. 2001;33(Suppl 6):S521–S527; discussion S8–9.

[108] Kay SJ, Fiatarone Singh MA. The influence of physical activity on abdominal fat: a systematic review of the literature. Obes Rev Off J Int Assoc Study Obes. 2006;7(2):183–200. doi:10.1111/j.1467-789X.2006.00250.x

[109] Ohkawara K, Tanaka S, Miyachi M, Ishikawa-Takata K, Tabata I. A dose-response relation between aerobic exercise and visceral fat reduction: systematic review of clinical trials. Int J Obes (2005). 2007;31(12):1786–1797. doi:10.1038/sj.ijo.0803683

[110] Rana JS, Arsenault BJ, Després JP, Côté M, Talmud PJ, Ninio E, et al. Inflammatory biomarkers, physical activity, waist circumference, and risk of future coronary heart disease in healthy men and women. Eur Heart J. 2011;32(3):336–344. doi:10.1093/eurheartj/ehp010

[111] Akbartabartoori M, Lean ME, Hankey CR. Relationships between cigarette smoking, body size and body shape. Int J Obes. 2005;29(2):236–243. doi:10.1038/sj.ijo.0802827

[112] Shimokata H, Muller DC, Andres R. Studies in the distribution of body fat. III. Effects of cigarette smoking. JAMA. 1989;261(8):1169–1173. doi:10.1001/jama.1989.03420080089037

[113] Canoy D, Wareham N, Luben R, Welch A, Bingham S, Day N, et al. Cigarette smoking and fat distribution in 21,828 British men and women: a population-based study. Obes Res. 2005;13(8):1466–1475. doi:10.1038/oby.2005.177

[114] Saarni SE, Pietilainen K, Kantonen S, Rissanen A, Kaprio J. Association of smoking in adolescence with abdominal obesity in adulthood: a follow-up study of 5 birth cohorts of Finnish twins. Am J Public Health. 2009;99(2):348–354. doi:10.2105/AJPH.2007.123851

[115] Clair C, Chiolero A, Faeh D, Cornuz J, Marques-Vidal P, Paccaud F, et al. Dose-dependent positive association between cigarette smoking, abdominal obesity and body fat: cross-sectional data from a population-based survey. BMC Public Health. 2011;11:23.

[116] Kim JH, Shim KW, Yoon YS, Lee SY, Kim SS, Oh SW. Cigarette smoking increases abdominal and visceral obesity but not overall fatness: an observational study. PLoS One. 2012;7(9):e45815. doi:10.1371/journal.pone.0045815

[117] Chiolero A, Faeh D, Paccaud F, Cornuz J. Consequences of smoking for body weight, body fat distribution, and insulin resistance. Am J Clin Nutr. 2008;87(4):801–809.

[118] Olinto MT, Willett WC, Gigante DP, Victora CG. Sociodemographic and lifestyle characteristics in relation to dietary patterns among young Brazilian adults. Public Health Nutr. 2011;14(1):150–159. doi:10.1017/S136898001000162X

[119] Tian J, Venn A, Otahal P, Gall S. The association between quitting smoking and weight gain: a systemic review and meta-analysis of prospective cohort studies. Obes Rev Off J Int Assoc Study Obes. 2015;16(10):883–901. doi:10.1111/obr.12304

[120] Filozof C, Fernandez Pinilla MC, Fernandez-Cruz A. Smoking cessation and weight gain. Obes Rev Off J Int Assoc Study Obes. 2004;5(2):95–103. doi:10.1111/j.1467-789X.2004.00131.x

[121] Pisinger C, Jorgensen T. Waist circumference and weight following smoking cessation in a general population: the Inter99 study. Prev Med. 2007;44(4):290–295. doi:10.1016/j.ypmed.2006.11.015

[122] Kahn HS, Tatham LM, Rodriguez C, Calle EE, Thun MJ, Heath CW, Jr. Stable behaviors associated with adults' 10-year change in body mass index and likelihood of gain at the waist. Am J Public Health. 1997;87(5):747–754. doi:10.2105/AJPH.87.5.747

6

Nutrition Labelling: Educational Tool for Reducing Risks of Obesity-Related Non-communicable Diseases

Visith Chavasit, Wantanee Kriengsinyos, Mayuree Ditmetharoj, Manasuwee Phaichamanan, Kangsadan Singsoong, Prapaisri Sirichakwal and Araya Rojjanawanicharkorn

Abstract

Food and nutrition education is globally recognized as the most efficient tool for reducing the risks of non-communicable diseases (NCDs). For decades, different nutrition labelling formats found on the back of food packages have been used as educational tools to provide information on amounts of nutrients for preventing both under- and over-nutrition. However, these traditional panels have proven to be ineffective for consumer education due to their complexity. Other systems, so-called 'Simplified Nutrition Labelling', which are normally shown on the front of a food package, were then introduced as 'Front-of-Pack, FOP' labelling. These labelling panels normally contain only the nutrients that relate to NCDs and that should be limited for consumption. At least four types of FOP nutrition labelling panels exist, namely, nutrient specific, summary indicator, food group information and hybrids. These panels using different patterns provide consumers with three types of information: non-evaluative, evaluative or interpretative and conclusive. In this chapter, the advantages and disadvantages of different types of nutrition labelling are discussed, especially their roles in reducing the risk of obesity-related NCDs in a population.

Keywords: nutrition labelling, front-of-pack, non-communicable diseases, nutrition education, nutrition in transition

1. Introduction

Currently, nutrition in transition can be found globally even in most developing countries. Declining under-nutrition is occurring in parallel with increases in over-nutrition, obesity and non-communicable diseases (NCDs). A double burden of malnutrition is now affecting the world population's quality of life.

For decades, nutrition education has been recognized as a preventive strategy for the sustainable reduction of both under- and over-nutrition. International organizations have developed guidelines for healthy eating that countries have adopted for preparing more practical food-based dietary guidelines (FBDGs). More simplified FBDGs were later developed in different graphical designs according to national cultures and eating contexts. These FBDGs have been modified periodically by including additional factors other than foods that affect the nutrition and health statuses of population.

Industrially-produced foods are the other important sources of nutrients for people especially in more developed countries. An attempt in using industrial food products as an education tool for populations exists in terms of nutrition labelling, which indicates the amounts of certain selected nutrients on food package.

The traditional nutrition labelling panel, which contains amounts of nutrients that reduce risks of under- and over-nutrition, has been mandated in many countries. Data on these traditional nutrition labelling panels are normally tabulated and located on the back of food package or so called 'Back of Pack, BOP' nutrition labelling panel. After several years of implementation, the traditional BOP nutrition labelling panels were found to be inefficient tools for educating consumers, due to such causes as their hidden location on shelves, complicated information and unattractive design. Consumers generally did not use the panel, and it did not attract industries to reformulate their recipes towards healthier nutrient profiles. A more effective nutrition educational tool is now needed as the problems of overweight, obesity and non-communicable diseases have become serious nutrition issues worldwide, especially among the people of low socio-economic classes and with less education.

A simplified nutrition label in graphic format was introduced in the 1960s intentionally to conquer over-nutrition, and later more designs and types were widely developed. Among these differences, the common agreement was on the nutrients used for criteria development, which were basically related to non-communicable diseases, for example fat, sodium and sugar. In addition, this simplified nutrition labelling panel was located on the front of food package or so called 'Front-of-Pack, FOP' nutrition labelling panel. These panels of different types and different degrees of informativeness have been recognized differently by different groups of stakeholders within the food system. Most FOP nutrition labelling panels are still implemented on a voluntary basis. In this chapter, the logic behind the development of traditional and simplified nutrition labelling panels are discussed as well as their uses in many countries.

2. Global nutrition in transition

For decades in many parts of the world, protein energy malnutrition (PEM) and micro-nutrient deficiencies have been significant health burdens. Consequently, tremendous investments have been made in programs to alleviate these under-nutrition issues. However, most malnutrition scenarios arise not just from a lack of sufficient, adequately nutritious and safe food. A host of other interacting processes also play a role, for example healthcare, education, sanitation and hygiene, agriculture, trade, access to resources, women empowerment and more [1]. Consequently, a multidisciplinary approach involving different stakeholders, such as public health, agriculture, education and local authorities, must be implemented with the involvement of communities. The applied knowledge of these stakeholders as well as strong contributions and the cooperation of communities are important requirements for the production and consumption of nutritious and safe foods. For example, improvements in human quality of life, via efficient sanitation and nutrition programs, can successfully reduce morbidity and mortality due to nutrient deficiencies and communicable diseases. Over the past four decades, this multidisciplinary approach has been tested and implemented on a large scale in several developing countries. Thailand is one such success story where PEM among under-5 year old children was drastically reduced after 20 years of implementing this approach (**Figure 1**).

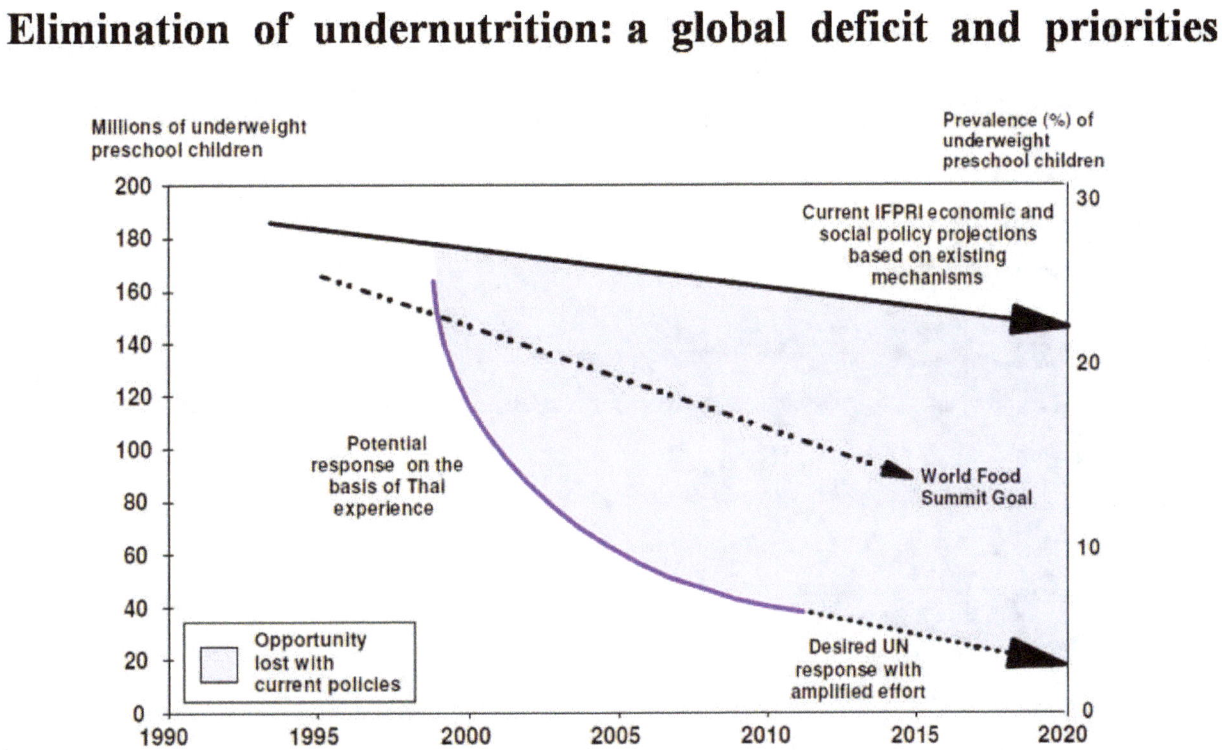

Figure 1. The World Food Summit Goal in reducing underweight problem in school children, the current situation of most countries and the Thailand's experience. *Source*: Ending malnutrition by 2020: an agenda for change in the millennium. Final Report to the ACC/SCN by the Commission on the nutrition challenges of the twenty-first century.

Among many supporting factors, food and nutrition education is one of the keys to success. As information is modified and simplified to fit community contexts, understandable messages and practical guidance can be passed to consumers. In the case of Thailand, the messengers were village health volunteers—at a ratio of 1 volunteer per 10 households—who distributed important nutrition information all over the country. Effective communication proved to be a powerful tool for altering consumer behaviours in the food system.

It must be recognized, however, that economic development is also a significant factor for success in solving a country's under-nutrition challenges. It can allow a country to invest more in nutrition and increase people's access to nutritious and safe foods. Under-nutrition problems in many countries have shown improvement as national economies have grown in strength (**Figure 2**). As a consequence of economic development, potentially more nutritious, safe and energy-rich foods can be available, affordable and accessible by people of varying socio-economic statuses. Economic development and industrialization provide more food choices in marketplaces, which have changed food environments in many countries.

The roles of food industries nowadays have also become more significant in the daily diets of the world's populations, and not always for the better. Globalization and modernization have drastically changed people's lifestyles in developing countries that formerly had a more balanced way of living. Traditional and imported energy-rich foods can be easily accessed in fresh markets, convenience stores, supermarkets, food vendors, local restaurants and multinational franchise restaurants due to better logistics, more modern and economical agricultural and

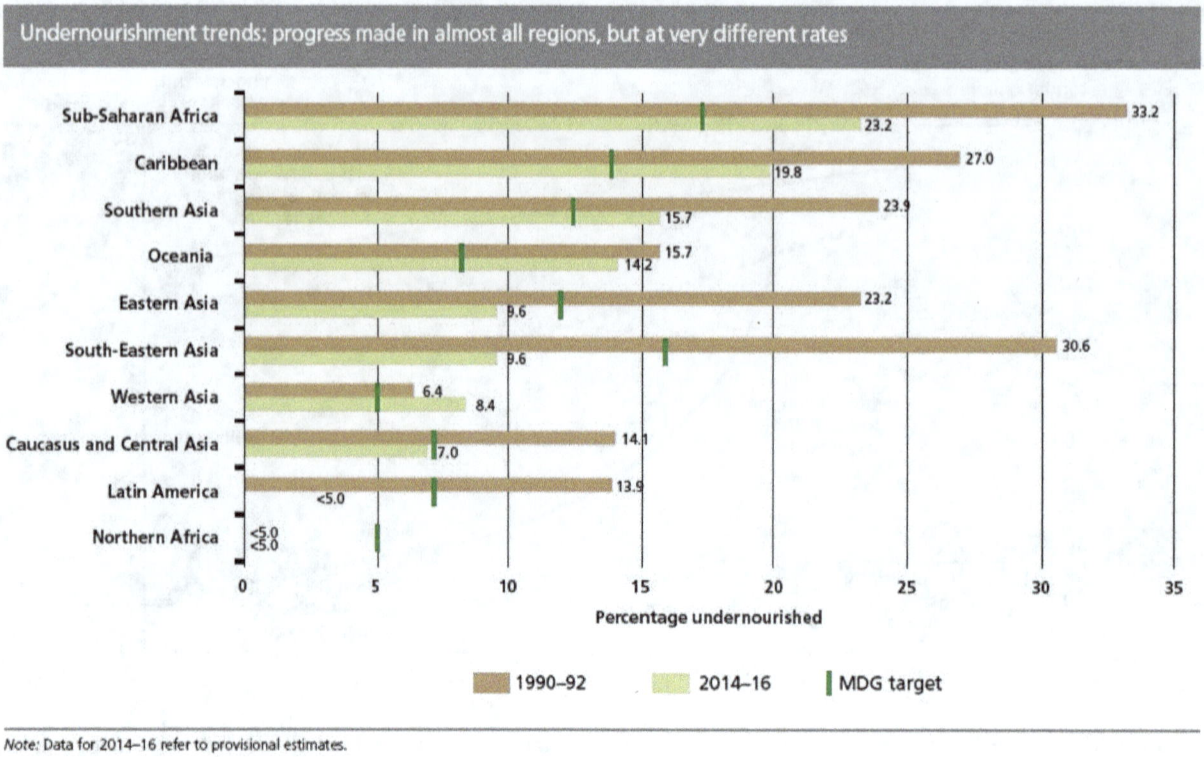

Figure 2. World situation on protein energy malnutrition (PEM) problem. *Source*: http://www.fao.org/hunger/key-messages/en/.

industrial production technologies and free trade agreements. Unfortunately, though, messages from food businesses can, in part, be based on fact, but they can also contain misleading information. Deceptive food advertisements and sales promotions can create an unhealthy food environment for consumers by promoting the excessive consumption of energy-, sugar-, saturated fat- and sodium-rich foods. In such an environment, physically easy or sedentary lifestyles, which result in low physical activity and less energy expenditure in everyday life, promote unbalanced nutrition. A mentally stressful lifestyle, furthermore, can cause a negative impact on non-communicable diseases.

Allied, often well-meaning, government health programs can also affect a population's nutritional status. For example, successful family planning programs have led to very low population fertility rates in many countries (lower than 2.1). Due to lower birth rates as well as better public health care, these countries have steadily seen a decline in working age people and a growing elderly population (**Figure 3**). As the ratio of elderly people increases, these countries are faced with an ageing society with the expectation that a longer life will also be a healthy life. However, non-communicable diseases often come to the forefront, since they are found more often in older age population groups who are physiologically prone to the diseases, especially among overweight and obese individuals. Changes in food availability, lifestyle and population profiles, therefore, can exacerbate expanding problems of NCDs. The increase in NCDs in developing countries—where under-nutrition used to be the main nutrition problem but has improved—can partly be explained by using Barker's theory, as well. Some persons found within a population affected by NCDs were born malnourished and were low-birth-weight newborns. Their bodies adapted to an environment that was chronically short of food. In adulthood and living in a more affluent environment, they become more prone to metabolic disorders, such as obesity and type II diabetes [2].

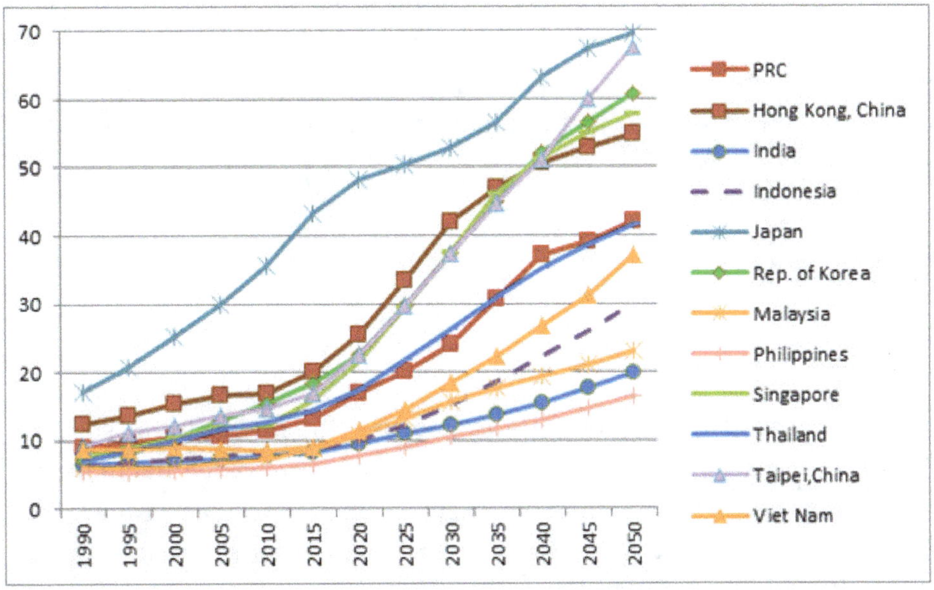

Figure 3. The trend of the ratio (%) of the population aged 65 and over to the working-age population (aged 15–64) through the year 2050. *Source*: http://www.asiapathways-adbi.org/2015/02/why-do-we-need-financial-education-in-asia/.

While under-nutrition in the form of PEM and micro-nutrient deficiencies remains unsolved in many developing countries, unfortunately the challenge of over-nutrition has also rapidly emerged, thus presenting the world with a double-burden in terms of malnutrition. Incidences of overweight, obesity and diet-related NCDs, which were mainly found in more affluent developed countries, are now growing in many developing countries at an alarming rate. The worldwide prevalence of obesity more than doubled between 1980 and 2014. Globally, NCDs are now the leading causes of death. Cardiovascular diseases, diabetes, cancer and chronic respiratory diseases caused up to 68% of deaths in 2012 [3]. Almost three-quarters of all NCD deaths occur in low- and middle-income countries [4]. Four major risk factors have been primarily responsible for the rise in NCDs are tobacco use, physical inactivity, alcohol use and unhealthy diets [5]. The rapid rise in NCDs is predicted to impede poverty reduction in low-income countries, particularly by increasing household costs associated with health care. Vulnerable and socially disadvantaged people become ill and die sooner than people of higher socio-economic status, since they are at higher risk of being exposed to harmful products, such as tobacco or unhealthy food, and have limited access to health services. To lessen the impact of NCDs on individuals and society, a comprehensive approach is needed that requires all sectors, including health, finance, foreign affairs, education, agriculture, planning and others, to work together to reduce the risks associated with NCDs, as well as promote interventions to prevent and control them. A global action plan for the prevention and control of NCDs 2013–2020 was initiated by WHO and member states. This plan aims to reduce the number of premature deaths from NCDs by 25% by 2025 [6].

Malnutrition, in every form, presents significant threats to human health. Today the world faces a double burden of malnutrition that includes both under-nutrition and over-nutrition, especially in developing countries (**Table 1**). Hunger and inadequate nutrition contribute to early deaths among mothers, infants and young children, and impaired physical and brain development in young children. Meanwhile, growing rates of overweight and obesity are linked to a rise in life-threatening chronic diseases (e.g. hypertension, stroke, cardiovascular disease, diabetes, cancer) that are difficult to treat in places with limited resources and already overburdened health systems. Nutrition problems that emerge in either direction impair individual productivity, which slow down national growth. The cost of malnutrition is approximately 3.5 trillion USD per year [7].

3. Guideline for healthy eating

3.1. Balanced diet

Consuming a healthy diet throughout life is one key for maintaining strength and good health. Eating a wide variety of foods in the right proportions can achieve and maintain healthy body weight and prevent malnutrition of all forms as well as a range of NCDs. Foods from nature provide both nutrients and non-nutrients that benefit human health. The basic elements, or nutritional requirements, for a healthy diet must include the right amounts of energy, protein, fat, carbohydrates, vitamins, minerals and water for the body. These requirements, in fact, differ for different individuals and at different life stages. However, sets of

Under-nutrition	Over-nutrition
- About 104 million children under age 5 worldwide (2010) are underweight and 171 million stunting - More than one-third of preschool-age children globally are Vitamin A deficient	- About 1.5 billion people are overweight worldwide, of whom 500 million are obese (2008) - About 43 million children under age 5 were overweight in 2010
- Maternal under-nutrition, leads to poor foetal development and higher risk of pregnancy complications - 13 million children are born with low birth weight or prematurely due to maternal under-nutrition and other factors	- Growing rates of maternal overweight are leading to higher risks of pregnancy complications and heavier birth weight and obesity in children
- Maternal and child under-nutrition account for more than 10% of the global burden of disease - Under-nutrition contributes to about one-third of all child deaths	- At least 2.6 million people die each year as a result of being overweight or obese

Source: WHO Nutrition Challenges 2014, http://www.who.int/nutrition/challenges/en/August 12, 2016.

Table 1. Impacts from double burden malnutrition in the world as quoted by World Health Organization in 2010.

nutrient requirements have been established for general populations living in many countries. These sets go by different names, such as Dietary Reference Intake (DRI) in the United States and Canada, Dietary Reference Values (DRV) in the United Kingdom, etc. The human body needs different nutrients for different functions in differing amounts. Carbohydrate, fat and protein—known as 'macronutrients'—are required in much larger amounts than minerals and vitamins that are called 'micro-nutrients'. In addition, the human body's physiological function is also regulated by non-nutrient substances that are found naturally in food. Consequently, the term 'balanced diet' must contain the right amounts of the right kinds of nutrients and non-nutrients. Nutrient and non-nutrient requirements for a healthy diet are, in fact, quite individualized, since they relate to genetics, age, gender, physical activity and health status of an individual.

3.2. Food-based dietary guidelines

Information contained in the FAO/WHO recommendations on energy, protein and nutrient requirements is quite abstract and difficult for consumers to understand. Consequently, a simplified message was developed in terms of Food-Based Dietary Guidelines (FBDG) by transforming nutrients into food groups for better understanding. In the Cyprus meeting in 1995, FAO and WHO in collaboration with experts developed eating guidelines for healthy lifestyles for preventing under-nutrition, over-nutrition and unsafe food consumption [8]. These guidelines serve as principles for countries to adopt and adapt as their own guidelines. Upon implementation, a guideline can be periodically revised in line with current scientific evidence. Over 100 countries worldwide have developed their own FBDGs that are suitable for their own nutrition situations, food availability, culinary cultures and eating habits. From the simplified message, FBDGs have been developed into more consumer-friendly formats, especially in terms of graphic design. Examples of graphical FBDGs from different countries are shown in **Figure 4**. Many of the designs are specific to the cultures of implementing countries. In addition, a design can also be modified if it proves to be an ineffective tool for consumer education, especially for preventing NCDs. For example, the USA's graphical

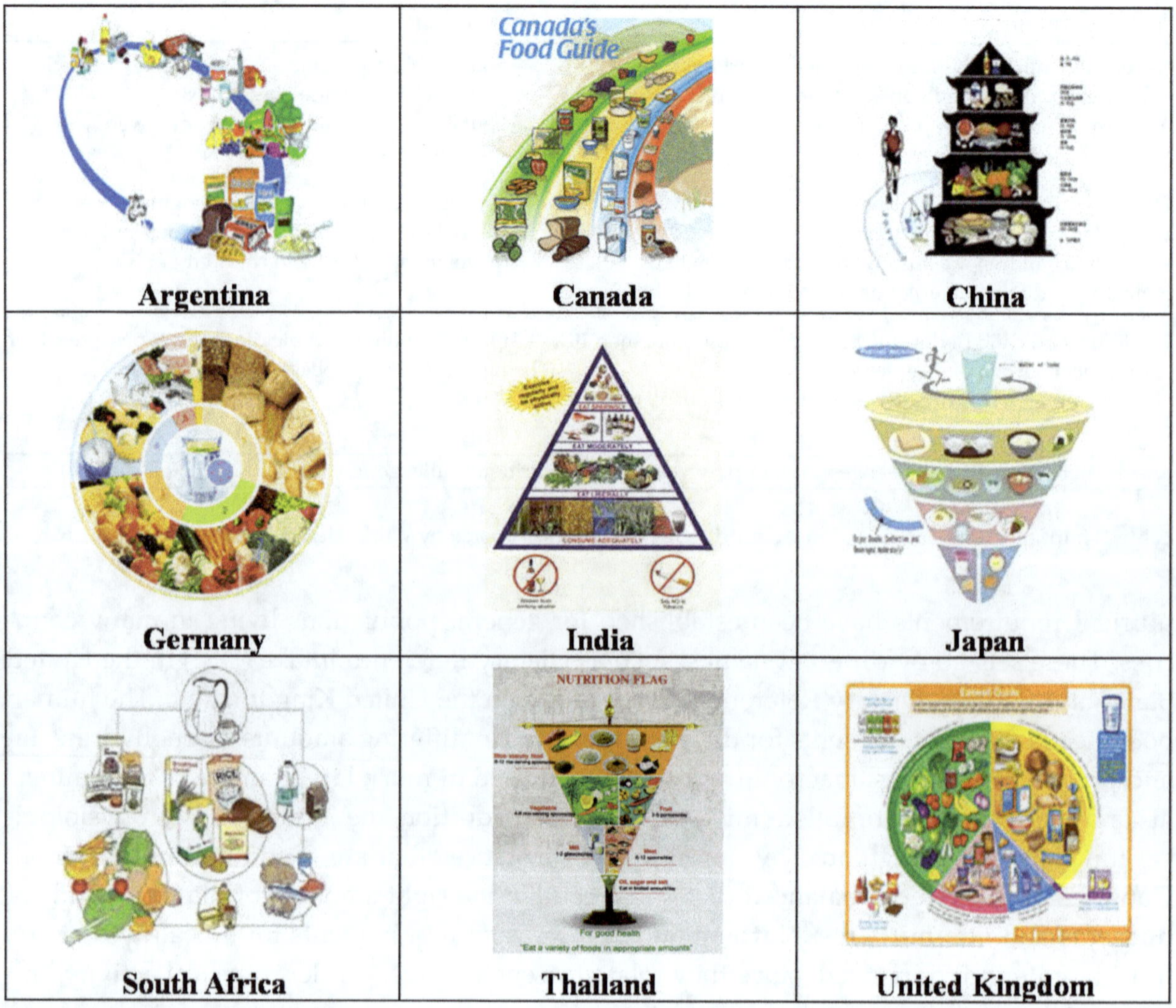

Figure 4. Examples of graphical FBDGs implemented in different countries. *Source*: http://www.fao.org/nutrition/nutrition-education/food-dietary-guidelines/en/.

FBDG was changed from a pyramid pattern into a plate pattern (**Figure 5**). In addition, many countries later included exercise in their graphical FBDGs, since food alone cannot lead to a healthy life. Messages on the graphical FBDGs of every country are similarly shown as food groups, not nutrients, which general consumers can more easily understand.

3.3. Nutrient reference values for nutrition labelling

In 1941, the Food and Nutrition Board first developed a set of recommended nutrient requirements known as recommended dietary allowances or RDAs. These allowances were meant to provide 'nutrients beyond enough' for civilians and military personnel, since the values included a 'margin of safety' [9]. The established values for a nutrient can be different for different requirements due to age and gender. These RDAs were subsequently revised every 5–10 years until 1997 when dietary reference intake (DRI) was introduced in order to broaden the existing RDA system. The DRI consisted of a set of four reference values: (i) estimated average requirements (EARs) wherein the average nutrient intake satisfies the needs of 50%

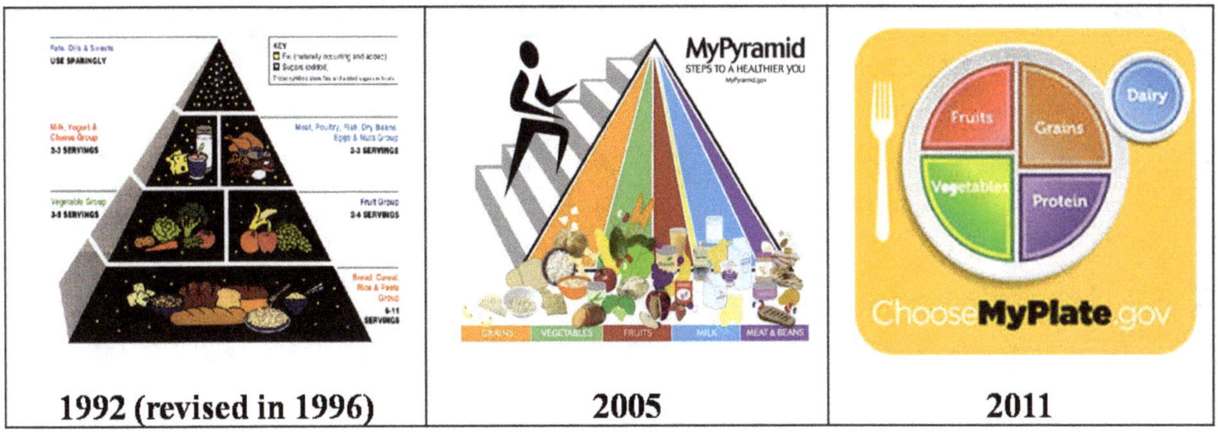

Figure 5. Series of changes in USA's graphical FBDGs. *Source*: http://www.cnpp.usda.gov.

of healthy individuals, (ii) recommended dietary requirements (RDA) or nutrient amounts sufficient to meet the requirements of 97.5% of a population, (iii) adequate intake (AI) or the approximate value determined from observations or experiments on nutrient intake from a group or groups of healthy people (where there was no established RDA) and (iv) tolerable upper intake (UL) or the highest level of nutrient intake that is considered to be safe and causes no side effects in most people [10]. Since these sets of values were developed for specific purposes, they could be adopted directly for use as references among general consumers.

In 1985, CODEX grouped nutrients into a single set and established their reference values known as 'nutrient reference values-requirements (NRVs-R)' to be used for individuals aged older than 36 months as shown in **Table 2** [11]. Most of the NRVs-R values are similar to those listed in the RDA. The CODEX values are meant to be used as references in preparing nutrition labels for consumer education. It is expected that a consumer can decide the appropriateness of a food for his/her health by considering what percentage of a nutrient's daily requirement (%NRVs) can he/she obtain from eating a portion of a food. Percentage NRVs is meant to help consumers in making correct food choices for their health. Other than the term NRVs-R as defined by CODEX, other terminologies have been developed, such as daily value (DV) used by the U.S. Food and Drug Administration (USFDA) for their Nutrition Fact Panel (NFP). Moreover, nutrient reference values–non-communicable disease (NRVs-NCD) has also been specifically established by CODEX for consumer education in order to educate the risks of NCDs.

3.4. Nutrients related to the risks of NCDs

To prevent diet-related NCDs, WHO recommended healthy populations to limit their intake of saturated fat, *trans* fat, cholesterol, sugar, sodium and total energy, while ensuring adequate intakes of carbohydrate, protein and dietary fibre [12, 13]. Nutrient intake goals for preventing NCDS are shown in **Table 3**. Similarly, the FBDGs of most countries recommend limiting the consumption of fat, sugar or salt, as well as foods and beverages high in energy. For fat, concern is placed on not only the quantity but also the quality of fat consumed, especially saturated fats and *trans* fat. In addition, and based on convincing evidence, CODEX

Nutrients	Values of NRV-R
Vitamins	
Vitamin A (μg)	800*
Vitamin D (μg)	5**
Vitamin C (μg)	60
Vitamin K (μg)	60
Thiamin (mg)	1.2
Riboflavin (mg)	1.2
Niacin (mg NE)	15**
Vitamin B6 (mg)	1.3
Folate (μ DFE)	400
Folic acid (μg)	200
Vitamin B12 ((μg)	2.4
Pantothenate (mg)	5
Biotin (μg)	30
Minerals	
Calcium (mg)	1000
Magnesium (mg)	300
Iron (mg)	14
Zinc (mg)	15
Iodine (μg)	150**
Copper	Value to be established
Selenium	Value to be established
Protein	50

* For the declaration of β-carotene (provitamin A) the following conversion factor should be used: 1 μg retinol = 6 μg β-carotene.

**Nutrient reference values for vitamin D, niacin and iodine may not be applicable for countries where national nutrition policies or local conditions provide sufficient allowance to ensure that individual requirements are satisfied.

Table 2. A set of numerical values of nutrient requirements (NRV-R) that are based on scientific data for purposes of nutrition labelling and relevant claims.

established NRVs-NCD that recommended limiting saturated fat and sodium—two main nutrients for lowering risks of NCDs—to not higher than 20 g and 2000 mg/day, respectively [11]. *Trans* fat is classified as the worst quality fat with recommended consumption at less than 1% of total energy. *Trans* fat increases blood low-density lipoprotein (bad) cholesterol as well as decreases high-density lipoprotein (good) cholesterol. The USFDA stated that partially hydrogenated oils (PHOs) are the primary dietary source of artificial *trans* fat in processed foods and must not be classified as 'generally recognized as safe' or GRAS for use in human food [14]. In contrast, increased intake of fruits, vegetables, whole grains and nuts is

Dietary factor	1989 WHO study group recommendations	2002 Joint WHO/FAO expert consultation recommendations (CODEX)	Rationale for Joint WHO/ FAO expert consultation recommendations
Total fat	15–30%	15–30%	Obesity/CVD/diabetes
Saturated fatty acids (SFAs)	0–10%	<10%	Diabetes/CVD
Polyunsaturated fatty acids (PUFAs)	3–7%	6–10%	CVD
n-6 PUFAs	55–75%	5–8%	CVD
n-3 PUFAs	0–10%	1–2%	CVD
Trans fatty acids		<1%	CVD
Monounsaturated fatty acids (MUFAs)		By difference[a]	
Total carbohydrate	55–75%	55–75%[b]	
Free sugars[c]	0–10%	<10%	Obesity/dental diseases
Complex carbohydrate	50–70%	No recommendation	
Protein	10–15%	10–15%[d]	
Cholesterol	0–300 mg	<300 mg/d	CVD
Sodium chloride (sodium)[e]	<6 g/d	<5 g/d (<2 g/d)	
Fruits and vegetables	≥ 400 g/d	≥400 g/d	CVD/cancer
Pulses, nuts and seeds	≥ 30g/d (as part of the 400 g of fruit and vegetables)		
Total dietary fibre	27–40 g/d	From food[f]	Obesity/diabetes/
Non-starch polysaccharides (NSP)	16–24 g/d	From food[f]	CVD/cancer

Notes: [a]This is calculated as total fat – (SFAs + PUFAs + *trans* fatty acids).
[b]The percentage of total energy available after taking into account that consumed as protein and fat, hence the wide range.
[c]The term 'free sugars' refers to all monosaccharides and disaccharides added to foods by the manufacturer, cook or consumer, plus sugar naturally present in honey, syrups and fruit juices.
[d]The suggested range should be seen in the light of the Joint WHO/FAO/Consultation on Protein and Amino Acid Requirements in Human Nutrition, held in Geneva from 9 to 16 April 2002.
[e]Salt should be iodized appropriately. The need to adjust salt iodization, depending on observed sodium intake and surveillance of iodine status of the population, should be recognized.
[f]Wholegrain cereals, fruits and vegetables are the preferred sources of NSP. The recommended intake of fruits and vegetables and consumption of wholegrain foods is likely to provide >20 g per day of NSP (>25 g per day of total dietary fibre).
*Adapted from Diet, nutrition and the prevention of chronic diseases. Report of a joint WHO/FAO expert consultation (WHO Technical Report Series 916) [13].

Table 3. Recommendations for nutrient intakes in population by WHO and CODEX* (% of total energy, unless otherwise stated).

recommended by all organizations for preventing NCDs. An average intake of a minimum of 400 g of fruits and vegetables per day, or five servings, is recommended for preventing the risks of NCDs, such as heart disease, cancer, diabetes and obesity [13]. Eating a variety of vegetables and fruits clearly ensures an adequate intake of potassium and most micro-nutrients, dietary fibre and a host of essential non-nutrient substances. The consumption of fruits and vegetables can replace foods high in saturated fats, sugar or salt.

Balanced eating at all life stage, beginning with conception, is crucial for preventing chronic diseases. Over the last two decades, growing evidence has shown that *in utero*, infant and young child under-nutrition are directly linked to vulnerability to adult NCDs [2, 15]. Consequently, public health and nutrition interventions during the first 1000 days of life, or from conception to 2 years of age, are encouraged.

It is globally accepted that deaths related to NCDs can be partly reduced by investments to promote healthy diets following WHO's recommended eating pattern among populations. Appropriate information via food and nutrition labelling, as well as restrictions on the marketing of unhealthy foods, are major interventions to promote healthy diets [16] (**Figure 6**).

4. Nutrition labelling

Consumer education is an efficient tool for addressing malnutrition challenges. However, it must use effective messages, delivered by effective media and under the right environment. Nutrition labelling on packaged foods is widely used as an educational tool to provide consumers with nutrition information about specific food products. It is intentionally used as

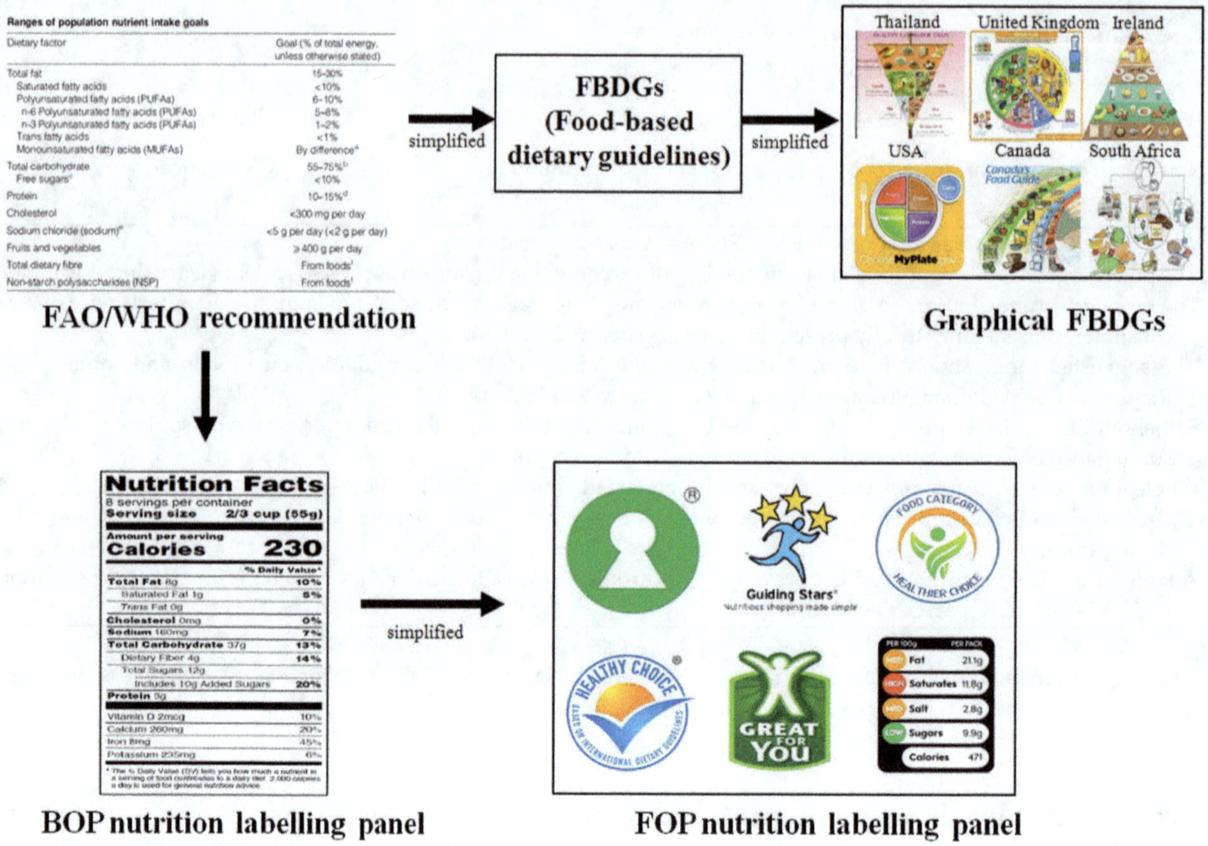

Figure 6. From healthy eating recommendations to different interventions for consumer education.

a tool for enabling general consumers to select foods that are appropriate for their health. Ideally, nutritionally educated consumers should be the demand for creating a healthy-food environment. Moreover, nutrition labelling is also used as a marketing tool for the food industry in terms of product reformulation and market expansion of packaged food products around the world [11, 17].

According to the CODEX Guidelines on Nutrition Labelling (CAC/GL 2-1985), the nutrient declaration should be mandated for all pre-packaged foods if nutrition or health claims are made. Two formats exist for the nutrition labelling panel, namely, a traditional format and a graphical format [17]. Nutrition labels using the traditional format are normally located on the back side of food packages, while graphical format panels use a simplified format and are located on the front side of a food package.

4.1. Traditional format nutrition labelling

The traditional format normally reports factual information about the nutrients found in a food item. The patterns/panels and nutrients included vary among countries or regions depending upon priority nutrition issues. A basic panel contains a nutrient declaration and supplementary information. For the nutrient declaration, essential key elements include amounts of energy, protein, carbohydrates, sugars, fat, saturated fat and sodium, as well as vitamins and minerals. Under certain circumstances, a nutrient may be declared differently. For example, most nutrition panels identify sodium (in milligrams) as a nutrient, except in the EU nutrition labelling panel that identifies it as a food item in terms of 'salt in grams'. Surprisingly, the explanation for this difference is for the same purpose, which is to avoid consumer confusion and for their better understanding. In fact, in the CODEX Guidelines on Nutrition Labelling, national authorities can choose to use the term 'salt' instead of the term 'sodium'. This issue highlights an interesting challenge for national authorities in developing educational strategies for public awareness, especially in how to understand and use nutritional labelling most effectively (**Figure 7**). Furthermore, the energy value and nutrient amounts can be expressed based on different reference units, i.e. per 100 g or 100 mL or per serving or per package, with percentages of nutrient reference values, particularly for vitamins and minerals. This situation might be due to different logics used during panel development. In fact, different reference units provide consumers with different views of information and usefulness. A reference unit of per 100 g or 100 ml compares nutritional properties between food products of the same category; whereas, a reference unit of per serving or per package is intended to inform consumers about the amounts of energy and nutrients obtained in one eating.

Some nutrition panels also contain information on the percentage that a certain amount of a consumed nutrient can fulfil in terms of daily requirements. Simply put for consumers, 'what percent of my daily requirements does this nutrient fulfil if consumed in a specific amount, recommended serving, or serving size?' This information is shown as percent nutrient reference values (%NRVs) or percent daily intake (%DI). Unfortunately, this information does not always appear in every panel format even though it is a useful guide for consumers.

Supplementary information located below the nutrition fact information usually consists of certain reference numbers on daily requirements of the nutrients which have been used for

Nutrition Facts

Serving Size 2/3 cup (55g)
Servings Per Container About 8

Amount Per Serving	
Calories 230	Calories from Fat 72
	% Daily Value*
Total Fat 8g	**12%**
Saturated Fat 1g	**5%**
Trans Fat 0g	
Cholesterol 0mg	**0%**
Sodium 160mg	**7%**
Total Carbohydrate 37g	**12%**
Dietary Fiber 4g	**16%**
Sugars 1g	
Protein 3g	
Vitamin A	10%
Vitamin C	8%
Calcium	20%
Iron	45%

* Percent Daily Values are based on a 2,000 calorie diet. Your daily value may be higher or lower depending on your calorie needs.

	Calories:	2,000	2,500
Total Fat	Less than	65g	80g
Sat Fat	Less than	20g	25g
Cholesterol	Less than	300mg	300mg
Sodium	Less than	2,400mg	2,400mg
Total Carbohydrate		300g	375g
Dietary Fiber		25g	30g

(a) USA

Energy	kJ/kcal
Fat	g
of which	g
- saturates,	g
- mono-unsaturates,	g
- polyunsaturates,	
Carbohydrate	g
of which	g
- sugars	g
- polyols,	g
- starch,	
Fibre	g
Protein	g
Salt	g
Vitamins and minerals	mg or µg

(b) EU

NUTRITION INFORMATION

Servings per package: (insert number of servings)
Serving size: g (or mL or other units as appropriate)

	Average Quantity per Serving	% Daily Intake* (per Serving)	Average Quantity per 100g (or 100mL)
Energy	kJ (Cal)	%	kJ (Cal)
Protein	g	%	g
Fat, total	g	%	g
– saturated	g	%	g
Carbohydrate	g	%	g
– sugars	g	%	g
Sodium	mg (mmol)	%	mg (mmol)
Vitamin C	mg	%RDI	mg
Calcium	mg	(per serving)	mg
		%	
		%	

*Percentage daily intakes are based on an average adult diet of 8700 kJ.

(c) Australia

NUTRITION INFORMATION

Servings per package: 25
Serving size: 15 g

	Average Quantity per Serving	Average Quantity per 100 g
Energy	384 kJ	2560 kJ
Protein	4.4 g	29.3 g
Fat, total	7.6 g	50.7g
– saturated	1.5 g	10.0 g
Carbohydrate	2.0 g	13.3 g
– sugars	0.9 g	6.0 g
Sodium	41 mg	273 mg

Figure 7. Examples of nutrition labelling panels.

evaluating the percent contribution to needs of those nutrients. This supplementary information is optional under the CODEX and can be included if it can provide consumers with better information [11]. Recently, the US has changed its traditional nutrition labelling panel format to remove certain complicated information in the nutrient list [18] (**Figure 8**).

Nutrition labelling is regulated differently in different countries in terms of being mandatory or voluntary. Due to increasing concerns about overweight, obesity and NCDs, many countries are making nutrition labelling mandatory for all packaged food items. This stance is in line with the most current CODEX amendment to the Guidelines on Nutrition Labelling. This amendment recommends that nutrient declaration should be mandatory for all pre-packaged

Nutrition Facts
Serving Size 2/3 cup (55g)
Servings Per Container About 8

Amount Per Serving	
Calories 230	Calories from Fat 72
	% Daily Value*
Total Fat 8g	**12%**
Saturated Fat 1g	**5%**
Trans Fat 0g	
Cholesterol 0mg	**0%**
Sodium 160mg	**7%**
Total Carbohydrate 37g	**12%**
Dietary Fiber 4g	**16%**
Sugars 1g	
Protein 3g	
Vitamin A	10%
Vitamin C	8%
Calcium	20%
Iron	45%

* Percent Daily Values are based on a 2,000 calorie diet. Your daily value may be higher or lower depending on your calorie needs.

	Calories:	2,000	2,500
Total Fat	Less than	65g	80g
Sat Fat	Less than	20g	25g
Cholesterol	Less than	300mg	300mg
Sodium	Less than	2,400mg	2,400mg
Total Carbohydrate		300g	375g
Dietary Fiber		25g	30g

Nutrition Facts
8 servings per container
Serving size 2/3 cup (55g)

Amount per serving	
Calories	**230**
	% Daily Value*
Total Fat 8g	**10%**
Saturated Fat 1g	**5%**
Trans Fat 0g	
Cholesterol 0mg	**0%**
Sodium 160mg	**7%**
Total Carbohydrate 37g	**13%**
Dietary Fiber 4g	**14%**
Total Sugars 12g	
Includes 10g Added Sugars	**20%**
Protein 3g	
Vitamin D 2mcg	10%
Calcium 260mg	20%
Iron 8mg	45%
Potassium 235mg	6%

* The % Daily Value (DV) tells you how much a nutrient in a serving of food contributes to a daily diet. 2,000 calories a day is used for general nutrition advice.

Figure 8. Comparison between original and new nutrition facts label of the United states *Source*:http://www.fda.gov/Food/GuidanceRegulation/GuidanceDocumentsRegulatoryInformation/LabelingNutrition/ucm385663.htm.

foods, although nutrition or health claims are not made [11, 19]. Such implementation can be found in the United States, Canada, Australia and New Zealand, amongst other countries, where all pre-packaged foods, except for some certain food items, are mandated for nutrition labelling. Under regulation (EU) No. 1169/2011 of the European Parliament and of the Council of 25 October 2011, nutrition labelling will be mandatory for all pre-packaged foods in European Union (EU) countries from December 13, 2016. In ASEAN countries, nutrition labelling is still voluntary unless a nutrition or health claim is made.

Traditional nutrition labelling panels are not effective nutrition education tools for general consumers, because consumers rarely use them to make informed food choices [20]. Cowburn and Stockley conducted a systematic review on consumer understanding and use of nutrition labelling. Their research showed that while a high number of consumers read nutrition label panels, in reality the effect of the panels on their food choice decisions was low. In particular, food panels that were more complex in terms of format hindered consumer understanding, interpretation and use of the panels [20]. Similarly, Hammond and co-workers conducted a systematic review of nutrition labels on packaged foods in seven developed and developing countries. They highlighted that while overall prevalence of nutrition label use amongst the general population in each country was generally high, it still varied across subgroups. However, in terms of understanding, many consumers had difficulty in interpreting the quantitative information due to reading frequency, level of education, nutrition knowledge and health status. Moreover, graphical formats were preferred, such as healthy symbols on front-of-pack (FOP) labels. Nevertheless, both systematic reviews concluded that nutrition labelling was a constructive and cost-effective intervention that can contribute to make informed food choices. They also recommended that governments should try to find the most appropriate and effective format that consumers can most easily access and understand [21]. Under these circumstances, national authorities and non-governmental organizations in many countries intend to simplify their current nutrition labelling panels into the easiest formats possible to increase their use and promote healthier food choices and eating habits.

4.2. From 'traditional' to 'graphical'

Although the number of persons affected by over-nutrition has grown, along with NCDS, few of the most recognized intervention strategies have included providing effective consumer education and creating a healthy food environment. Nonetheless, simplification of the traditional nutrition labelling panels has sparked the interest of many governments and non-governmental organizations. To reduce consumer confusion in using the panels, greater attention has been placed on those nutrients that have proven to be potential risk factors for NCDs and excluding other nutrients usually listed on traditional nutrition labelling panels. Emphasis is being placed on guiding consumers to make quicker, easier and more accurate buying decisions. Likewise, food industries must be inspired and have greater opportunities to develop products with better nutrition profiles and introduce them into the market at affordable prices for consumers. In terms of format, a large area is often times needed to display the traditional nutrition labelling panel that is on the back of a food package or back-of-pack (BOP), which hinders visibility and legibility. As an important consequence, the traditional format may not encourage food industries to reformulate their products to have better nutrient profiles. Consequently, governments and non-governmental organizations have been working towards simplified nutrition labelling to help consumers identify and make healthier food choices at a glance.

4.3. Graphical format nutrition labelling

Initial interest in simplified nutrition labelling emerged in the late 1960s and was first developed by a non-profit organization (the American Heart Association) in 1987, followed by a government sector (Swedish Food Administration) in 1989 in the form of heart check and green keyhole symbols, respectively (**Figure 9**). The simplified nutrition labelling panel was in a graphical format and located on the front of food packages or front-of-pack. The FOP nutrition labelling panel became interesting and friendly for consumers.

Different FOP nutrition labelling panels were later developed in many parts of the world and managed by different organizations, for example, food industries, government agencies, non-profit organizations, food retailers and non-industry experts. To reduce panel complexity,

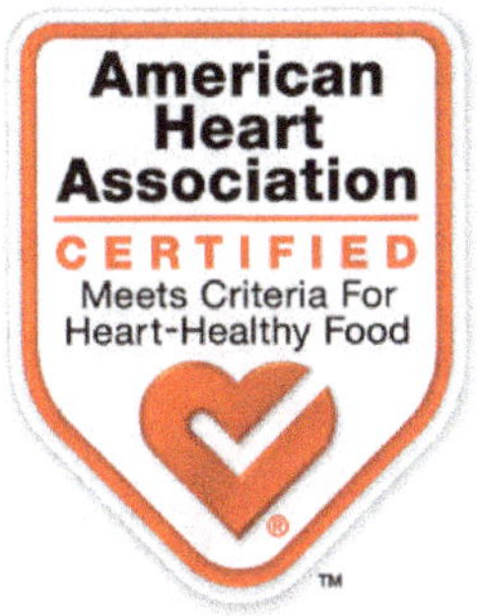
American
Heart
Association
CERTIFIED
Meets Criteria For
Heart-Healthy Food

(a) US- Heart Check Mark

(b) Norway – Green Keyhole

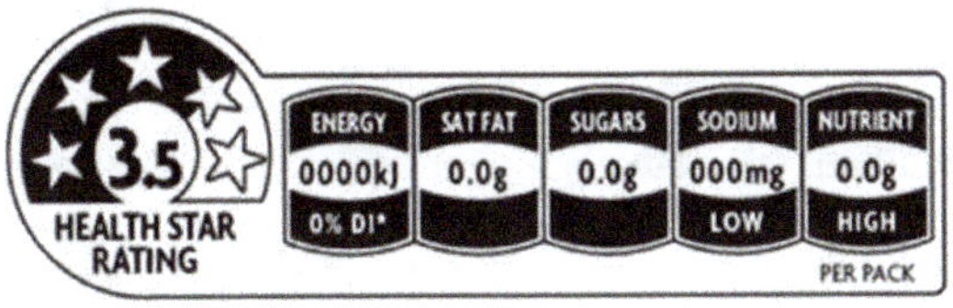

(c) Australia - Health star rating

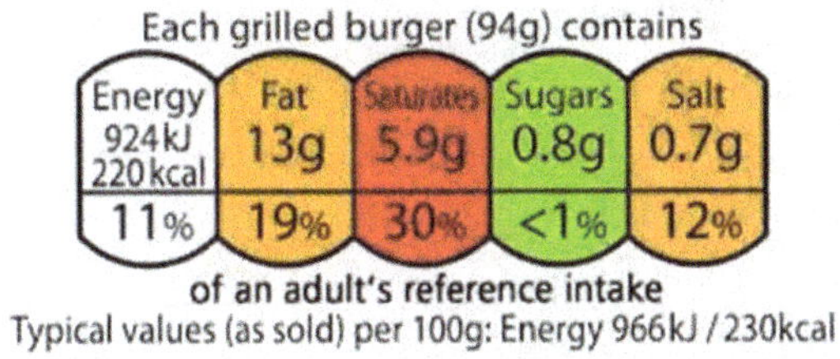

(d) UK – Traffic light label

Figure 9. Examples of Front-of-Pack nutrition labelling panels. *Source*: (a) http://www.heart.org/HEARTORG/HealthyLiving/HeathyEating/Heart-CheckMarkCertification/Heart-Check-Mark-Certification_UCM_001179_SubHomePage.jsp?pid=7bc18bff66f34f909&pcid=MP; (b) http://www.livsmedelsverket.se/en/food-and-content/labelling/nyckelhalet/; (c) http://healthstarrating.gov.au/internet/healthstarrating/publishing.nsf/content/home; (d) https://www.gov.uk/government/uploads/system/uploads/attachment_data/file/300886/2902158_FoP_Nutrition_2014.pdf.

they contained information on 'undesirable' or 'disqualified' nutrients including energy, fat, saturated fat, *trans* fat, sugar and sodium. In some cases, more 'desirable' or 'qualified' nutrients were also included, such as dietary fibre or those nutrients that reduce the risks of NCDs. Van Der Bend et al. studied 40 FOP nutrition labelling panels in use around the world and they noted that undesirable nutrients as well as dietary fibre were the most common elements contained in the panels [22] (**Table 4**).

The standards for these nutrients in foods or food products can be interpreted based either on serving size, 100 g/ml, 100 kcal/kJ, daily value or a combination. Which standard is used depends upon the one that consumers best understand and/or the one that is most agreeable to the food industry. The design in terms of message, size, characteristics and panel location should be one that consumers can easily see, remember and understand. However, it should not make false or exaggerated claims about a product. The values used to establish criteria are normally based on internationally recognized health guidelines as well as the unique characteristics of food products. The established criteria usually are found as either independent qualifying/disqualifying thresholds or relative to what is found in commercial products. The different designs used in FOP nutrition labelling panels may require consumer input to determine what is absolutely (non-directive), partly (semi-directive) or not at all (directive) needed [22].

Nutrient	Percentage (%) use in FOP nutrition labelling panels
Dietary fibre	62.5
Protein	35
Calcium	30
Saturated fatty acids	75
Total sugar	62.5
Total fat	62.5
Sodium	62.5
Energy	52.5
Trans fatty acids	37.5
Cholesterol	30

Table 4. Percentages of nutrients normally found mentioning on the FOP nutrition labelling panels.

According to The Strategic Counsel, Toronto, Canada, at least 158 FOP nutrition labelling panels are being implemented and these are divisible into four types, nutrient specific, summary indicator, food group information and hybrids [23]. Examples of these FOP nutrition labelling panels are shown in **Table 5**.

1. *Nutrient specific*: This type of FOP panel contains four to five types of nutrients that should be limited in order to reduce the risk of NCDs, that is energy, fat, saturated fat, sugar and sodium. The information shown is generally in amounts of nutrients per serving, which is not always the case and depending on a country's context. In some instances, per 100 g or 100 ml or per package are also used. Percentages of daily requirement or maximum consumption limits per day of the nutrients are additional information shown on these panels. The presentation pattern can be shown as a sequence of rows or as a pie chart. The pattern is presented either in monochrome or multi-chrome (normally consisting of three colours similar to a traffic light).

2. *Summary indicator*: A summary indicator is represented only by a symbol that may or may not imply good health. To have a summary indicator shown on the front of a food package, the nutrient profile of the food must pass the established nutrition standard for that food, usually through comparisons on the nature of such food or food product. The criteria mostly depend on the amount of undesirable nutrients removed, reduced or contained.

3. *Food group information*: This type of FOP nutrition labelling panel is based on the existence of certain food groups or food items that should be consumed in greater amounts to reduce the risk of NCDs. The terminologies used for identifying food items on the panel are normally similar to those recommended in a country's food-based dietary guidelines and aiming for better consumer understanding.

4. *Hybrids*: More than one type of FOP nutrition labelling panel can be shown on the same package, which should provide additional information on different aspects to increase

	Nutrient specific	Summary indicator	Food group information	Hybrids
Non-evaluative				
Nutrient	monochrome GDA			
food group content			Food group information • My Pyramid • "Great For You" icon (Walmart) • whole grains council stamp	
Evaluative or interpretative				
Ordinal rating scale		• Health Star Rating – Australia • Nu Val		
Classification	• Multichrome GDA • Traffic light			In affiliated with the Singapore HCS
Conclusive				
Qualifying or disqualifying threshold criteria		• Healthier Choice (Choices Program) • Keyhole • Healthier Choice (TH)		• Health Star Rating – Australia • Singaporean Healthier Choice Symbol
Relative criteria		• Healthier Choice (TH)		

Source: Van Der Bend et al. [22], www.healthierlogo.com.

Table 5. Examples of each type of FOP nutrition labelling panels..

consumer understanding. For example, a summary indicator panel provides information for purchasing decisions, while an additional nutrient specific type panel explains the beneficial nutrient profile of the product.

Within the same type of FOP nutrition labelling panel, messages can provide different levels of information. A deeper informative message should have a higher impact on consumer decision-making, especially for those with health concerns. However, such a message must be developed through a process of evaluation, interpretation and conclusion as provided by different sectors, that is government, NGOs, food businesses, consumer protection agency and academics.

The degree of informativeness can be ranked at three levels.

1. *Non-evaluative or non-directive*: The information shown on monochrome FOP nutrient specific and food group information panels are based on this level of informativeness. Fact-based information on nutritive values of the selected nutrients is shown. The input is only on selecting certain information from traditional BOP nutrition labelling panels and reporting it in a simplified format or indicating what beneficial natural food group the product contains. Consequently, all foods can have a monochrome nutrient specific type of FOP panel with no need for further screening or evaluation by any party, as long as a complete data set for the required nutrients exists. At this level of informativeness, a FOP nutrient specific panel is suitable for more knowledgeable consumers since there is limited guidance. Additional information, such as percent contribution to the recommended daily intake, may not be understandable by most consumers as well. For food group information panels, the food group that is recommended for greater consumption is already visible. Hence, it should be easy for consumers to make a decision.

2. *Evaluative or interpretative or semi-directive*: Nutrition criteria are normally developed for categories of foods based on the FAO/WHO recommendations for energy, protein and nutrient requirements and using the nutrition criteria of four to five undesirable nutrients for meals, snacks and beverages. The criteria are usually developed into three levels of risk classification for each nutrient of each food category, that is high risk, potentially high risk and low risk. The multi-chrome FOP nutrient specific type panel is an example of a product at this level of informativeness. The amount and percent recommended daily intake of nutrients are listed with the NCDs risk evaluation. The risk evaluation result is indicated as colours, and usually as traffic light colours where red, amber and green indicate high, potentially high and low risk, respectively. Consumers can classify a food or a food product as good or bad depending upon the numbers of red, amber and green colours presented. The FOP summary indicator panel at this level is being implemented in Australia and the USA. Australia's Star® and the United States' Nu Val® are good examples of the use of this level for ordinal rating, wherein the risk evaluation is presented as number of stars or a full score of 100, respectively. The more stars there are, or the higher the score, the healthier the products. The application of this level of informativeness, either in the FOP nutrient specific or summary indicator type, still requires consumers to make independent judgments.

3. *Conclusive or directive*: A holistic nutrition standard for each food or food product is developed at this level of informativeness in either a positive or negative direction with the aim of reducing the risks of NCDs. Similar to the evaluative and interpretative levels, development must involve academicians and stakeholders. However, the criteria implemented at this level must provide a clear judgment in terms of qualified/disqualified or pass/non-pass in order to allow the use of a specific symbol on a product's FOP. Normally, the nutrition standard is specifically developed for each food product with regard to its nature, which may be as a threshold value or ability to reduce the undesirable nutrient(s) associated with NCDs risk that are normally high in such food or food product. Criteria can be developed based on reference values found in food products of the same type or group that are available in the market. These can be single or multiple criteria depending on the nature of the product. In practice, the criteria can be ideal, but they must also be feasible for food industries. For example, the nutrition standard for fish sauce is <6000 mg of sodium per 100 ml, which is a 30% reduction from what is normally found in the market (9000 mg per 100 ml). The nutrition standard for beverages is <6% sugar, which is a 50% reduction from 12% in generally marketed beverages. Sodium and sugar represent single criterion that have been developed relative to commercial products. An example of multiple criteria is milk, wherein the nutrition standard includes no sugar added and <1.5% fat. These criteria are independently developed as threshold values. The input of this informativeness level results in products that are deemed to be nutritionally healthier than others of the same type or group that are available in the market. Only products that pass screening with their nutrition standards qualify for these specific symbols. Most summary indicator types are developed at this level of informativeness.

4.4. A note of caution

A simplified FOP nutrition labelling panel aims to ease the lives of consumers by providing decision-making guidance based on scientific evidence. However, consumers tend to interpret panels that contain higher levels of informativeness in terms of 'claims'. Consequently, the processes used for nutrition standard development, as well as consumer communication, must be conducted carefully and take into account the available international standard found in the Codex Alimentarius on nutrition and health claims. For example, the green colour on a multi-chrome FOP nutrient specific type panel can be understood as a 'nutrition claim'. An FOP summary indicator can be understood either as a nutrition or health claim in terms of its environmental factors. An FOP summary indicator with a description of a food category and dominate nutrient (either higher or lower) can be interpreted as a nutrition claim, while ones with no description can be understood either way. Take, for example, the first two symbols on the green key hole and heart check symbol FOP nutrition labelling panels. Even though these two different symbols might have been developed from the same criteria found in a nutrient profile, they may affect consumer recognition differently. Since the green keyhole symbol was issued by the government authority that controls food quality and safety, it may be interpreted by consumers as a nutrition or health claim. Consequently, it is necessary for the government or issuing organization to either provide adequate information that the symbol has been issued based on the product's nutrient profile, not health impact, or indicate the FOP nutrition labelling panel is a hybrid type comprised of other types of FOP nutrition labelling, such as GDAs. Furthermore, consumers may interpret a symbol issued by a professional health association as a health claim. For the heart check symbol, the product might be interpreted in terms of lowering the risk for cardiovascular diseases. Consequently, harmonization of established standards with local and international standards and regulations should also be taken into consideration.

4.5. Outcome and expectation

While traditional BOP nutrition labelling panels are mandatory in most countries, the FOP nutrition labelling panels are implemented mainly on a voluntary basis. The exception is the monochrome Guideline Daily Amounts (GDAs) panel that is preferred by the food industry and has become mandated in some countries. After nutrition standards have been developed and accepted, the food industry is the first stakeholder that is actively involved. Products that have met their nutritional standards should be promoted first. Product development research should be performed continuously in order to offer more product choices in the market by changing composition and/or reformulating using new ingredients and/or replacers. In addition, new products with acceptable nutrient profiles can also be introduced into the market. **Figure 10** indicates the numbers of food products that have been sorted, reformulated and developed with regard to the Choice International® criteria.

Reduction in packaging size to fit with minimum serving size can also improve a product's nutrient profile as well as consumer behaviour. Consumers tend to eat a larger amount of food if that food is served/packaged in a larger serving size. To launch a qualified food

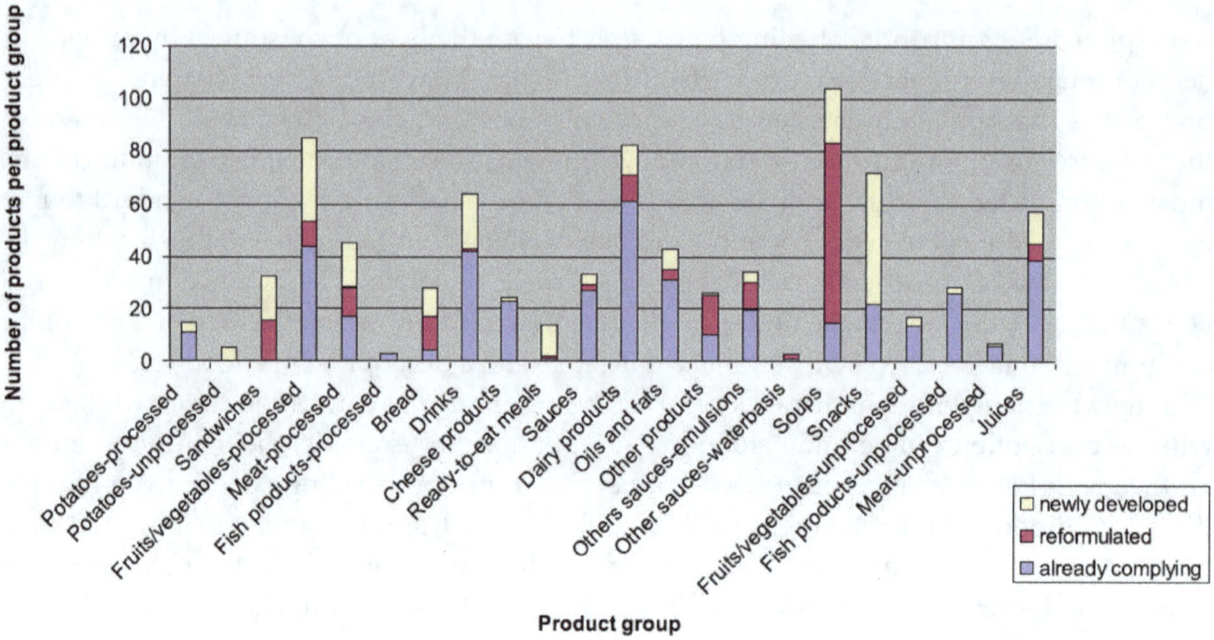

Figure 10. Total numbers of products that were newly developed, reformulated or already complaint with the Choice International® criteria (slide 26 Canada slide). *Source*: Ellis L Vyth et al. (2010) [24].

product (original, reformulated, newly developed) in the market, costs due to labelling changes is unavoidably increase. Hence, there must be a grace period for utilizing left-over packages and printing new ones. The concept used for advertising and promoting the FOP nutrition labelling panel must then include NCD risk, the purpose of which is for consumer education. For most consumers, sensory quality is an important issue and oftentimes more important than nutritional quality. The most conservative strategy is to improve the nutrient profile of a product but still maintain its original sensory quality. This may involve replacing normally-used ingredients with substitutes or replacers for salt, sugar or fat. Consumer behaviours may not change for the better if those undesirable nutrients are not replaced with acceptable ones. Since change in consumer eating behaviours towards better nutrition is the paramount goal, the promotion message sometimes must guide consumers to partly modify their sensory preference in order to gain better nutrition. However, this is a difficult process and takes time, but it must be urgently started. Marketing and logistics strategies are equally important as part of the promotion strategy, since the products must be widely available for consumers at affordable prices. If both main players—consumers and the food industry—satisfactorily respond to a program, the outcomes should have beneficial impacts for health and marketing.

Table 5 also indicates that external factors (i.e. community, culture) and internal factors (i.e. individual) can influence expected outcomes. Inputs from government and non-governmental agencies on several important issues, such as nutrition education, preventive medical care policy, support for nutritious food production and promotion in relationship to the food culture, are examples of external factors that can significantly influence to stakeholders. For consumers at the demand side, their buying decisions can also be influenced by individual factors, such as educational background, socioeconomic status, health status and awareness.

The program's outcomes should initially benefit consumers and food industries in terms of availability of nutritious foods in the market and increased product sales, respectively. In the long-term, it is expected that the information that is provided through the FOP nutrition labelling panel should serve as a nutrition education tool for changing consumers' eating behaviours, especially in terms of preference for undesirable nutrients.

A number of studies have evaluated the impacts of FOP nutrition labelling on consumer and industrial sides. Methodologies, such as self-reporting and focus groups, have been used to evaluate understanding and use of the FOP nutrition labelling panel among consumers in terms of their food purchasing decisions. Observational studies estimated the impact of FOP nutrition labelling panel on consumers' selection. Indicators, such as increased numbers of qualified product sales as well as reformulated and newly developed products in the market, were used to determine the impact of FOP nutrition labelling among industries. In addition, the impact of FOP nutrition labelling on nutrient intake and health outcomes can be evaluated from national food consumption and national nutrition surveys [25].

Many studies have shown that the FOP nutrition labelling panel has been quite helpful to consumers and their food choice decisions [25, 26]. Moreover, the simpler format for FOP nutrition labelling panels (e.g. Healthier Choice Tick, Smileys and Stars) is more effective than complex ones (e.g. Multiple Traffic Light, Wheel of Health, GDA scores), since consumers can more

<table>
<tr><th colspan="2">1st Example: Thailand's Healthier Choices for Meal</th></tr>
<tr><td>Character:</td><td>Source: http://healthierlogo.com/</td></tr>
<tr><td>Criteria:</td><td>Based on scorings of 4 desirable nutrients: protein, fiber, calcium, and iron, and 4 undesirable nutrients: total fat, saturated fat, total sugar, and sodium. The score ranges from 0-5 (0 – worst to 5 – best) regarding the content of each nutrient per 100 kcal, in which the full score is 40.
The qualifying thresholds are: (i) Energy per serving is 250-500 kcal, (ii) Score for each undesirable nutrient is > 0, and (iii) Total score is ≥ 20.</td></tr>
<tr><td>Type:</td><td>Summary indicator; Multiple criteria; Informativeness: Conclusive (Qualifying or disqualifying threshold)</td></tr>
<tr><td>Managing organization:</td><td>Government, Non-profit organization</td></tr>
<tr><th colspan="2">2nd Example: Thailand's Monochrome Guideline Daily Amounts (GDAs)</th></tr>
<tr><td>Character:</td><td>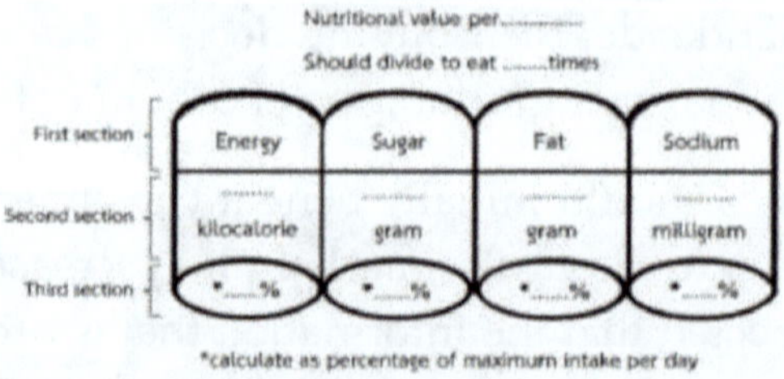

Source: Attachment to the Announcement of the Ministry of Public Health (No. 374) B.E.2559 (2016) Re. Food products Required to bear Nutrition Labelling and energy value, sugar, fat, sodium on the labels of some kinds of foods Guideline Daily Amounts, GDA Labelling</td></tr>
<tr><td>Criteria:</td><td>The panel consists of energy value, contents of undesirable nutrients, and percentages of recommended daily intake (%DI) per package. This FOP nutrition labelling panel is presently applied in snack foods, chocolate and similar products, certain bakery products, instant noodles and porridge, and chilled and frozen ready-to-eat meals.</td></tr>
<tr><td>Type:</td><td>Nutrient specific; No specific criteria; Informativeness: Non-evaluative (Nutrient)</td></tr>
<tr><td>Managing organization:</td><td>Government</td></tr>
</table>

3rd **Example**: United Kingdom's Multichrome Guideline Daily Amounts

Character:

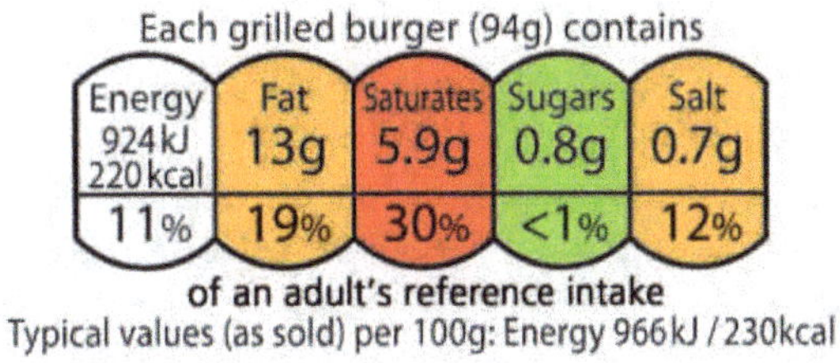

Source:
https://www.gov.uk/government/uploads/system/uploads/attachment_data/file/300886/2902158_FoP_Nutrition_2014.pdf

Criteria:

The energy value and contents of undesirable nutrients as well as their percentages in terms of adult reference intake (%RI) are shown on the panel as per one serving. However, the evaluation using color coding is performed based on the criteria shown in the table below after the values have been converted into per 100 g or 100 ml.

Text	LOW	MEDIUM	HIGH	
Colour code	Green	Amber	red	
Fat	≤ 3.0g/100g	> 3.0g to ≤ 17.5g/100g	> 17.5g/100g	> 21g/portion
Saturates	≤ 1.5g/100g	> 1.5g to ≤ 5.0g/100g	> 5.0g/100g	> 6.0g/portion
(Total) Sugars	≤ 5.0g/100g	> 5.0g and ≤ 22.5g /100g	> 22.5g/100g	> 27g/portion
Salt	≤ 0.3g/100g	> 0.3g to ≤ 1.5g/100g	>1.5g/100g	>1.8g/portion

(Department of Health, the Food Standards Agency, and devolved administrations in Scotland, Northern Ireland and Wales in collaboration with the British Retail Consortium, 2013, p.14)

Type: Nutrient specific; Multiple criteria; **Informativeness:** Evaluative and Interpretative (classification)

Managing organization: Government

4th **Example**: Australia's Health Star Rating (HSR)

Character:

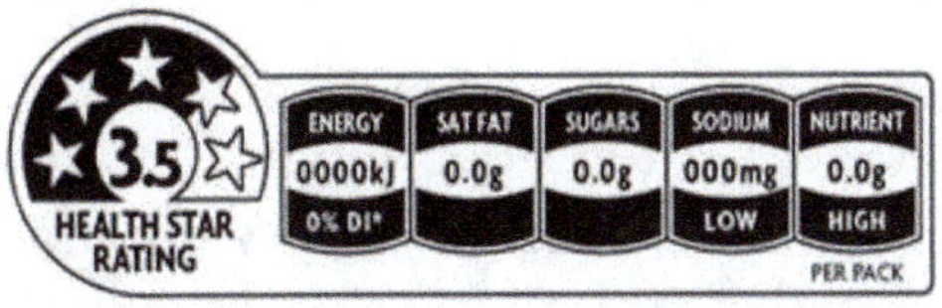

Source: http://healthstarrating.gov.au/internet/healthstarrating/publishing.nsf/content/home

Criteria:	Energy value, 3 undesirable nutrients, and 2 desirable nutrients (i.e., protein and fibre) indicated in one capsule as "nutrient" are shown on the panel as per package or per serving or per 100 g or 100 ml. However, the amounts are then converted into per 100 g or 100 ml and scored using established scoring criteria with a full score of 5.0 points. The calculated score is shown as numerically and in a darkened zone. The amount of nutrient per 100 g or 100 ml is evaluated for the "nutrient claim" message.
Type:	Hybrid; Multiple criteria; **Informativeness:** Evaluative and interpretative (Ordinal rating scale)
Managing organization:	Government
5th Example: USA's whole grains council stamp	
Character:	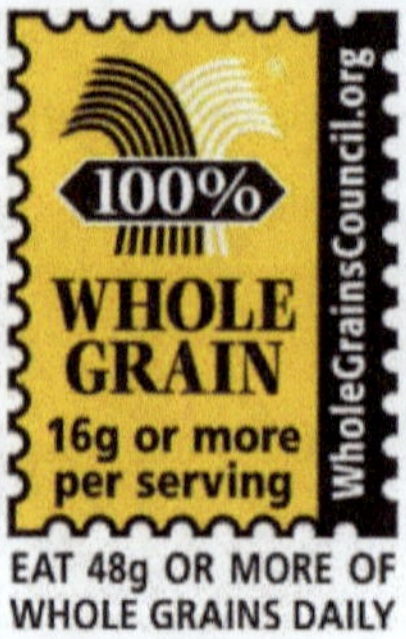 (a) **100 % Stamp** 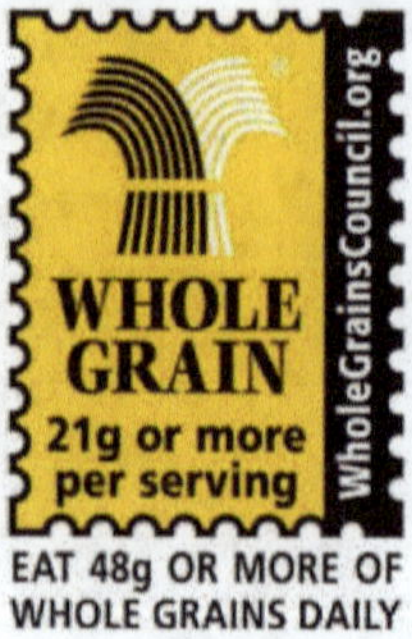 (b) **Basic Stamp** Source: http://wholegrainscouncil.org/whole-grain-stamp
Criteria:	**(a) 100% Stamp** – Product contains only whole grains of at least 16 g per serving. **(b) Basic stamp** - Product contain whole grain of at least 8 g per serving.
Type:	Food group information; Single criteria; **Informativeness**: Non-Evaluative (food group content)
Managing organization:	Non-government (Whole Grains Council)

Table 6. Examples of the implemented front- of pack nutrition labelling panels.

quickly select healthier food choices [27]. Furthermore, FOP nutrition labelling panels implemented by national authorities have more credibility. The wide variety of FOP nutrition labelling panels of different designs and criteria that are being implemented worldwide, however, can be confusing for consumers, which leads to misinterpretation and hinder their effectiveness [28]. Consequently, it has been suggested that a single format should be implemented. Before beginning the panel harmonization process, the use of a simple visual model, the so-called 'Funnel

Model' that was developed by Van Der Bend et al. can be effectively used to evaluate available FOP nutrition labelling panels on the market worldwide. The model aims to illustrate, describe and compare all existing FOP nutrient profiling systems based on qualifying and disqualifying ingredients, reference units, purposes of use, methodological approaches, types of organizations and directivity [22]. Moreover, it also provides an overview of the different characteristics of each FOP in use. The model then can be used as a tool for situation analysis and provide efficient information for establishing a single format of FOP nutrition labelling panel (**Table 6**).

4.6. Range of applications

The main purpose of FOP nutrition labelling panel is to enable consumers to select pre-packaged food products that have better nutrient profiles in reducing the risks of NCDs. Another indirect benefit, which should also be a main purpose, is to educate consumers and improve their daily eating behaviours. Industries can use established nutrition standards as one of the criteria for product development. Since NCDs have become a global nutrition challenge, international and national government agencies tend to implement certain strategies for controlling unhealthy food products in the market, especially those high in fat, sugar and sodium. High taxation for food products that contain excessive amounts of fat, sugar or sodium is one strategy that has been used in some countries. Policy-makers can use the standard in the FOP nutrition labelling panel as a guideline to impose higher taxes, such as sugar a tax on sugary drinks. Regarding WHO concerns on the marketing of foods and beverages to children, the FOP nutrition labelling panel can be used as a screening tool for foods and beverages to be sold in schools and areas nearby, as well as for advertisements aimed at children. Foods and beverages that pass the nutrition standard can be included in the country's FBDGs, which is the guideline for the general population. Moreover, the FOP nutrition labelling panel can also be used for product promotion in international trade, wherein a better nutrient profile can add value to exported products, especially since the panel has been mutually recognized.

Author details

Visith Chavasit[1*], Wantanee Kriengsinyos[1], Mayuree Ditmetharoj[2], Manasuwee Phaichamanan[2], Kangsadan Singsoong[2], Prapaisri Sirichakwal[1] and Araya Rojjanawanicharkorn[2]

*Address all correspondence to: vchavasit@gmail.com

1 Institute of Nutrition, Mahidol University, Nakhonpathom, Thailand

2 Food and Drug Administration, Nonthaburi, Thailand

References

[1] Webb P. Nutrition and the Sustainable Development Goals: An opportunity for real progress. SCN NEWS. 2015; Nutrition and the post-2015 development agenda seizing the opportunity (41):11-19. Geneva, Switzerland: United Nations System Standing Committee on Nutrition; 2015.

[2] Barker DJP. Fetal growth and adult disease. BJOG: An International Journal of Obstetrics & Gynaecology. 1992;99(4):275–6.

[3] WHO. Global status report on noncommunicable diseases. Geneva, Switzerland: World Health Organization; 2014.

[4] WHO. Fact sheet: Noncommunicable Diseases. World Health Organization; 2015. Available from http://www.who.int/mediacentre/factsheets/fs355/en/

[5] Lim SS, Vos T, Flaxman AD, Danaei G, Shibuya K, Adair-Rohani H, et al. A comparative risk assessment of burden of disease and injury attributable to 67 risk factors and risk factor clusters in 21 regions, 1990–2010: a systematic analysis for the Global Burden of Disease Study 2010. Lancet (London, England). 2012;380(9859):2224–60.

[6] WHO. Global Action Plan for the Prevention and Control of NCDs 2013–2020. Geneva, Switzerland: World Health Organization; 2013. 103 p.

[7] FAO. FAO's Role in Nutrition. 2016. Available from: http://www.fao.org/nutrition/en/

[8] Tontisirin K. Historical overview of food-based dietary guidelines. In FAO/WHO Technical Consultation on National Food-based Dietary Guidelines: Geneva, Switzerland: World Health Organization; 2006. pp. 7–8.

[9] IOM. How Should the Recommended Dietary Allowances Be Revised? Washington, DC: National Academies Press; 1994.

[10] IOM. Reference Intakes for Energy, Carbohydrate, Fiber, Fat, Fatty Acids, Cholesterol, Protein, and Amino Acids. Washington, DC: National Academies Press; 2002.

[11] Codex Alimentarius Commission. Codex Guidelines for Nutritional Labelling (CAC/GL 2-1985). Rome, Italy; 2013. Available from http://www.fao.org/ag/humannutrition/33309-01d4d1dd1abc825f0582d9e5a2eda4a74.pdf.

[12] WHO. WHO Technical Report Series No. 797. Geneva: World Health Organization; 1990.

[13] WHO. Diet, Nutrition and the Prevention of Chronic Diseases. Report of a Joint WHO/FAO Expert Consultation. Geneva, Switzerland: World Health Organization; 2003.

[14] USFDA. The FDA takes step to remove artificial trans fats in processed foods. 2015. Available from http://www.fda.gov/NewsEvents/Newsroom/PressAnnouncements/ucm451237.htm

[15] Gluckman PD, Hanson MA, Buklijas T. A conceptual framework for the developmental origins of health and disease. Journal of Developmental Origins of Health and Disease. 2010;1(01):6–18.

[16] Beaglehole R, Bonita R, Horton R, Adams C, Alleyne G, Asaria P, et al. Priority actions for the non-communicable disease crisis. The Lancet. 377(9775):1438-47.

[17] Hawkes C. 4-Government and voluntary policies on nutrition labelling: a global overview. In: Innovations in Food Labelling. Janice Albert, Ed. Cambridge: Woodhead Publishing; 2010. pp. 37–58.

[18] USFDA. Changes to the Nutrition Facts Label. In: USFDA, editor. 2016. Available from http://www.fda.gov/Food/GuidanceRegulation/GuidanceDocumentsRegulatoryInformation/LabelingNutrition/ucm385663.htm

[19] EUFIC. Global Update on Nutrition Labelling Brussels, Belgium: the European Food Information Council; 2015.

[20] Cowburn G, Stockley L. Consumer understanding and use of nutrition labelling: a systematic review. Public health nutrition. 2005;8(1):21–8. PubMed PMID: 15705241. eng.

[21] Campos S, Doxey J, Hammond D. Nutrition labels on pre-packaged foods: a systematic review. Public health nutrition. 2011;14(8):1496–506. PubMed PMID: 21241532.

[22] Van Der Bend D, Van Dieren J, Marques MDV, Wezenbeek NL, Kostareli N, Rodrigues PG, et al. A simple visual model to compare existing front-of-pack nutrient profiling schemes. European Journal of Food Research & Review. 2014;4(4):429.

[23] Schermel A, Emrich TE, Arcand J, Wong CL, L'Abbé MR. Nutrition marketing on processed food packages in Canada: 2010 Food Label Information Program. Applied Physiology, Nutrition, and Metabolism. 2013;38(6):666–72.

[24] Vyth EL, Steenhuis IH, Roodenburg AJ, Brug J, Seidell JC. Front-of-pack nutrition label stimulates healthier product development: a quantitative analysis. Int J Behav Nutr Phys Act. 2010 Sep 8;7:65. doi: 10.1186/1479-5868-7-65.

[25] Borgmeier I, Westenhoefer J. Impact of different food label formats on healthiness evaluation and food choice of consumers: a randomized-controlled study. BMC Public Health. 2009;9:184. PubMed PMID: PMC2702386.

[26] Sacks G, Rayner M, Swinburn B. Impact of front-of-pack 'traffic-light' nutrition labelling on consumer food purchases in the UK. Health Promotion International. 2009 December 1, 2009;24(4):344–52.

[27] Feunekes GI, Gortemaker IA, Willems AA, Lion R, van den Kommer M. Front-of-pack nutrition labelling: testing effectiveness of different nutrition labelling formats front-of-pack in four European countries. Appetite. 2008;50(1):57–70.

[28] Draper AK, Adamson AJ, Clegg S, Malam S, Rigg M, Duncan S. Front-of-pack nutrition labelling: are multiple formats a problem for consumers? The European Journal of Public Health. 2013;23(3):517–21.

7

Physical Activity and Obesity in Adults

Hidetaka Hamasaki

Abstract

Both obesity and physical inactivity are global health problems responsible for the risk increment of non-communicable diseases. Obese individuals usually cannot perform the recommended level of physical activity because of their low physical fitness and comorbidities. The purpose of this chapter is summarizing and evaluating the effects of physical activity on obesity. The author also focuses on the association between non-exercise activity thermogenesis (NEAT) and obesity. The author has reviewed 13 systematic reviews and meta-analyses of randomized controlled trials investigating the effects of physical activity on obesity. Exercise is essential for the management of obesity. However, exercise alone is not sufficient for long-term weight loss and improving cardiovascular disease (CVD) risk factors. Diet seems to be more effective for treating obesity than exercise. On the other hand, exercise improves cardiorespiratory fitness and skeletal muscle fitness, which leads to prevent sarcopenic obesity in the elderly. Exercise therapy should be performed in conjunction with diet therapy to improve obesity. NEAT is the main determinant of variability in daily energy expenditure, which considerably contributes to weight change in humans. The current evidence regarding NEAT is limited; however, NEAT appears to be effective for the management of metabolic diseases as well as weight loss. To reveal the optimal mode of physical activity and to elucidate the effects of NEAT on health beyond weight lowering, further well-designed studies are warranted.

Keywords: obesity, physical activity, exercise, systematic review and meta-analysis, non-exercise activity thermogenesis

1. Introduction

Obesity prevalence rapidly increases in the world. A recent epidemiological study reported that an estimated 1.46 billion adults were overweight (body mass index (BMI) > 25 kg/m^2), and 502 million adults were obese (BMI > 30 kg/m^2) [1]. Such global obesity pandemic has serious health problems. Obesity is an established risk factor for type 2 diabetes, cancers, and cardiovascular diseases (CVD), which cause large disease burden in many low-income countries as well as high-income countries [2]. Meanwhile, physical inactivity is also a global health problem responsible for the risk increment of non-communicable diseases such as type 2 diabetes, coronary heart disease, and breast and colon cancers [3]. If physical inactivity disappears, the life expectancy of humans would rise by 0.68 years [3]. The American College of Sports Medicine and the American Heart Association have recommended that obese individuals engage in moderate-intensity aerobic physical activity for at least 30 minutes for 5 days per week, or vigorous-intensity aerobic physical activity for at least 20 minutes for 3 days per week [4]. However, obese individuals have usually physical, social, and psychological barriers to perform the recommended level of physical activity [5], it is quite difficult to resolve these two major health problems worldwide; obesity and physical inactivity pandemic. Nevertheless, a large number of clinical studies investigating the effects of physical activity on obesity have been conducted, and the evidence has been accumulated. This review is aimed at summarizing the current literature related to physical activity and obesity, and evaluating the effects of physical activity on obesity. This review will help clinicians, researchers, and obese individuals in the management of obesity. In addition to the literature review, the author focuses on the association between non-exercise activity thermogenesis (NEAT) and obesity to explore the possibility of applying NEAT to the treatment of obesity.

2. Methods

The author searched the English literature on physical activity and obesity using PubMed/MEDLINE and Cochrane Database of Systematic Reviews in the last 5 years (from June 2011 to May 2016). The author reviewed systematic reviews and meta-analyses of randomized controlled trials (RCTs) in principle. The search terms were "physical activity or exercise", "obesity", "systematic review", and "meta-analysis". The search returned 175 published articles. If the study participants were younger than 18 years, pregnant and women in the perinatal, and study outcomes were not related to weight loss, metabolic diseases, and CVD risk factors, the studies were excluded from this review. The titles and abstracts of the identified articles were reviewed to determine their relevance. Thirteen articles met the criteria for this review.

3. Results

3.1. The effect of lifestyle intervention on obesity

Obviously, the first-line treatment for obesity is lifestyle habit improvement. Peirson et al. [6] updated the previous review of the effectiveness of behavioral and pharmacologic interventions for treating obesity in adults. Of 68 identified studies, eight studies were diet interventions, four studies were exercise interventions, 10 studies were diet plus exercise interventions, and 19 studies were lifestyle modifications. The exercise intervention had −1.49 kg reduction in weight, and the diet plus exercise intervention had −3.83 kg reduction in weight, respectively. Interventions by exercise alone did not achieve the greater reduction in weight, while interventions by diet alone showed the largest reduction in weight compared with the control group. However, the quality of evidence rating of these interventions was low. Additionally, this meta-analysis showed improvements in metabolic parameters in behavioral intervention subjects; TC (−0.10 mmol/L), low-density lipoprotein cholesterol (LDL-C) (−0.14 mmol/L), fasting blood glucose (−0.14 mmol/L), systolic blood pressure (−1.76 mmHg), and diastolic blood pressure (−1.60 mmHg). The incidence of type 2 diabetes was also less in the behavioral intervention group than in control group (risk ratio = 0.55, absolute risk reduction = 8.88%). No significant difference between behavioral and pharmacologic interventions for obesity-related outcomes was observed, although the potential adverse effects occurred more frequently in pharmacologic interventions than behavioral interventions. This result is of importance. Lifestyle intervention including an increase in physical activity is a safer and highly effective strategy for the management of obesity. However, this review also showed that the effectiveness of physical activity alone on obesity was small.

Behavioral weight management interventions can achieve weight reduction by 8–10%; however, most obese individuals regain weight after interventions end. A systematic review reported that the effect of extended care on weight-loss maintenance resulted in an additional 3.2 kg weight loss than normal care [7]. Dombrowski et al. [8] systematically reviewed the long-term effects of non-surgical treatments for weight-loss maintenance. Among 45 eligible studies, the weighted average age and BMI before interventions were 47.3 years and 35.2 kg/m^2, respectively. The weighted average weight loss across studies was −10.8 kg during the initial weight loss treatment (ranged from 2 to 12 months). The physical activity recommendations for weight loss were various. The most common recommendation was walking. Physical activity frequency varied from three to five times per week with a 20–30 minutes session; however, physical activity intensity was not described in detail. Most studies did not provide details of physical activity interventions. For weight-loss maintenance, recommendations for physical activity promoted a general increase in physical activity in most studies. Some studies provided specific recommendations such as walking, resistance training, and exercise classes. Extended behavioral/lifestyle management showed a mean weight change of −1.56 kg at 12 months, −1.96 kg at 18 months, and −1.48 kg at 24 months. However, there were no evidence of effectiveness for physical activity interventions and adding aerobic exercise or physical activity such as walking to a dietary intervention. Similarly, Johansson et al. [9] evaluated the effects of diet, exercise, or anti-obesity drugs on weight-loss maintenance after low-calorie diet interventions. A total of 20 RCTs met the criteria, which included three exercise (one of the three studies investigated the effect of both diet and exercise) intervention studies. The mean age and BMI of participants ranged from 28 to 48 years and from 27.9 to 41.6 kg/m^2, respectively. After the weight-loss intervention using very-low-calorie diet (<800 kcal/day) or low-calorie diet (800–1000 kcal/day), the studies randomly assigned participants to a weight-loss maintenance intervention group or a control group. Exercise interventions were resistance training, walking, and arthritis-adapted knee exercises. Exercise did not improve weight-loss maintenance, and a significant heterogeneity among studies was observed. When included two studies that focused on the only exercise, weight-loss maintenance was improved; weighted mean difference was 1.6 kg with 8 months of maintenance phase duration. However, if the unsupervised follow-up (median follow-up duration: 24 months) was included in the analysis, weight-loss maintenance was not improved; the weighted mean difference was −0.7 kg. Going on a diet without physical activity instructions seems to be quite difficult.

Several systematic reviews have examined the effectiveness of workplace physical activity interventions [10,11] and eHealth using the internet and smartphones [12], or interactive computer-based interventions [13] on obesity. They are effective for weight loss and weight maintenance than no behavioral intervention. However, there is insufficient evidence for improving obesity by such interventions. Daily physical activity in workplace and home besides structured exercise plays a crucial role in the management of obesity [14]. Hence, to elucidate the role of daily physical activity, NEAT is important in controlling body weight. The details are described later.

Table 1 shows a summary of published systematic reviews of the effectiveness of lifestyle interventions on obesity.

Authors, year	Number of studies	Summary of inclusion and exclusion criteria	Physical activity	Results
Peirson et al., 2014 [6]	68 RCTs	Subjects: BMI ≥25 kg/m², <40 kg/m² Study duration: no restrictions Outcomes: changes in weight, WC and BMI Language: English or French Surgical treatments were excluded	No detailed description	The exercise intervention: −1.49 kg The diet plus exercise intervention: −3.83 kg Behavioral intervention: TC −0.10 mmol/L, LDL-C −0.14 mmol/L, FBG −0.14 mmol/L, SBP −1.76 mmHg, DBP −1.60 mmHg The incidence of type 2 diabetes↓ No significant differences between behavioral and pharmacologic interventions for obesity were found
Dombrowski et al., 2014 [8]	45 RCTs	Subjects: BMI ≥30 kg/m², weight loss >5% of body weight at baseline within 24 months Study duration: ≥12 months Outcomes: weight change during the weight loss phase and maintenance treatment period Language: any language Surgical treatments and alternative interventions were excluded	Walking Exercise classes	The initial weight loss treatment: −10.8 kg Extended behavioral/lifestyle management: −1.56 kg at 12 months, −1.96 kg at 18 months, and −1.48 kg at 24 months No evidence of effectiveness for physical activity interventions and adding aerobic exercise or physical activity such to a dietary intervention

Authors, year	Number of studies	Summary of inclusion and exclusion criteria	Physical activity	Results
		Subjects with mental disorders were excluded		
Johansson et al., 2014 [9]	20 RCTs	Subjects: treatment with a very-low-calorie diet (<800 kcal/day) or low-calorie diet (<1000 kcal/day) Study duration: no restrictions Outcomes: weight change during the calorie restriction phase and the weight-loss maintenance phase Language: English	Resistance training Walking Arthritis-adapted knee exercises	The weighted mean difference was 1.6 kg with 8 months of maintenance phase duration The weighted mean difference was −0.7 kg if the unsupervised follow-up was included in the analysis

RCT, randomized controlled trial; BMI, body mass index; WC, waist circumference; TC, total cholesterol; LDL-C, low-density lipoprotein cholesterol; FBG, fasting blood glucose; SBP, systolic blood pressure; DBP, diastolic blood pressure.

Table 1. Systematic reviews and meta-analyses investigating the effects of lifestyle interventions on obesity.

3.2. Diet or exercise: comparing the effectiveness of management option for obesity

Which then is more effective for long-term weight loss, diet or exercise? There are four systematic reviews of RCTs to assess the effect of weight loss method on long-term change in weight and CVD risk factors. Schwingshackl et al. [15] compared the long-term effectiveness of (1) diet plus exercise vs. diet, (2) diet plus exercise vs. exercise, and (3) diet vs. exercise in overweight or obese individuals. Twenty one RCTs met the criteria and were analyzed. The mean age and BMI of subjects varied from 35 to 70 years and from 25.6 to 38.2 kg/m^2, respectively. Among eligible trials, 17 trials compared diet plus exercise vs. diet, 11 trials compared diet plus exercise vs. exercise, and 14 trials directly compared diet vs. exercise. Exercise interventions include aerobic exercise (walking, jogging, circuit training) and resistance training with the intensity of 50–85% of maximal heart rate. The weighted mean differences in change of body weight (−1.38 kg), waist circumference (−1.68 cm), waist-to-hip ratio (−0.01 U), and fat mass (−1.65 kg) were more significant in diet plus exercise group than in diet only group. The diet plus exercise group also had a more significant increase in cardiorespiratory fitness represented by maximal oxygen uptake (VO_2max) (3.61 mL/kg/min) and HDL-C (1.62 mg/dL), and a decrease in TG (−10.08 mg/dL) and diastolic blood pressure (−1.2 mmHg). When comparing diet plus exercise group with exercise only group, body weight (−4.13 kg), waist circumference (−3 cm), waist-to-hip ratio (−0.01 U), and fat mass (−3.6 kg) had more distinctive reductions in diet plus exercise group than in exercise only group. The weighted mean difference in change of VO_2max (2.13 mL/kg/min) was larger in diet plus exercise group. TC (−11.36 mg/dL), LDL-C (−10.03 mg/dL), systolic blood pressure (−2.84 mmHg), and diastolic blood pressure (−2.06 mmHg) changed more substantially by diet plus exercise interventions compared with exercise only interventions. Direct comparison between the effectiveness of diet and exercise revealed that diet interventions were more effective for reductions in body weight (−2.93 kg), fat mass (−2.2 kg), HDL-C (−0.96 mg/dL), and systolic blood pressure (−2.19 mmHg). However, the significant difference in change of cardiorespiratory fitness was not observed. This systematic review found that a combination of diet and exercise intervention was more effective in improving obesity-related anthropometric parameters, lipid profile, and blood pressure. Exercise is less effective for improving obesity than diet. However, the authors could not conclude which treatment is more effective for HDL-C. Washburn et al. [16] compared the effect of energy restriction, aerobic and resistance exercise, and various combinations of them on long-term (≥12 months) weight loss and metabolic parameters. A total of 20 studies were included in quantitative synthesis. Seven studies were selected for the review of the effectiveness of diet vs. exercise. Aerobic exercise included various modes such as walking/jogging, treadmill or cycle ergometer, and Nordic Track exercise machine. When subjects were engaged in exercise, two trials were supervised, two trials were partially supervised, and three trials were not supervised. Exercise intensity, frequency, and duration were also various. The median age and BMI for exercise groups were 58.1 years and 28.9 kg/m^2, respectively. The median weight loss for five out of seven trials with long-term comparisons was 7.2% in diet groups and 2.4% in exercise groups. Waist circumference reduced by 1.9 cm in exercise groups and 3.7 cm in diet groups. The median long-term change in fat mass was −6.1 kg by diet interventions and −0.6 kg by aerobic exercise interventions. A long-term trial evaluated the change in metabolic parameters such as lipid profile and blood pressure; however, no significant differences between groups were reported. Three trials provided data on weight change in follow-up periods of 6 months, 12 months, and 18 months. Briefly, weight regains in the diet and exercise groups were 77 and 148% of their weight loss, respectively. Diet tends to be more effective for long-term weight loss than exercise. Adding aerobic exercise to diet results in greater weight loss than diet alone. However, in most trials of exercise for obesity, the exercise intensity, frequency, and duration is not well-controlled and physical activity level is not accurately measured, prescribed exercise level is also insufficient for significant weight loss [17]. Therefore, exercise protocol should probably be standardized to perform "head-to-head" comparison of diet vs. exercise in obesity. For example, energy expenditure by exercise should be objectively measured (e.g., using accelerometry or doubly labeled water method) to match the energy deficit by diet interventions.

Johns et al. [18] examined the effectiveness of combined behavioral weight management programs in comparison with diet only or physical activity only programs on weight loss. Eight studies were included in the analysis, four of which included both diet only and physical activity only arms. Seven studies compared a combined program with diet only intervention, and five studies compared a combined program with physical activity intervention. The mean age and BMI of subjects ranged from 32 to 70 years and from 29.2 to 37.3 kg/m^2, respectively. As is common in clinical studies investigating weight change, there were more female subjects than male subjects. Physical activity interventions were various; however, most studies advised moderate to vigorous intensity physical activity (e.g., brisk walking, using upstairs, step aerobics) three to five times per week. Seven studies had supervised exercise sessions, and two studies performed resistance training as well as aerobic exercise. Weight loss at 3–6 months was significantly higher in combined programs than in physical activity alone interventions (mean difference = −5.33 kg) Weight loss at 12 months was also higher in combined programs than in physical activity alone interventions (mean difference = −6.29 kg). Measurement of physical activity was reported in four trials; step count, VO_2max, and a 400 m walking time. No significant differences in the improvement of physical activity were reported in two studies; however, one trial reported an increase of step count, and the other reported a greater improvement in VO_2max by combined behavioral weight management programs compared with physical activity alone interventions. Weight management by physical activity alone is less effective than combined weight management programs in both short- and long-term. Miller et al. [19] investigated the specific effects of exercise on physical function, fitness, and body composition in obesity during diet interventions alone than the combination of diet and exercise interventions. Fourteen studies were included in this systematic review. The mean age and BMI of subjects across all trials ranged from 37 to 75 years and 31 to 37 kg/m^2, respectively. Ten studies included older individuals and postmenopausal women. The duration of trials ranged from 3 to 12 months. Exercise interventions included aerobic exercise, resistance training, or both of them. Aerobic exercise was mostly performed at moderate to vigorous intensities (65–85% maximum heart rate) and for 90–225 minutes per week. Resistance training was typically performed 2–3 sets of 8–12 repetitions at approximately 65–85% of one repetition maximum. All aerobic exercise groups showed a significant improvement in VO_2max than in energy restriction alone. All exercise interventions demonstrated improvement in upper and/or lower extremity muscle strength. On the other hand, all energy restriction groups showed no significant change or decrease in muscle strength following weight loss. Fat mass loss between diet alone groups and diet plus exercise groups was not different in the studies that showed similar weight loss. The lean mass loss in diet alone groups and diet plus exercise groups ranged from 0.4 ± 1.0 kg to 4.1 ± 1.9 kg and from 0.5 ± 1.1 kg to 3.4 ± 2.0 kg, respectively. Six trials reported that skeletal muscle mass loss was smaller in diet plus exercise groups than that in diet alone groups. Adding exercise to energy restriction for obese individuals has beneficial effects for physical fitness and body composition. Exercise is crucial for lifestyle modifications in the improvement of cardiorespiratory fitness and body composition in obese individuals. **Table 2** summarizes published systematic reviews that compared the effectiveness of diet with exercise.

Authors, year	**Number of studies**	**Summary of inclusion and exclusion criteria**	**Exercise**	**Results**
Schwingshackl et al., 2014 [15]	21 RCTs	Subjects: BMI ≥25 kg/m^2 Study duration: ≥12 months Outcomes: BW, WC, WHR, FM, TC, LDL-C, HDL-C, TG, SBP, DBP, VO_2max Language: no restrictions Participants with coronary heart disease were excluded	Partly supervised Aerobic exercise (jogging, walking, flexibility, circuit training) Resistance training 50–85% of maximal heart rate	Diet + exercise vs. diet: BW −1.38 kg, WC −1.68 cm, WHR −0.01 U, FM −1.65 kg, HDL-C 1.62 mg/dL, TG −10.08 mg/dL, DBP −1.2 mmHg, VO_2max 3.61 mL/kg/min Diet + exercise vs. exercise: BW −4.13 kg, WC −3 cm, WHR −0.01 U, FM −3.6 kg, TC

Authors, year	Number of studies	Summary of inclusion and exclusion criteria	Exercise	Results
				−11.36 mg/dL, LDL-C −10.03 mg/dL, SBP −2.84 mmHg, DBP −2.06 mmHg, VO_2max 2.13 mL/kg/min Diet vs. exercise: BW −2.93 kg, FM −2.2 kg, HDL-C −0.96 mg/dL, SBP −2.19 mmHg
Washburn et al., 2014 [16]	20 RCTs	Subjects: BMI ≥25 kg/m^2, age ranged from 18 to 65 years Study duration: ≥6 months Outcomes: BW, body composition, TC, HDL-C, LDL-C, TG, insulin, glucose, HbA1c, blood pressure Language: English	Aerobic exercise: walking/jogging, treadmill or cycle ergometer, and Nordic Track exercise machine	Diet vs. exercise: weight loss 7.2% vs. 2.4%, WC −1.9 cm vs. −3.7, FM −6.1 kg vs. −0.6, weight regain 77% vs. 148%
Johns et al., 2014 [18]	8 RCTs	Subjects: BMI ≥25 kg/m^2, BMI ≥2 kg/m^2 in Asian populations Study duration: ≥12 months Outcomes: weight change Language: any language Studies in pregnant women, participants with eating disorders, and specific diseases were excluded	Moderate to vigorous intensity physical activity (e.g., brisk walking, using upstairs, step aerobics) three to five times per week. Supervised sessions Two studies performed resistance training as well as aerobic exercise	BWMPs vs. physical activity alone: mean difference −5.33 kg at 3–6 months, −6.29 kg at 12 months
Miller et al., 2013 [19]	14 RCTs	Subjects: BMI ≥30 kg/m^2 Study duration: no description Outcomes: body composition (by DXA and MRI), cardio-respiratory fitness Language: English	Aerobic exercise: at moderate to vigorous intensities and for 90–225 minutes per week Resistance training: 2–3 sets of 8–12 repetitions at approximately 65–85% of one repetition maximum	Exercise: VO_2max↑, extremity muscle strength↑ Energy restriction: VO_2max→ Skeletal muscle mass loss was smaller in diet plus exercise groups than that in diet alone groups

RCT, randomized controlled trial; BMI, body mass index; BW, body weight; WC, waist circumference; WHR, waist-to-hip ratio; FM, fat mass; TC, total cholesterol; LDL-C, low-density lipoprotein cholesterol; FBG, fasting blood glucose; HbA1c, hemoglobin A1c; SBP, systolic blood pressure; DBP, diastolic blood pressure; BWMP, behavioral weight management program; DXA, dual-energy X-ray absorptiometry; MRI, magnetic resonance imaging.

Table 2. Systematic reviews and meta-analyses comparing the effects of exercise interventions with diet interventions on obesity.

3.3. The effect of isolated exercise on obesity

There are two systematic reviews evaluating the effects of isolated exercise on weight loss and lipid profile. Kuhle et al. [20] conducted a systematic review and meta-analysis to appraise the evidence regarding the effect of aerobic exercise and/or resistance training on body composition and serum lipids in older individuals. Nine RCTs were included in the analysis. Studies enrolling patients with diabetes, cognitive impairment, and cardiovascular disease were

with moderate to vigorous intensity based on 50–80% of maximal heart rate and resistance training with an increase in weight load depending on individuals' muscle strength were performed. Exercise significantly reduced BMI (−1.01 kg/m^2) and waist circumference (−3.09 cm). However, exercise did not statistically change LDL-C levels in older subjects. In addition, data on TG and HDL-C were insufficient for analysis. This review is notable for focusing on the effect of exercise on obesity in individuals over the age of 60 years. Sarcopenic obesity, which is defined as the age-related decrease in muscle mass and increase in fat mass [21], increase the risk of mortality as well as disability [21, 22]. Sarcopenic obesity is an important issue for countries in which society is aging. Losing weight without loss of lean body mass will not be achieved by only exercise. Exercise programs in combination with dietary interventions such as protein supplements will be required to combat sarcopenic obesity in older individuals.

Thorogood et al. [23] evaluated the isolated efficacy of aerobic exercise (without energy restriction) programs on weight loss in overweight and obese individuals. Six trials met the inclusion/exclusion criteria of their review. The mean age of subjects ranged from 19 to 72 years. The mean BMI of subjects was unclear because three trials did not report baseline BMI. Exercise included various modes such as walking, jogging, cycle ergometer, aerobics, mini-trampoline, and rowing ergometer. Exercise was performed with the intensity of 40–85% maximum heart rate and 40–70% VO_2max. Exercise durations were 120–240 minutes per week. The mean difference of weight between the exercise groups and the control groups ranged from 0.8 to −2.5 kg. Two studies reported weight gain in the exercise groups (0.5 kg and 0.6 kg, respectively). However, the exercise groups had significant weight loss in all 6- and 12-month exercise programs. Additionally, exercise was beneficial for waist circumference reduction in all 6- and 12-month exercise interventions. Five studies reported a significant decrease in systolic and diastolic blood pressure, and the mean differences ranged from −1.7 to −5.6 mmHg and −0.8 to −3.0 mmHg, respectively. Four out of six trials reported a decrease in TC levels (−1.6 to −18.2 mg/dL), and five trials also reported a decrease in TG levels (−8.9 to −36.5 mg/dL) by aerobic exercise. Pooled analysis revealed that 6- and 12-month aerobic exercise programs were associated with a decrease in weight (−1.6 kg and −1.7 kg, respectively), a reduction in waist circumference (−2.12 cm and −1.95 cm, respectively). At 6 months, aerobic exercise programs had beneficial effects on blood pressure and TC; however, the number of studies was insufficient for performing pooled analysis at 12 months. This systematic review shows that 6–12 month moderate-intensity aerobic exercise programs have modest benefits to obesity, but isolated aerobic exercise is not sufficiently effective for weight loss. The authors recommend that exercise therapy be performed in conjunction with diet therapy to improve obesity.

3.4. Comparison of the effectiveness for obesity between aerobic exercise and resistance training

One systematic review directly compared the effectiveness of aerobic exercise and resistance training for visceral adipose tissue [24]. A total of 35 studies met the eligibility criteria. The mean age of subjects ranged from 28 to 83 years. Eighteen studies had obese subjects, 15 had overweight subjects, and study participants of two studies were within normal weight. The most common mode of aerobic exercise was cycle ergometer, and resistance training on a weight machine was most commonly prescribed. The intensity of aerobic exercise ranged from 40 to 55% (expressed as a percentage of maximum heart rate or VO_2peak) in initial weeks, which progressed to 60–90% in the final week. The most common intensity of aerobic exercise was moderate intensity: 60–75% of maximal heart rate. The intensity of resistance training expressed as one repetition maximum ranged from 30 to 100%. The frequency of aerobic exercise was commonly 3–5 days per week. The frequency of resistance training was commonly 2–3 days per week. Six studies combined aerobic exercise and resistance training. We should have a particular concern about dietary intake during the study period. Indeed, diet was not controlled in ten studies, and eight studies did not report on diet. When compared aerobic exercise therapy with control, a significant pooled effect size (ES) was found (ES = −0.33; 95% CI, −0.52 to −0.14, $p < 0.01$). However, the pooled ES for progressive resistance training therapy when compared with control was not significant (ES = 0.09: 95% CI, −0.17 to 0.36, $p = 0.49$). Heterogeneity among studies was observed in both analyses. The pooled ES for the comparison between aerobic exercise and resistance training therapy did not reach statistical significance, which tended to favor aerobic exercise (ES = 0.23; 95% CI, −0.02 to 0.50, $p = 0.07$). Moreover, the combined aerobic exercise and resistance training therapy was not significantly effective for reducing visceral fat tissue compared with control. This review suggests that not resistance training but aerobic exercise is relatively effective for improving visceral fat obesity; however, exercise intervention alone is insufficient for ameliorating obesity.

3.5. The effect of weight loss on glycemic control and the prevention of obesity

Franz et al. [25] investigated the effect of lifestyle weight-loss interventions on glycemic control in overweight and obese patients with type 2 diabetes. A total of 11 trials were eligible for meta-analysis. The mean weight at baseline with weight loss <5% and ≥5% were 98.4 kg and 99.9 kg, respectively. Unfortunately, only three weight-loss intervention trials [26–28] measured and reported physical activity (goal setting: 175 minutes per week of physical activity), although physical activity was recommended as a lifestyle intervention. The effect of physical activity on glycemic control in obese patients with type 2 diabetes was not described in this review. Moreover, no significant beneficial effects on hemoglobin A1c (HbA1c), lipid profile, and blood pressure were reported by this meta-analysis. However, two trials that included regular physical activity intervention and frequent contact with health professionals reported beneficial effects on HbA1c, lipid profile, and blood pressure. The Mediterranean-style diet study group in newly diagnosed patients with type 2 diabetes reported a decrease in HbA1c of 1.2%, TC of 15.1 mg/dL, TG of 39.0 mg/dL, systolic blood pressure of 2.3 mmHg, and diastolic blood pressure of 4.0 mmHg, and an increase in HDL-C of 3.9 mg/dL [28]. The intensive lifestyle intervention in the LooK AHEAD trial reported a decrease in HbA1c of 0.6%, LDL-C of 4.4 mg/dL, TG of 29.3 mg/dL, systolic blood pressure of 9.9 mmHg, and diastolic blood pressure of 3.1 mmHg, and an increase in HDL-C of 3.4 mg/dL [26, 29]. This review concluded that over 5% of weight loss is necessary for beneficial effects on glycemic control, lipid profile, and blood pressure. Not only energy restriction but energy expenditure, namely regular physical activity, is essential for improving metabolic diseases in obese patients with type 2 diabetes.

Considering that the number of obese individuals is rapidly increasing, the prevention of weight gain in non-obese individuals is also important. Hebden et al. [30] reviewed RCTs of lifestyle interventions for preventing weight gain among healthy young (18–35 years) individuals. This systematic review excluded interventions for obese subjects (BMI ≥ 30 kg/m^2) because such subjects did not represent the general population. Eight studies were included in the analysis. The average BMI of subjects at baseline was <30 kg/m^2. Lifestyle interventions consisted of face to face or group sessions for weight control, dietary counseling, physical activity recommendations, and feedback by using the internet. Three out of eight studies performed supervised exercise sessions such as treadmill walking, resistance training, and walking/running measured by pedometer. Although the independent effect of physical activity on preventing weight gain was not described, the combined weighted mean weight change in lifestyle intervention subjects and controls were −0.87 kg and +0.86 kg, respectively. Interventions for longer than 4 months were associated with greater weight loss. However, the authors stated that the effectiveness of lifestyle intervention for preventing weight gain in young individuals was unclear because of the small number of subjects, short duration, and large heterogeneity of the studies. Further large-scale RCTs with standard lifestyle intervention methods are warranted to reveal the effect of lifestyle modification for preventing obesity.

4. Non-exercise activity thermogenesis (NEAT) and obesity

Many previous studies have shown that sedentary lifestyle and daily physical inactivity contribute to obesity [31–35]. A recent systematic review and meta-analysis showed that obesity was associated with higher all-cause mortality than normal weight [36], and physical inactivity is a crucial problem for the prevention and treatment of obesity. Increasing energy expenditure in daily life is essential. NEAT is the main determinant of variability in total daily energy expenditure [37]. It is defined as the energy expenditure due to physical activities besides volitional exercise and includes various activities in daily life such as walking for pleasure, going to work, gardening, doing housework, singing, and dancing [38]. NEAT covers a wide range of intensity that at times reaches to the recommended level for obese individuals [39]. The energy expenditure by sitting and watching television is no more than 9 kcal per hour, but gardening and cleaning reach higher levels of energy expenditure; 100–150 kcal per hour and 500 kcal/day, respectively [40]. Steeves et al. [41] conducted a randomized controlled pilot study to examine the 6-month effects of two interventions; stepping in house during TV commercials vs. walking 30 minutes per day in sedentary and obese individuals. Although no significant difference between groups were observed, daily steps increased, and time of TV viewing, dietary intake, body fat percentage, waist and hip circumference significantly decreased after both interventions. Only stepping during watching TV could be a feasible approach for improving obesity. In the modern world, walking in a break during work is effective for weight loss. Levine and Miller [42] investigated whether the change of work environment affect individuals' energy expenditure at workplace. The vertical workstation that allows obese workers to use a personal computer while walking on a treadmill was established. The mean energy expenditure while walking at workplace was 191 kcal per hour, which was significantly higher than energy expenditure while seated at work (72 kcal per hour). This amount of energy expenditure could be equal to a weight loss of 20–30 kg per year. Furthermore, they assessed the effect of using an office-place stepping device housed under a desk on workers' energy expenditure [43]. The mean increase of energy expenditure in obese office workers was 335 kcal per hour, which could be equal to a weight loss of 20 kg per year. Changing living environments to change sedentary behavior will increase NEAT and decrease body weight. Each NEAT is small; however, "Many a little makes a mickle." To increase NEAT should be effective for improving obesity (**Figure 1**). NEAT is intricately regulated by endocrine, genetic, and sociological factors [39]. Sarcolipin [44] and ventromedial hypothalamic melanocortin receptor [45] have been of current interest as new mediators of NEAT. Sarcolipin, which consists of 31 amino acids and is highly expressed in skeletal muscle, plays a role in energy expenditure. Sopariwala et al. [44] showed that sarcolipin overexpression mice are more resistant to fatigue and more physically active compared with wild type. This newly identified regulator may increase non-shivering thermogenesis in humans [45] and could be effective to increase energy expenditure and control weight gain in obese individuals [46]. The ventromedial hypothalamus also has an important role in regulating energy balance, and the brain melanocortin system not only decreases appetite but increases physical activity [45, 47]. Gavini et al. [48] showed that intra-ventromedial hypothalamus melanocortin receptor activation increased physical activity and induced the elevation of mRNA expression of mediators of energy expenditure such as uncoupling proteins, peroxisome proliferator-activated receptors, peroxisome proliferator-activated receptor gamma coactivator 1-α, and AMP-activated protein kinase. Modulating melanocortin receptors in the ventromedial hypothalamus may contribute to increase of NEAT. Identifying such novel mechanisms to increase energy expenditure is expected to be applied in the treatment of obesity. Moreover, the significant associations of NEAT with metabolic diseases such as type 2 diabetes, hypertension, and dyslipidemia have been identified [49–53]. NEAT intervention in addition to structured exercise prescription certainly improves obesity and metabolic diseases. To elucidate the effectiveness of NEAT for metabolic diseases, and further CVD, as well as obesity, well-designed longitudinal studies in humans are warranted. On the other hand, how to measure NEAT accurately under free-living (accelerometry, doubly labeled water method, or a completely new method?) and how to intervene NEAT (recommendation or supervised program?) are still unknown. The development of measurement and intervention method of NEAT will be needed to conduct such clinical studies.

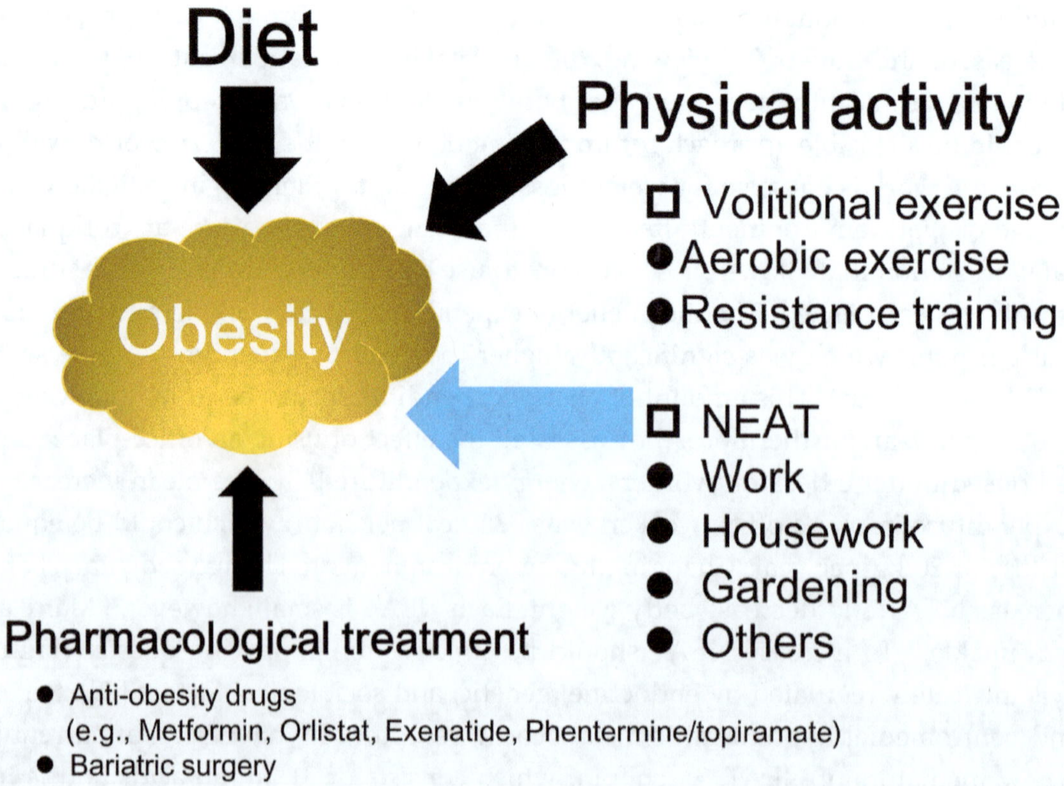
Diet
Physical activity
Volitional exercise
Aerobic exercise
Resistance training
Obesity
NEAT
Work
Housework
Gardening
Others
Pharmacological treatment
Anti-obesity drugs
(e.g., Metformin, Orlistat, Exenatide, Phentermine/topiramate)
Bariatric surgery

Figure 1. Obesity is treated with diet, physical activity, and pharmacologic therapy. Diet appears to be more effective for treating obesity than physical activity; therefore, physical activity intervention should be combined with dietary intervention in the management of obesity. Non-exercise activity thermogenesis (NEAT) beyond structured exercise may play a pivotal role in weight loss in obese individuals.

5. Conclusions

Exercise interventions are essential for the management of obesity. However, exercise alone is not sufficient for long-term weight loss and improving CVD risk factors. Diet seems to be more effective for treating obesity than exercise. On the other hand, exercise improves cardiorespiratory fitness and skeletal muscle fitness, which leads to prevent sarcopenic obesity in the elderly. Exercise therapy should be performed in conjunction with diet therapy to improve obesity. Although a number of systematic reviews have been conducted to assess the effectiveness of exercise for obesity, small number of subjects, short duration, and the heterogeneity of exercise modes between clinical studies makes it difficult to conclude. The optimal intensity, frequency, and duration of exercise to improve obesity and its comorbidities are not fully elucidated. In addition, NEAT is the main determinant of variability in daily energy expenditure, which considerably contributes to weight change in humans. The current evidence regarding NEAT is limited, but NEAT plays an important role for treating obesity. To my knowledge, there are no clinical studies which include "NEAT only" interventions besides volitional physical activity to investigate the effects of NEAT on obesity and metabolic diseases. This is a challenge for the future.

Author details

Hidetaka Hamasaki

Address all correspondence to: hhamasaki78@gmail.com

1 Department of Internal Medicine, National Center for Global Health and Medicine Kohnodai Hospital, Chiba, Japan

2 Hamasaki Clinic, Kagoshima, Japan

References

[1] Finucane MM, Stevens GA, Cowan MJ, Danaei G, Lin JK, Paciorek CJ, Singh GM, Gutierrez HR, Lu Y, Bahalim AN, Farzadfar F, Riley LM, Ezzati M; Global Burden of Metabolic Risk Factors of Chronic Diseases Collaborating Group (Body Mass Index). National, regional, and global trends in body-mass index since 1980: systematic analysis of health examination surveys and epidemiological studies with 960 country-years and 9.1 million participants. Lancet. 2011;377:557–567. DOI: 10.1016/S0140-6736(10)62037-5.

[2] Swinburn BA, Sacks G, Hall KD, McPherson K, Finegood DT, Moodie ML, Gortmaker SL. The global obesity pandemic: shaped by global drivers and local environments. Lancet. 2011;378:804–814. DOI: 10.1016/S0140-6736(11)60813-1.

[3] Lee IM, Shiroma EJ, Lobelo F, Puska P, Blair SN, Katzmarzyk PT; Lancet Physical Activity Series Working Group. Effect of physical inactivity on major non-communicable diseases worldwide: an analysis of burden of disease and life expectancy. Lancet. 2012;380:219–229. DOI: 10.1016/S0140-6736(12)61031-9.

[4] Haskell WL, Lee IM, Pate RR, Powell KE, Blair SN, Franklin BA, Macera CA, Heath GW, Thompson PD, Bauman A; American College of Sports Medicine; American Heart Association. Physical activity and public health: updated recommendation for adults from the American College of Sports Medicine and the American Heart Association. Circulation. 2007;116:1081–1093.

[5] Hills AP, Shultz SP, Soares MJ, Byrne NM, Hunter GR, King NA, Misra A. Resistance training for obese, type 2 diabetic adults: a review of the evidence. Obes Rev. 2010;11:740–749. DOI: 10.1111/j.1467-789X.2009.00692.x.

[6] Peirson L, Douketis J, Ciliska D, Fitzpatrick-Lewis D, Ali MU, Raina P. Treatment for overweight and obesity in adult populations: a systematic review and meta-analysis. CMAJ Open. 2014;2:E306–E317. DOI: 10.9778/cmajo.20140012.

[7] Middleton KM, Patidar SM, Perri MG. The impact of extended care on the long-term maintenance of weight loss: a systematic review and meta-analysis. Obes Rev. 2012;13:509–517. DOI: 10.1111/j.1467-789X.2011.00972.x.

[8] Dombrowski SU, Knittle K, Avenell A, Araújo-Soares V, Sniehotta FF. Long term maintenance of weight loss with non-surgical interventions in obese adults: systematic review and meta-analyses of randomised controlled trials. BMJ. 2014;348:g2646. DOI: 10.1136/bmj.g2646.

[9] Johansson K, Neovius M, Hemmingsson E. Effects of anti-obesity drugs, diet, and exercise on weight-loss maintenance after a very-low-calorie diet or low-calorie diet: a systematic review and meta-analysis of randomized controlled trials. Am J Clin Nutr. 2014;99:14–23. DOI: 10.3945/ajcn.113.070052.

[10] Power BT, Kiezebrink K, Allan JL, Campbell MK. Effects of workplace-based dietary and/or physical activity interventions for weight management targeting healthcare professionals: a systematic review of randomised controlled trials. BMC Obes. 2014;1:23. DOI: 10.1186/s40608-014-0023-3.

[11] Verweij LM, Coffeng J, van Mechelen W, Proper KI. Meta-analyses of workplace physical activity and dietary behaviour interventions on weight outcomes. Obes Rev. 2011;12:406–429. DOI: 10.1111/j.1467-789X.2010.00765.x.

[12] Hutchesson MJ, Rollo ME, Krukowski R, Ells L, Harvey J, Morgan PJ, Callister R, Plotnikoff R, Collins CE. eHealth interventions for the prevention and treatment of overweight and obesity in adults: a systematic review with meta-analysis. Obes Rev. 2015;16:376–392. DOI: 10.1111/obr.12268.

[13] Wieland LS, Falzon L, Sciamanna CN, Trudeau KJ, Brodney S, Schwartz JE, Davidson KW. Interactive computer-based interventions for weight loss or weight maintenance in overweight or obese people. Cochrane Database Syst Rev. 2012;8:CD007675. DOI: 10.1002/14651858.CD007675.pub2.

[14] Villablanca PA, Alegria JR, Mookadam F, Holmes DR Jr, Wright RS, Levine JA. Non-exercise activity thermogenesis in obesity management. Mayo Clin Proc. 2015;90:509–519. doi: 10.1016/j.mayocp.2015.02.001.

[15] Schwingshackl L, Dias S, Hoffmann G. Impact of long-term lifestyle programmes on weight loss and cardiovascular risk factors in overweight/obese participants: a systematic review and network meta-analysis. Syst Rev. 2014;3:130. DOI: 10.1186/2046-4053-3-130.

[16] Washburn RA, Szabo AN, Lambourne K, Willis EA, Ptomey LT, Honas JJ, Herrmann SD, Donnelly JE. Does the method of weight loss effect long-term changes in weight, body composition or chronic disease risk factors in overweight or obese adults? A systematic review. PLoS One. 2014;9:e109849. DOI: 10.1371/journal.pone.0109849.

[17] Donnelly JE, Blair SN, Jakicic JM, Manore MM, Rankin JW, Smith BK; American College of Sports Medicine. American College of Sports Medicine Position Stand. Appropriate

physical activity intervention strategies for weight loss and prevention of weight regain for adults; Med Sci Sports Exerc. 2009;41:459–471. DOI: 10.1249/MSS.0b013e3181949333.

[18] Johns DJ, Hartmann-Boyce J, Jebb SA, Aveyard P; Behavioural Weight Management Review Group. Diet or exercise interventions vs combined behavioral weight management programs: a systematic review and meta-analysis of direct comparisons. J Acad Nutr Diet. 2014;114:1557–1568. DOI: 10.1016/j.jand.2014.07.005.

[19] Miller CT, Fraser SF, Levinger I, Straznicky NE, Dixon JB, Reynolds J, Selig SE. The effects of exercise training in addition to energy restriction on functional capacities and body composition in obese adults during weight loss: a systematic review. PLoS One. 2013;8:e81692. DOI: 10.1371/journal.pone.0081692.

[20] Kuhle CL, Steffen MW, Anderson PJ, Murad MH. Effect of exercise on anthropometric measures and serum lipids in older individuals: a systematic review and meta-analysis. BMJ Open. 2014;4:e005283. DOI: 10.1136/bmjopen-2014-005283.

[21] Prado CM, Wells JC, Smith SR, Stephan BC, Siervo M. Sarcopenic obesity: a critical appraisal of the current evidence. Clin Nutr. 2012;31:583–601. DOI: 10.1016/j.clnu.2012.06.010.

[22] Zamboni M, Mazzali G, Fantin F, Rossi A, Di Francesco V. Sarcopenic obesity: a new category of obesity in the elderly. Nutr Metab Cardiovasc Dis. 2008;18:388–395. DOI: 10.1016/j.numecd.2007.10.002.

[23] Thorogood A, Mottillo S, Shimony A, Filion KB, Joseph L, Genest J, Pilote L, Poirier P, Schiffrin EL, Eisenberg MJ. Isolated aerobic exercise and weight loss: a systematic review and meta-analysis of randomized controlled trials. Am J Med. 2011;124:747–755. DOI: 10.1016/j.amjmed.2011.02.037.

[24] Ismail I, Keating SE, Baker MK, Johnson NA. A systematic review and meta-analysis of the effect of aerobic vs. resistance exercise training on visceral fat. Obes Rev. 2012;13:68–91. DOI: 10.1111/j.1467-789X.2011.00931.x.

[25] Franz MJ, Boucher JL, Rutten-Ramos S, VanWormer JJ. Lifestyle weight-loss intervention outcomes in overweight and obese adults with type 2 diabetes: a systematic review and meta-analysis of randomized clinical trials. J Acad Nutr Diet. 2015;115:1447–1463. DOI: 10.1016/j.jand.2015.02.031.

[26] Look AHEAD Research Group, Pi-Sunyer X, Blackburn G, Brancati FL, Bray GA, Bright R, Clark JM, Curtis JM, Espeland MA, Foreyt JP, Graves K, Haffner SM, Harrison B, Hill JO, Horton ES, Jakicic J, Jeffery RW, Johnson KC, Kahn S, Kelley DE, Kitabchi AE, Knowler WC, Lewis CE, Maschak-Carey BJ, Montgomery B, Nathan DM, Patricio J, Peters A, Redmon JB, Reeves RS, Ryan DH, Safford M, Van Dorsten B, Wadden TA, Wagenknecht L, Wesche-Thobaben J, Wing RR, Yanovski SZ. Reduction in weight and cardiovascular disease risk factors in individuals with type 2 diabetes: one-year results of the look AHEAD trial. Diabetes Care. 2007;30:1374–1383.

[27] Look AHEAD Research Group, Wing RR. Long-term effects of a lifestyle intervention on weight and cardiovascular risk factors in individuals with type 2 diabetes mellitus: four-year results of the Look AHEAD trial. Arch Intern Med. 2010;170:1566–1575. DOI: 10.1001/archinternmed.2010.334.

[28] Esposito K, Maiorino MI, Ciotola M, Di Palo C, Scognamiglio P, Gicchino M, Petrizzo M, Saccomanno F, Beneduce F, Ceriello A, Giugliano D. Effects of a Mediterranean-style diet on the need for antihyperglycemic drug therapy in patients with newly diagnosed type 2 diabetes: a randomized trial. Ann Intern Med. 2009;151:306–314.

[29] Wing RR, Lang W, Wadden TA, Safford M, Knowler WC, Bertoni AG, Hill JO, Brancati FL, Peters A, Wagenknecht L; Look AHEAD Research Group. Benefits of modest weight loss in improving cardiovascular risk factors in overweight and obese individuals with type 2 diabetes. Diabetes Care. 2011;34:1481–1486. DOI: 10.2337/dc10-2415.

[30] Hebden L, Chey T, Allman-Farinelli M. Lifestyle intervention for preventing weight gain in young adults: a systematic review and meta-analysis of RCTs. Obes Rev. 2012;13:692–710. DOI: 10.1111/j.1467-789X.2012.00990.x.

[31] Brown WJ, Miller YD, Miller R. Sitting time and work patterns as indicators of overweight and obesity in Australian adults. Int J Obes Relat Metab Disord. 2003;27:1340–1346.

[32] Mummery WK, Schofield GM, Steele R, Eakin EG, Brown WJ. Occupational sitting time and overweight and obesity in Australian workers. Am J Prev Med. 2005;29:91–97.

[33] Brown WJ, Williams L, Ford JH, Ball K, Dobson AJ. Identifying the energy gap: magnitude and determinants of 5-year weight gain in midage women. Obes Res. 2005;13(8):1431–1441.

[34] Blanck HM, McCullough ML, Patel AV, Gillespie C, Calle EE, Cokkinides VE, Galuska DA, Khan LK, Serdula MK. Sedentary behavior, recreational physical activity, and 7-year weight gain among postmenopausal U.S. women. Obesity (Silver Spring). 2007;15:1578–1588.

[35] Chau JY, van der Ploeg HP, Merom D, Chey T, Bauman AE. Cross-sectional associations between occupational and leisure-time sitting, physical activity and obesity in working adults. Prev Med. 2012;54:195–200. DOI: 10.1016/j.ypmed.2011.12.020.

[36] Flegal KM, Kit BK, Orpana H, Graubard BI. Association of all-cause mortality with overweight and obesity using standard body mass index categories: a systematic review and meta-analysis. JAMA. 2013;309:71–82. DOI: 10.1001/jama.2012.113905.

[37] Donahoo WT, Levine JA, Melanson EL. Variability in energy expenditure and its components. Curr Opin Clin Nutr Metab Care. 2004;7:599–605.

[38] Levine JA. Non-exercise activity thermogenesis (NEAT). Nutr Rev. 2004;62:S82–S97.

[39] Hamasaki H. Daily physical activity and type 2 diabetes: a review. World J Diabetes. 2016;7:243–251. doi: 10.4239/wjd.v7.i12.243.

[40] McCrady-Spitzer SK, Levine JA. Nonexercise activity thermogenesis: a way forward to treat the worldwide obesity epidemic. Surg Obes Relat Dis. 2012;8:501–506. DOI: 10.1016/j.soard.2012.08.001.

[41] Steeves JA, Bassett DR, Fitzhugh EC, Raynor HA, Thompson DL. Can sedentary behavior be made more active? A randomized pilot study of TV commercial stepping versus walking. Int J Behav Nutr Phys Act. 2012;9:95. DOI: 10.1186/1479-5868-9-95.

[42] Levine JA, Miller JM. The energy expenditure of using a "walk-and-work" desk for office workers with obesity. Br J Sports Med. 2007;41:558–561.

[43] McAlpine DA, Manohar CU, McCrady SK, Hensrud D, Levine JA. An office-place stepping device to promote workplace physical activity. Br J Sports Med. 2007;41:903–907.

[44] Sopariwala DH, Pant M, Shaikh SA, Goonasekera SA, Molkentin JD, Weisleder N, Ma J, Pan Z, Periasamy M. Sarcolipin overexpression improves muscle energetics and reduces fatigue. J Appl Physiol. 2015;118:1050–1058. DOI: 10.1152/japplphysiol.01066.2014.

[45] Bal NC, Maurya SK, Sopariwala DH, Sahoo SK, Gupta SC, Shaikh SA, Pant M, Rowland LA, Bombardier E, Goonasekera SA, Tupling AR, Molkentin JD, Periasamy M. Sarcolipin is a newly identified regulator of muscle-based thermogenesis in mammals. Nat Med. 2012;18:1575–1579. DOI: 10.1038/nm.2897.

[46] Maurya SK, Periasamy M. Sarcolipin is a novel regulator of muscle metabolism and obesity. Pharmacol Res. 2015;102:270–275. DOI: 10.1016/j.phrs.2015.10.020.

[47] Garfield AS, Lam DD, Marston OJ, Przydzial MJ, Heisler LK. Role of central melanocortin pathways in energy homeostasis. Trends Endocrinol Metab. 2009;20:203–215.

[48] Gavini CK, Jones WC, Novak CM.Ventromedial hypothalamic melanocortin receptor activation: Regulation of activity energy expenditure and skeletal muscle thermogenesis.J Physiol. 2016, in press. doi: 10.1113/JP272352.

[49] Hamasaki H, Yanai H, Mishima S, Mineyama T, Yamamoto-Honda R, Kakei M, Ezaki O, Noda M. Correlations of non-exercise activity thermogenesis to metabolic parameters in Japanese patients with type 2 diabetes. Diabetol Metab Syndr. 2013;5:26. DOI: 10.1186/1758-5996-5-26.

[50] Hamasaki H, Yanai H, Kakei M, Ezaki O, Noda M. Non-exercise activity thermogenesis is associated with markers for diabetic microangiopathy in Japanese female patients with type 2 diabetes. Int J Cardiol. 2013;168:4836–4837.

[51] Hamasaki H, Noda M, Moriyama S, Yoshikawa R, Katsuyama H, Sako A, Mishima S, Kakei M, Ezaki O, Yanai H. Daily physical activity assessed by a triaxial accelerometer is beneficially associated with waist circumference, serum triglycerides, and insulin resistance in Japanese patients with prediabetes or untreated early type 2 diabetes. J Diabetes Res. 2015;2015:526201. DOI: 10.1155/2015/526201.

[52] Hamasaki H, Yanai H, Kakei M, Noda M, Ezaki O. The association between daily physical activity and plasma B-type natriuretic peptide in patients with glucose intolerance: a cross-sectional study. BMJ Open. 2015;5:e006276. DOI: 10.1136/bmjopen-2014-006276.

[53] Hamasaki H, Yanai H, Kakei M, Noda M, Ezaki O. Higher daily energy expenditure by locomotive activities is favorably associated with cardiac autonomic nervous function and arterial stiffness. Int J Cardiol. 2015;194:70–71. DOI: 10.1016/j.ijcard.2015.05.094.

8

Obesity as a Growing Public Health Problem

Hülya Çakmur

Abstract

Obesity is one of the most important reasons for reduced life expectancy within the "modern" world. The prevalence of overweight and obesity continues to increase both in developing and in developed countries. It is common in every age group, from pediatric to geriatric individuals, which serve as our future and heritage in the universe. It was clearly seen in reported studies around the world that overweight and obesity are still growing epidemic health problems. It is well known that obesity results in impaired health and premature death. Obesity does not only impair the physical and mental health of people but also impairs economic wealth of most communities. The heavy burden of treatment cost and reductions in effective labor power leads to financial losses all over the world. Obesity has a higher morbidity rate than diseases emanating from underweight. Primarily, we have to find a reasonable and sustainable solution to this problem, in order to reach the longer life expectancy and more qualified life span in the twenty-first century. The policy makers in health services and health professionals in medicine have important roles to prevent and cure this "contemporary" epidemic. Additionally, the most crucial step for people is to get rid of the prevailing inertia and take personal responsibility for their health development.

Keywords: obesity, overweight, prevalence, public health, survey

1. Introduction

1.1. What is obesity and its health-related and economic consequences?

As far as we know, there was no obesity problem in the early age of life on Earth while the human being had lived as a hunter and gatherer. Unfortunately, improvements in agriculture, food processing, marketing, rural, and urban planning with low physical activity patterns, resulted in an "obese world" over time. The body weight is regulated by various physiological mechanisms that maintain the balance between energy intake and energy expenditure. Obesity occurs when the body consumes more calories than it burns, through overeating and underexercising [1]. Obesity could be defined as a final picture of abnormal, excessive fat accumulation in the body because of increased feeding and decreased physical activity [2]. When the body weight exceeds 20% above what is considered normal, according to standard age, height, and weight tables, it is defined as obesity [3]. Obesity is not only a cosmetic concern, but it is also a complex disorder, which increases the risk of impaired health. According to various studies, overweight and obesity are important contributing factors for the development a variety of mental and physical disorders [4, 5]. Excess bodyweight is the sixth most important risk factor contributing to the overall burden of disease, worldwide [6]. The obese individuals incur an elevated risk from all-cause mortality. It has been reported that obesity is the fifth leading risk factor for global deaths. The mortality rate from all causes in the obese population is at least 20% higher, compared to the normal-weighted society [7]. Information has been provided showing that obesity lead to several disorders including type 2 diabetes mellitus, high blood pressure, cardiovascular diseases, stroke, kidney disease, breathing problems, sleep apnea, osteoarthritis, malignancy, mental problems (such as clinical depression), anxiety, and eventually impaired health in general [8–11]. Since obesity tends to exert a global impact on inflammation, it increases the risk of many cancer types, such as breast, colon, endometrial, kidney, gallbladder, and liver cancers [12]. It has clearly been shown that obesity results in lowered quality of life, as well as a higher risk of premature death [5]. Overall quality of life could be diminished due to disability, depression, and social isolation of the obese person, besides impaired physical health. It has been proven that obesity markedly reduces life expectancy [13]. The severe consequences of obesity for physical health and emotional well-being already emerge in childhood [14], and it is well known that childhood obesity is the most serious public health problem, as children are more likely to become obese adults in their future life. Furthermore, it has been shown that overweight and obesity developed in childhood confers significant impact on both physical and psychological health in the future [1, 14, 15]. Overweight and obese children will also be exposed to higher risk of disability and premature death [16]. A vicious circle has been shown in children who are overfed, as they become overeating adults [15].

The childhood obesity has also been linked to cardiovascular disease risk during adulthood. This is compounded by the risk related to chronic hyperglycemia exposure in youth with type 2 diabetes mellitus [17]. The World Health Organization (WHO) reported that children in low- and middle-income countries are more vulnerable to inadequate prenatal, infant- and young-child nutritional states. And, at the same time, these kids are exposed to high-fat, high-sugar, high-salt, energy-dense, micronutrient-poor foods, which tend to be lower in cost and also lower in nutrient quality [18]. These dietary patterns, in conjunction with lower levels of physical activity, result in a sharp increase in childhood obesity, while undernutrition issues remain unsolved [18]. The obesity and overweight conditions are also pervasive among elderly people. It has been reported that obesity is also the problem of wealthy people. However, obesity now inversely affects the poor and uneducated people. It has been reported in several studies that obesity is higher in low social classes, amongst those on a low educational level, and within ethnic minority groups [7, 18]. WHO reported that children in developing countries incur a risk of obesity and inadequate nutrition, simultaneously [18]. The obesity and overweight are also pervasive among elderly people. The prevalence of obesity is rising progressively among older age groups [19], and it is well known that main complications of obesity in elderly people is the metabolic syndrome (with glucose intolerance, hypertension, and cardiovascular disease) [20, 21]. It is therefore not surprising that obesity increases the risk of heart failure in elderly. Other serious consequences of obesity in elderly people are the several cancer types, Alzheimer's disease, pulmonary dysfunction, osteoarthritis, obstructive sleep apnea syndrome, and functional inactivity [20, 22, 23]. It has been proven that inactivity, (mostly depending on obesity), aging, and comorbidity reduced quality of life are commonly leading to frailty and premature death in elderly people [3, 24]. The other dark side of obesity is the economy. It is obvious that obesity leads to many health problems, which can cost millions to treat.

Obese individuals are likely to have more medical and health problems [1]. Moreover, these reduce personal economic productivity, due to impaired health. It was reported that obese individuals have medical expenses that were approximately 30% greater than their normal weight peers [25]. Obesity is considered a top public health concern, due to the high level of morbidity and mortality in the United States [26]. It was reported that medical costs for obesity accounted for 40% of the healthcare budget in 2006. The medical care costs of obesity in the United States were estimated to be $147 billion in 2008. The annual nationwide productive costs of obesity-related absenteeism range between $3.38 billion ($79 per obese individual) and $6.38 billion ($132 per obese individual). Obesity affects 34% of children in the United States. For the pediatric healthcare delivery system, expenses were $179 per year higher in obese children versus children with a normal body mass index (BMI) [24]. Recently, it was reported that direct medical cost of overweight and obesity combined is approximately 5.0–10% of the United States healthcare spending [27]. The actual cost of obesity and related morbidity in developing countries have not been reported in any detail to date, but it is clear that prevalence of childhood and adulthood obesity is increasing in low-income countries, which lead to heavy treatment burden in their domestic budget.

1.2. Prevalence of overweight and obesity

Obesity threats public health more than communicable diseases in the present world. Overweight and obesity cause death in more people than those being underweight. The increased prevalence of obesity has occurred in the United States during the last 30 years [27], and according to WHO, the worldwide prevalence of obesity, more than doubled between 1980 and 2014 [18]. In 2014, more than 1.9 billion adults, 18 years and older, were overweight. Of these, over 600 million were obese [28]. Historically, at the beginning of the era, obesity was only the problem of rich people and the affluent countries. However, obesity is now dramatically increased in lower and middle-income countries. Rural-urban comparisons and migration studies provide evidence for an effect of modernization in increasing the prevalence of obesity [7]. Fifty percent of the adults are overweight and obese in many countries [15]. The "WHO-MONICA" study revealed markedly different prevalence patterns within Europe, ranging from 7% in Swedish men to 45% in women from Lithuania [28]. It was asserted, in a research report from China, that 55.6% of the population express central obesity [10]. Obesity prevalence in the United States ranged from 29 to 50% [28, 29], and around the world, rates of obesity are on the rise—since 1980, the global obesity rate has nearly doubled, and there are now over 200 million obese men and nearly 300 million obese women. However, the Japanese population is exempted from these trends [28].

Overweight and obesity affect every age group around the world. The National "Health and Nutrition Examination Survey" in the United States has reported that the prevalence of obesity is on the increase in all the pediatric age groups, in males and females, and in various ethnic and racial groups [1]. World Health Organization (WHO) reported that 39% of adults were overweight in the year 2014, especially in the urban area [18]. The more disturbing situation is that the 42 million children under the age of five were overweight or obese in the year 2013 [18]. The childhood overweight and obesity in developing countries have been 30% higher than in the developed countries [18], and childhood obesity has reached epidemic levels in developed countries! Twenty-five percent of children in the United States are overweight and 11% are obese [18, 30, 31]. Although there is a paucity of data on the prevalence of childhood obesity in developing countries, the worldwide prevalence of pediatric obesity has increased several-fold in recent years [18].

1.3. What is the common reason?

There is no single cause for overweight and obesity. The mechanism of obesity development is not fully understood, and it is believed to be a disorder with multiple causes. In the human body, excess energy is stored as fat in the adipose tissue, in order to be used in case of an energy deficit. Formerly, the focus on adipose tissue and adipogenesis (which means the development of fat cells) has been on obesity. The molecular and biological studies in adipose tissue have displayed unpredictable results. But, the negative image of adipose tissue has been turned around with the discovery of its crucial role in immune responses, glucose homeostasis, as well as thyroid biology and reproductive functions [32]. During the past two decades, it has been recognized that adipose tissue, which contains both white and brown adipocyte, is regulating energy balance and substrate metabolism [33, 34]. The white adipose tissue (WAT) is storing energy as triglycerides and is chiefly responsible for the obesity due to excess energy storage [35].

The regulation of energy intake and expenditure is a homeostatic process. Adipocytes secrete bioactive proteins, such as leptin, adiponectin, visfatin, omentin, tumor necrosis factor-α (TNF-α), cytokines, resistin, and retinol-binding protein 4, responsible for the regulation of overall energy homeostasis [32]. Therefore, obesity may be regarded as an inflammatory reaction in the human body, and consequently, WAT is mainly associated with obesity. The circulating inflammation-related adipokines are usually increased, as the adipose tissue expands [33]. However, the brown adipose tissue (BAT), which surrounds the hearth and large vessels during infancy, serve as important "furnaces" burning energy in the human body [35]. The amount of BAT decreases in adulthood as humans mature and can now only be found within white fat pads as scattered cells. The brown adipocytes are multilocular and contain less lipid than white adipocytes [32, 35], and BAT exerts a very important role in the regulation of energy turnover by increasing when the environment turns cold, as well as with catecholamine discharge [36]. This knowledge points to the fact that various factors may serve as internal and external "regulators" in either combatting or preserving obesity. Environmental factors, lifestyle preferences, emotional problems, and cultural environment play pivotal roles externally in the rising prevalence of obesity worldwide [15]. However, one fundamental cause of overweight and obesity is an energy imbalance between consumed and expended calories. Once overweight, then obesity takes place, when the body consumes more calories than it burns. Factors, such as inactivity, unhealthy diet, eating habits, family lifestyle, metabolism, and genetics play important roles in the development of overweight and obesity [1]. It was reported that over the 90% of obesity causes are idiopathic and <10% are associated with genetic and hormonal causes [1]. Various countries, from America to Europe, from the Middle East to North Africa, have reported that obesity is a major health issue [29–31, 37, 38]. It was documented that every country (from developed to developing) has own particular contributing factors to obesity, including the fast food chains, adopting western like eating, traditionally lack of exercises and more. However, they have reported that *low educational and socioeconomic level* as a common point.

1.4. What can be done?

The studies have shown that understanding the biology of adipogenesis might lead to an effective solution treating the obesity epidemic. Researchers are specifically asserting that a manipulation of adipocyte biology, via enhancement of leptin and adiponectin synthesis, would be a sounder strategy combatting the obesity epidemic [32]. They reported that reactivation of BAT in adult humans is a potentially viable solution for successfully treating the obesity epidemic [32]. Almost all researchers agree that prevention is the key strategy for controlling the current epidemic of obesity. However, obesity prevention is one of the greatest public health challenges in the twenty-first century. The International Obesity Task Force (IOTF) has been working with this purpose for a long time [18]. Although 50% of the adults are overweight and obese in many countries, obesity and overweight are preventable and curable [7, 18]. It is well known that heavy children incur an increased risk of being overweight adults, and it is harder for them to reduce excessive weight, once it becomes established [39]. For this reason, prevention of obesity, especially in the low age group, is the key strategy for controlling this epidemic problem. The weight control must be constituted in early childhood [15]. Prevention may include primary prevention of overweight or obesity, secondary prevention or prevention of weight regains following weight loss, and avoidance of more weight increase in obese persons unable to lose weight [15]. There is no doubt that the primary prevention is the main strategy for controlling this growing public health problem. Supportive environments and communities are fundamental in shaping people's choices and preventing obesity [15]. However, the clinical and epidemiological evidence demonstrated that lifestyle factors, like physical activity and nutrition, should be efficient to some degree to prevent and treat overweight and obesity in the adult population [2, 8]. As part of the intervention strategies and staff in early life, parents should be primarily enlightened for the results of their act on their children. Management of obesity in children differs from adults and focusing on the prevention of weight gain is more important rather than weight loss during childhood.

Effective health service should be established for the top priority groups, i.e., the children and adolescents. As the prevalence of overweight and obesity is higher in low-income and uneducated people, the educational program should be implemented by institutions like schools and the media. Obesity and its comorbidities necessitate careful clinical assessment to identify underlying factors to allow coherent management. Effective long-term weight loss depends on permanent changes in dietary quality, energy intake, and activity [6]. There is no concern about personal responsibility being crucial for ongoing healthy life. For this reason, WHO describes the actions to support healthy diets and regular physical activity. WHO suggests that people should limit energy intake from total fats and sugars and increase consumption of fruits and vegetables, as well as legumes, whole grains, and nuts, at an individual level. People can engage in regular physical activity (60 min a day for children and 150 min per week for adults) [18]. WHO also emphasizes that individual responsibility can only have its full effect where people have access to a healthy lifestyle. Therefore, at the societal level, it is important to support individuals through sustained political commitment. It is clear that the responsibility could be awakened with enhanced knowledge. The awareness derived from information may force people to take responsibility with their life. All weight management strategies need to educate people about healthy lifestyle. Weight management, to be achieved chiefly by behavior techniques that focus on lifestyle, includes dietary measures and physical activity. The public health policies should be established to prevent and avoid overweight and obesity in every age group. With this purpose, the policy makers in public health services should build sustainable strategies for a healthy environment for physical activity and non-processed (raw) food for healthy diet. WHO has developed the "Global Action Plan for the prevention and control of noncommunicable diseases 2013–2020." The countries commit to advance the implementation of the WHO Global Strategy on Diet, Physical Activity and Health, including, where appropriate, through the introduction of policies and actions aimed at promoting healthy diets and increasing physical activity in the entire population [18]. The government's role in obesity has largely focused on interventions and policies, such as national surveillance, obesity education and awareness, grant-based food subsidy programs, zoning for food access, school-based nutrition programs, dietary guidelines, nutrition labeling, and food marketing and pricing policies. Over the last 50 years, the childhood obesity problem has caught researcher's attention. Although they agree that prevention is basic, one still needs to understand why childhood obesity is a common problem, from east to west, and poverty to affluent countries around the world. Moreover, the low and middle-income countries experience a double burden of diseases derived from malnutrition and western like fast-food nutrition, simultaneously. To prevent the epidemic and find a sustainable solution for the childhood obesity problem primarily, it should be understood why children develop obesity. There is no doubt that unexpected changes in society's way of living affect children's lifestyle and well-being deeply. What are the changes in adult life, regarding the facilitation of reducing the incidence of obesity in their children? In order to shed some light on the problem in question, researchers, policy makers, doctors, healthcare providers, and finally, the whole society must think again on societal norms and man's way of living. The lifestyle of human beings changed fundamentally in the twenty-first century, due to developing technology, agricultural changes, food processing, and marketing. The most striking change in human behavior is getting too familiar with a lifestyle ruled by technology. As a result, the essential chain between production and consumption disappeared. People's behavior about consumption without sound skepticism reflects on their children. Children's nature is prone to activity. Everybody has observed his or her unlimited energy. However, this "modem" way of living has repressed the "life energy" of children and turned it into "virtual energy". A new approach is required for combatting the childhood epidemic obesity problem, since the present problem is environmental and not genetic. The frequency of "obesity" gene expression has not increased in the population, but the children's environment has changed. Combatting the childhood obesity epidemic can be achieved with changing in societal norms. Children are hermeneutical entities like adults, and they need durable role models in their lives. Therefore, preventing the childhood obesity depends on the prevention of adulthood obesity. Society must be reconstructed and rid themselves of the vicious circle of overeating, overconsuming, inactivity, technology, impaired biorhythms, sleepiness, and finally meaningless activities. People will have to retrieve a sound purpose and meaning in their lives. There are two possible ways of fighting the obesity epidemic; reforming social norms or modifying people's organ/cellular phenotypes, introducing a predefined diet and exercise program.

2. Conclusion

Lifestyle preferences, cultural environment, education, socioeconomic level, and environmental factors, play pivotal roles in the rising prevalence of obesity worldwide. It is important to emphasize that all of the given causes for the increased levels of obesity are predicated. It is essential to build sustainable strategies for a healthy lifestyle. The most crucial step for people is to take personal responsibility for their health. There is no doubt that the primary prevention is the main strategy for controlling this growing public health problem.

3. Key points

- Overweight and obesity cause death of more people than underweight and communicable diseases.
- Overweight and obesity reduce life expectancy.
- Overweight and obesity impair health and reduce quality of life.
- More than half of the population in the world is overweight and obese.
- The worldwide prevalence of obesity more than doubled between 1980 and 2014.
- Obesity in children is a major health concern in the developed world.
- Almost a quarter of children around the world are overweight and obese.
- Forty-two million children under the age of five are overweight or obese.

- Obesity affects 34% of children in the United States.
- Overweight and obese children are being overweight and obese when becoming adults.
- The prevalence of overweight and obesity is higher in poor and uneducated people.
- Education is the most important step for challenging obesity.
- Primary prevention is essential for challenge obesity.
- The policy makers in health services, and health professionals in medicine, play important roles in preventing and curing this "contemporary" epidemic.
- People should take personal responsibility for their health development.
- Combatting the childhood obesity epidemic can be achieved by changing social norms.
- Obesity is preventable.

Author details

Hülya Çakmur

Address all correspondence to: hulyacakmur@gmail.com

Department of Family Medicine, School of Medicine, University of Kafkas, Kars, Turkey

References

[1] Xu S, Xue Y: Pediatric obesity: causes, symptoms, prevention and treatment. Exp Ther Med. 2016;11:15–20. doi:10.3892/etm.2015.2853

[2] Garaulet M, Ordovás JM, Madrid JA: The chronobiology, etiology and pathophysiology of obesity. Int J Obes. 2010;34:1667–1683. doi:10.1038/ijo.2010.118

[3] Wolin KY, Petrelli JM: Obesity; Greenwood, 2009. Greenwood Press, Santa Barbara, CA, 2009. ISBN 10: 0313352763/ISBN 13: 9780313352768.

[4] Luppino FS, de Wit LM, Bouvy PF, Stijnen T, Cuijpers P, Penninx BW, Zitman FG: Overweight, obesity, and depression: a systematic review and meta-analysis of longitudinal studies. Arch Gen Psychiatry. 2010;67:220–229. doi:10.1001/archgenpsychiatry.2010.2

[5] Onyike CU, Crum RM, Lee HB, Lyketsos CG, Eaton WW: Is obesity associated with major depression? Results from the third national health and nutrition examination survey. Am J Epidemiol. 2003;158:1139–1147. doi:10.1093/aje/kwg275

[6] Haslam DW, James WP: Obesity. Lancet. 2005;366:1197–1209. doi:10.1111/j.1467-789X.2009.00708

[7] Kobyliak N, Abenavoli L, Falalyeyeva T, Oleksandr V, Belemets N, Beregova T, Bodnar P, Spıvak M: Prevention of NAFLD development in rats with obesity via the improvement of pro/antioxidant state by cerium dioxide nanoparticles. Clujul Med. 2016;89:229–235. doi:10.15386/cjmed-632

[8] Landsberg L, Aronne LJ, Beilin LJ, Burke V, Igel LI, Lloyd-Jones D, Sowers J: Obesity-related hypertension: pathogenesis, cardiovascular risk, and treatment-A position paper of the Obesity Society and the American Society of Hypertension. Obesity. 2013;1:8–24. doi:10.1002/oby.20181

[9] Mokdad AH, Ford ES, Bowman BA, Dietz WH, Vinicor F, Bales VS, Marks JS: Prevalence of obesity, diabetes, and obesity-related health risk factors. JAMA. 2003;289:76–79. doi:10.1001/jama.289.1.76

[10] Zhang P, Wang R, Gao C, Jiang L, Lv X, Song Y, Li B: Prevalence of central obesity among adults with normal BMI and ıts association with metabolic diseases in Northeast China. PLoS One. 2016;11(7):e0160402. doi:10.1371/journal.pone.0160402

[11] Çakmur H, Ardıç S: Investıgatıon of obesıty and depressıon ın a sample of Turkısh elderly adults. Turkish J Geriatr. 2015;2:115–122.

[12] Kolb R, Sutterwala FS, Zhang W: Obesity and cancer: inflammation bridges the two. Curr Opin Pharmacol. 2016;29:77–89. doi:10.1016/j.coph.2016.07.005

[13] Dombrowski SU, Avenell A, Sniehott FF: Behavioural interventions for obese adults with additional risk factors for morbidity: systematic review of effects on behaviour, weight and disease risk factors. Obes Facts. 2010;3:377–396. doi:10.1159/000323076

[14] Tabibzadeh P, Mewes R: Thin mother, obese child? A review of early risk factors for obesity in offspring. Curr Opin Psychiatry. 2016;29:309–315. doi:10.1097/YCO.0000000000000268

[15] Daniels SR, Arnett DK, Eckel RH, Gidding SS, Hayman LL, Kumanyika S, Robinson TN, Scott BJ, St Jeor S, Williams CL: Overweight in children and adolescents: pathophysiology, consequences, prevention, and treatment. Circulation. 2005;111:1999–2012. doi:10.1161/01.CIR.0000161369.71722.10

[16] Reilly JJ, Kelly J: Long-term impact of overweight and obesity in childhood and adolescence on morbidity and premature mortality in adulthood: systematic review. Int J Obes. 2011;35:891–898. doi:10.1038/ijo.2010.222

[17] Bacha F, Gidding SS: Cardiac abnormalities in youth with obesity and Type 2 Diabetes. Curr Diab Rep. 2016;16:62. doi:10.1007/s11892-016-0750-6

[18] WHO, Global Strategy on Diet, Physical Activity and Health Solarex. [Internet]. 2014. Available from: http://www.who.int/features/factfiles/obesity/en/ [Accessed: 2016-04-12].

[19] Porter Starr KN, Bales CW: Excessive body weight in older adults: concerns and recommendations. Clin Geriatr Med. 2015;31:311–326. doi:10.1016/j.cger.2015.04.001

[20] Mathus-Vliegen EMH, Basdevant A, Finer N, Hainer V, Hauner H, Micic D, Maislos M, Roman G, Schutz Y, Tsigos C, Toplak H, Yumuk V, Zahorska-Markiewicz B: Prevalence, pathophysiology, health consequences and treatment options of obesity in the elderly: a guideline. Obes Facts. 2012;5:460–483. doi:10.1159/000341193

[21] Koster A, Stenholm S, Alley DE, Kim LJ, Simonsick EM, Kanaya AM, Visser M, Houston DK, Nicklas BJ, Tylavsky FA, Satterfield S, Goodpaster BH, Ferrucci L, Harris TB: Body fat distribution and ınflammation among obese older adults with and without metabolic syndrome. Obesity. 2010;18:2354–2361. doi:10.1038/oby.2010.86

[22] Hauser W, Schmutzer G, Brahler E, Schiltenwolf M, Hilbert A: The impact of body weight and depression on low back pain in a representative population sample. Pain Med. 2014;15:1316–1327. doi:10.1111/pme.12458

[23] Boudreau M, Bacon SL, Ouellet K, Jacob A, Lavoie KL: Mediator effect of depressive symptoms on the association between BMI and asthma control in adults. Chest. 2014;146:348–354. doi:10.1378/chest.13-1796

[24] Çakmur H: Frailty among elderly adults in a rural area of Turkey. Med Sci Monit. 2015;1:1232–1242. doi:10.12659/MSM.893400

[25] Withrow DA, Alter D: The economic burden of obesity worldwide: a systematic review of the direct costs of obesity. Obes Rev. 2011;12:131–141. doi:10.1111/j.1467-789X.2009.00712

[26] Wolf AM, Finer N, Allshouse AA, Pendergast KB, Sherrill BH, Caterson I, Hill JO, Aronne LJ, Hauner H, Radigue C, Amand C, Despres JP: PROCEED: prospective obesity cohort of economic evaluation and determinants: baseline health and healthcare utilization of the US sample. Diabetes Obes Metab. 2008;10:1248–1260. doi:10.1111/j.1463-1326.2008.00895

[27] Tsa AG, David F. Williamso DF, Glick HA: Direct medical cost of overweight and obesity in the United States: a quantitative systematic review. Obes Rev. 2011;12:50–61. doi:10.1111/j.1467-789X.2009.00708

[28] Berghöfer A, Pischon T, Reinhold T, Apovian CM, Sharma AM, Willich SN: Obesity prevalence from a European perspective: a systematic review. BMC Public Health. 2008;8:200. doi:10.1186/1471-2458-8-200

[29] von Ruesten A, Steffen A, Floegel A, Van der A DL, Masala G, Tjonneland A, Halkjaer J, Palli D, Wareham NJ, Ruth JF, Loos RJF, Sørensen TIA, Boeing H: Trend in obesity prevalence in European adult cohort populations during follow-up since 1996 and their predictions to 2015. PLoS One. 2011;6:e27455. doi:org/10.1371/journal.pone.0027455

[30] Blondin KJ, Giles CM, Cradock AL, Gortmaker SL, Long MW: US States' childhood obesity surveillance practices and recommendations for ımproving them, 2014–2015. Prev Chronic Dis. 2016;13:E97. doi:10.5888/pcd13.160060

[31] Ogden CL, Carroll MD, Curtin LR, McDowell MA, Tabak CJ, Flegal KM: Prevalence of overweight and obesity in the United States, 1999-2004. EJAMA. 2006;295:1549–1555. doi:10.1001/jama.295.13.1549

[32] Rosen ED, Spiegelman BM: Adipocytes as regulators of energy balance and glucose homeostasis. Nature. 2006;444:847–853. doi:10.1038/nature05483

[33] Trayhurn P: Endocrine and signalling role of adipose tissue: new perspectives on fat. Acta Physiol Scand. 2005;184:285–293. doi:10.1111/j.1365-201X.2005.01468

[34] Giorgino F, Laviola L, Eriksson JW: Regional differences of insulin action in adipose tissue: insights from *in vivo* and *in vitro* studies. Acta Physiol Scand. 2005;183:13–30. doi:10.1111/j.1365-201X.2004.01385

[35] Gesta S, Tseng YH, Kahn CR: Developmental origin of fat: tracking obesity to its source. Cell. 2007;131:242–256. doi:10.1016/j.cell.2007.10.004

[36] Lefterova MI, Lazar MA: New developments in adipogenesis. Trends Endocrinol Metab. 2009;20:107–114. doi:10.1016/j.tem.2008.11.005

[37] Rashidi A, Mohammadpour-Ahranjani B, Vafa MR, Karandish M: Prevalence of obesity in Iran. Obes Rev. 2005;6:191–192. doi:10.1111/j.1467-789X.2005.00174

[38] Erem C:Prevalence of overweight and obesity in Turkey. IJC Metab Endocr. 2015;8:38–41. doi:10.1016/j.ijcme.2015.07.002

[39] Monasta L, Batty GD, Cattaneo A, Lutje V, Ronfani L, Van Lenthe FJ, Brug J: Early-life determinants of overweight and obesity: a review of systematic reviews. Obes Rev. 2010;11:695–708. doi:10.1111/j.1467-789X.2010.00735

9

The Brain, the Environment, and Human Obesity: An Evolutionary Perspective on the Difficulty with Maintaining Long-Term Weight Loss

Bruce M. King

Abstract

The dramatic increase in obesity within one or two generations cannot possibly be due to a change in genetics. It is the processing, distribution, and availability of foods that have changed, not the brain. For most people, in the presence of pleasant tasting (high calorie) foods, the brain's reward circuitry overwhelms the satiety signals. For 2 million years, overeating (on the occasional basis when that was possible) had adaptive value, and it has only been since the rise of an omnipresent obesogenic environment that such behavior has become maladaptive, resulting in widespread obesity. Long-term weight loss is, at minimum, a two-part process: (1) initial weight loss and (2) relapse prevention. All weight loss programs (diet, pharmacology, or surgical) work in the short run, but none used alone have proven widely effective in the long term. After initial weight loss, relapse is common because until recently interventions failed to consider our evolutionary history and thus have underestimated the sensory/reward aspects of feeding behavior. Strongly heritable behavioral characteristics that differentiate obesity-prone individuals from others (e.g., food cue responsiveness, satiety responsiveness) have now been identified and can potentially be targeted to help people learn how to better interact with an obesogenic environment.

Keywords: obesity, brain satiety mechanisms, evolutionary pressures, heritable traits, obesogenic environment

1. Introduction: The brain and regulation of food intake

Up until at least 1973, the brain was believed to act much like a thermostat in its regulation of food intake and body weight. Hundreds of studies had shown that damage to the ventromedial hypothalamus (VMH) resulted in hyperphagia and obesity in a wide variety of species including humans and that lesions of the adjacent lateral hypothalamus (LH) resulted in aphagia and weight loss [1]. Female rats with large VMH lesions frequently doubled their body weight within 30 days [2]. In 1954, Eliot Stellar used these two nuclei as the model example for his dual-center hypothesis for motivated behavior [3]. The LH was the "excitatory center," activation of which caused the organism to eat. Food intake provided some (unknown at that time) manner of glucostatic, lipostatic, and/or thermostatic feedback to the VMH, the "inhibitory center," which then inhibited the LH, resulting in cessation of feeding. The underlying principal was homeostasis, i.e., food intake decreased when body weight exceeded some stable state (set point) and increased when body weight fell below this set point (see [4] for a history of set point theory). The weight changes observed after lesions were generally attributed to a resetting of the set point [5].

So compelling was the evidence, and model, that the leading researchers of human obesity of that era directly compared obese humans to obese rats with VMH lesions [6–8]. Similarities in patterns of food intake, hyperreactivity to the sensory qualities of food (e.g., taste), and unwillingness to work for food were particularly noted. Researchers concluded that obese individuals had "a weak ventromedial hypothalamus" [6, p. 450] and that "the obesity of rats and men has a common physiological locus in the ventromedial hypothalamus" [8, p. 143].

The simplicity of the dual-center model was abandoned in the 1970s when, first, it was found that transection of the ventral noradrenergic bundle at the level of the midbrain resulted in overeating and obesity [9] and, second, when a few years later it was discovered that lesions of the hypothalamic paraventricular nucleus (PVN) also produced hyperphagia and obesity [10, 11]. The next 30 years of research (with lab rats) focused on the role of the PVN and arcuate nuclei [12] and circulating levels of leptin and insulin, hormones that are released in proportion to body fat content [13]. Mice that have mutations in the gene for leptin (ob/ob) become markedly obese [14]. Other brain structures were also found to play a role in the regulation of food intake and body weight, including the posterodorsal amygdala [15, 16]. The model had become more complex, but the underlying principal was still believed to be energy homeostasis [13, 17] and the related concept of set point (or settling point). Human obesity was explained, at least in part, as a malfunction of the system, e.g., resistance to leptin [18].

The studies with rats confined in small cages and fed a single standard lab chow diet have contributed greatly to our understanding of brain mechanisms regulating individual meal parameters [19], but how well do they explain regulation of body weight in free-living humans? The answer is not very well. Similar to lab rats, humans do not overeat when offered a bland diet ad libitum [20], but many researchers have noted that homeostatic controls appear to be absent in environments with an abundance of good-tasting foods [13, 18, 21–26]. In fact, in a long series of studies, de Castro and colleagues determined that only 14% of the variance in the daily food intake of free-living humans could be explained by brain homeostatic mechanisms [27]. As stated by Cameron and Doucet [21], "...when given a barrage of anorexigenic signals, humans still manage to overconsume even at gluttonous levels" (p. 183).

The prevalence of overweight and obese individuals in the United States has nearly tripled since 1980 [23]. One third of adults are overweight (BMI > 25 kg/m^2), and over one third more are clinically obese (BMI > 30 kg/m^2) [28]. Researchers have projected that at least 42–44% of Americans will be obese by 2030 [29, 30]. This is a substantial increase since 1960 when only about one in five Americans was overweight [31]. Any explanation for the regulation of body weight in humans must be able to account for this dramatic increase in obesity in just a few-decade time. It is highly unlikely that the modern obesity pandemic is due to recent pathology in genetics, metabolism, or the brain homeostatic (inhibitory) controls of feeding behavior [22]. Two thirds of the American population could not suddenly have become leptin resistant.

In actuality, the brain is reacting to present-day environmental stimuli exactly in the manner in which it evolved during 2 million years of environmental selective pressures since the appearance of the genus *Homo* [23]. Considerable evidence has accrued that in obesity-prone individuals, it is the reward circuitry of the brain, not the hypothalamic homeostatic nuclei, that developed during human evolution which control feeding behavior when there is an abundance of good-tasting foods [21]. As expected, initial brain fMRI studies found activation of hypothalamic nuclei in response to changes in glucose and insulin levels [32–34]. However, more recent brain fMRI studies also reveal hyperactivation of the cortico-limbic-striatal structures in the reward circuitry of obese children and adults in response to pleasant food stimuli (see Refs. [35–37] for reviews). Genetically obesity-prone children display hyperactivation of the reward circuitry before they become obese [38, 39]. Previously obese adults who have dieted and lost their excess weight continue to show hyperactivity in the reward circuits in response to food [40]. It must be noted that brain fMRI studies of obesity are still in their initial stages, and attempts to identify the specific reward circuitry associated with obesity are inconsistent [37].

One thing is certain: the brain's reward circuitry is not homeostatic, i.e., there is no upper-level body weight set point at which it shuts down [41]. In short, the brain developed as an organ attracted to energy-dense rewards. For many people, the sensory/reward aspects of food simply overwhelm the homeostatic satiety signals [18, 23].

2. The environment and obesity

Until about 8000 BC, all humans lived in small nomadic, hunter-gatherer tribes [42, 43]. King [23] has reviewed the anthropological research showing that for the previous 2 million years, there were certainly periods (short and/or prolonged) of food shortages. It would have been advantageous to store energy as fat to survive periods of deprivation and have energy to hunt and thus, when food was plentiful, to consume more calories than was required just to satisfy short-term inter-meal deficits in energy [21, 25, 44]. In a restricted environment, this would have resulted, at most, in a moderately overweight phenotype.

In short, the modern societal practice of "three meals plus snacks every day is abnormal from an evolutionary perspective" [45, p. 16,647]. Interestingly, recent research has shown that intermittent fasting not only reduces body weight [45–48] but improves clinical health indicators [45, 47, 48] and may reduce processes leading to diseases such as diabetes, heart disease, and certain cancers [45, 47].

What has changed is not the brain, but the environment [23, 26]. The anthropological record reveals that the switch from hunting-gathering to farming as the primary source of food (with a greater reliance on carbohydrates than lean meat) began 10,000 years ago [49, 50]. The use of salt (and probably herbs and spices) to flavor foods dates back to at least the Bronze Age [51], but sugar was not widely available until the 1500s [52]. However, it was the industrialization of the food supply (i.e., the processing and distribution of food) in the last half of the twentieth century that has had the most dramatic impact on how today's humans eat [26, 53, 54].

The availability of high-calorie foods (e.g., carbohydrates and fats) has markedly increased in the United States since the 1970s [55]. One of the most obvious changes that began in the 1970s, at about the same time as the prevalence of obesity began to rapidly increase, was the proliferation of fast-food restaurants. McDonald's opened in 1955, had 1000 restaurants in 1968, and today has over 36,000 restaurants in over 100 countries. Burger King opened in 1954, had 275 restaurants in 1967, and today has 13,000 restaurants in 79 countries. Wendy's opened in 1969 and today has over 6850 restaurants. Similarly, today, Kentucky Fried Chicken has over 19,400 restaurants, Pizza Hut over 11,000, Taco Bell over 6500, Arby's over 3300, Chick-fil-A over 1950, and Church's Chicken nearly 1700 restaurants. Most of them have drive-up windows. Altogether, sales at the US fast-food restaurants increased from $16.2 billion in 1975 to about $110 billion by 2004 [56] with a corresponding increase in American's proportional consumption of calories in the form sweetened drinks and such foods as cheeseburgers and pizza [57, 58]. Add to fast-food restaurants an increase in cafeteria and full-menu restaurants, convenience stores, and dispensing machines, and the end result is an obesogenic environment: a high density of high-calorie food sources that require little energy expenditure for consumers to access.

Numerous studies have found a positive association between the geographical density of fast-food restaurants and prevalence of obesity [59–64] or obesity and the frequency with which individuals eat at restaurants [65–70; see also 71]. Compared to normal-weight persons, overweight and obese individuals consume larger meals when eating away from home [72]. Many studies have also found that when groups of people move from areas of the world where the prevalence of obesity is low to an obesogenic environment (e.g., the United States), they gain weight and eventually display the same prevalence of obesity as is found among those who were born in the obesogenic environment [73; see 24 for a review]. Freshman students often gain excess weight during the first few weeks of attending college [74]. One third of American adults may not (yet) be overweight, but many of them live in areas (e.g., very rural) that are not obesogenic.

As with any genetic trait (e.g., height), there is diversity, and some people are more obesity prone than others [18, 75–77]. Obese individuals are less responsive to homeostatic satiety mechanisms [76–78] and are much more responsive to external feeding stimuli than are normal-weight people [7, 24, 27, 77, 79]. The latter includes not only the taste and texture of food but also social cues (e.g., number of others eating, the sight of and variety of foods, portion size, time of day). Compared to others, obese individuals have a strong tendency to discount delayed food rewards in favor of immediate rewards [80–83].

Studies with twins reveal that appetite (responsiveness to food cues) and satiety responsiveness are highly heritable behavioral characteristics [27, 76, 77, 79], as is cognitive restraint, which is generally less for obese individuals [27, 84, 85]. These heritable behavioral characteristics emerge early in life [76], and while they do not cause obesity directly, they result in individuals being more susceptible to overeating in an obesogenic environment [18, 77, 86]. Not everyone has these heritable traits, but based on the obesity statistics, a large majority of humans do have them. At present, at least 32 genetic loci associated with BMI have been identified [87].

In summary, obesity is the result of interaction between genetic risks and the environment. The brain reward circuitry that evolved during 2 million years of our hunter-gatherer ancestry has resulted in many humans being more responsive to environmental food stimuli than they are to caloric/homeostatic stimuli [7, 21, 23, 24, 27, 75–77]. In the words of one group of researchers, humans have "fat brains [and] greedy genes" [79].

3. Interventions to reduce obesity

As the prevalence of obesity has increased, the number and variety of weight loss programs have increased almost exponentially. Using the key terms "obesity," "humans," and "weight loss," Medline indicates 67 publications in the time period 1965–1974 and 13,904 publications from 2006 to 2015. Today, Americans spend over $60 billion a year on attempts to lose weight [88]. The medical cost of treating adult obesity in the United States is between $147 and $210 billion per year [30].

All diets work—in the short run. They may differ in the types of food recommended to eat, but when fewer calories are consumed than expended, the result is weight loss. Most overweight and obese individuals have successfully dieted for a few weeks and many for a few months, but in the long run, the success rate of behavioral therapies alone has proven to be very modest at best. Most dieting individuals do not maintain their weight loss [89, 90]. This was first noted nearly 60 years ago:

"Most obese patients will not remain in treatment. Of those who do remain in treatment, most will not lose significant poundage, and of those who do lose weight, most would regain it promptly" [91, p. 87].

Results with pharmacologic treatment of obesity alone have proven equally disappointing [92–94]—individuals achieve meaningful weight loss only when the medication is accompanied by additional lifestyle interventions [95] and maintain the weight loss (usually modest) only as long as they remain on the drugs [96]. Mean excess weight loss for extremely obese individuals who have undergone bariatric surgery is only about 50% ([97]; see [98, 99] for reviews), with many others losing substantially less weight (see [100] for a review), and still others eventually regaining much of their excess weight [101]. (Note: the author is not underestimating the health benefits of a 50% loss of excess weight.)

Long-term weight loss is, at minimum, a two-part process: (1) initial weight loss and (2) relapse prevention. The relapse rate is high because it is normal for the evolved brain's reward circuitry to direct humans to overeat when good-tasting/high-calorie foods are available [23]. Regardless of how weight loss is initially achieved (diet, pharmacology, and/or surgical intervention), sending the client back into an omnipresent obesogenic environment with a few behavioral-cognitive instructions (e.g., counting calories; monitoring carbohydrates, fats, and portion size; eating slowly; more exercise) has not worked long term for most people [89–91, 101].

For many individuals who have recently lost weight, relapse prevention will mean, in part, learning how to reduce food cue responsiveness [76]. Obese individuals are more easily tempted by pleasant-tasting food when it is easily available than are lean individuals [8], an aspect of the greater responsiveness to external stimuli. Today, the obesogenic environment is omnipresent—in the workplace, in schools, throughout the community, and in the media. Weight-loss interventions have failed because, historically, they have put the responsibility almost exclusively on the individual. In 2012, the Institute of Medicine [102] concluded that government, industry, the community, the media, and medicine must be part of a multifaceted approach (e.g., an increase in social marketing, as was done with smoking) to help individuals address how to limit and deal with an ever-increasing obesogenic environment [22, 26, 88, 103–105].

4. Conclusions

In free-living humans living in an obesogenic environment, there is little evidence in support of an upper limit set point around which body weight is regulated in a homeostatic fashion. For most people, the brain's reward circuitry plays the dominant role in feeding behavior. Living in a restricted environment with periods of food deprivation, it was necessary for survival for *Homo erectus* and *Homo sapiens* to consume as much pleasant-tasting food as possible when it was available. Only recently have high-calorie foods become widely available, but the brain still responds to pleasant-tasting foods in a manner that was adaptive for the hunter-gatherers that existed in our ancestral past. After excess weight loss, relapse is high because the brain's normal response is to direct humans to overeat in the presence of an abundance of foods. For obesity interventions to be successful, long-term strategies, both individual and collective, need to better address relapse prevention, and an important component of this must include how to limit and interact with an obesogenic environment.

Author details

Bruce M. King

Address all correspondence to: bking2@clemson.edu

Department of Psychology, Clemson University, Clemson, SC, USA

References

[1] King BM. The rise, fall, and resurrection of the ventromedial hypothalamus in the regulation of feeding behavior and body weight. Physiology & Behavior. 2006; 87: 221-244. DOI: 10.1016/j.physbeh.2005.10.007

[2] King BM., Gaston MG. Reappearance of dynamic hyperphagia during the static phase in medial hypothalamic lesioned rats. Physiology & Behavior. 1977; 18: 945-950. DOI: 10:1016/0031-9384(77)90205-0

[3] Stellar E. The physiology of motivation. Psychological Review. 1954; 61: 5-22. DOI: 10.1037/h0060347

[4] Berridge KC. Motivation concepts in behavioral neuroscience. Physiology & Behavior. 2004; 81: 179-209. DOI: 10.1016/j.physbeh.2004.02.004

[5] Hoebel BG, Teitelbaum P. Weight regulation in normal and hypothalamic hyperphagic rats. Journal of Comparative and Physiological Psychology. 1966; 61: 189-193. DOI: 10.1037/h0023126

[6] Nisbett RE. Hunger, obesity, and the ventromedial hypothalamus. Psychological Review. 1972; 79: 433-453. DOI: 10.1037/h0033519

[7] Schachter S. Obesity and eating. Science. 1968; 161: 751-756. DOI: 10.1126/science.161.3843.751

[8] Schachter S. Some extraordinary facts about obese humans and rats. American Psychologist. 1971; 26: 129-144. DOI: 10.1037/h0030817

[9] Ahlskog JE, Hoebel BG. Overeating and obesity from damage to a noradrenergic system in the brain. Science. 1973; 182: 166-169. DOI: 10.1126/science.182.4108.166

[10] Aravich PF, Sclafani A. Paraventricular hypothalamic lesions and medial hypothalamic knife cuts produce similar hyperphagia syndromes. Behavioral Neuroscience. 1983; 97: 970-983. DOI: 10.1037/0735-7044.97.6.970

[11] Leibowitz SF, Hammer NJ, Chang K. Hypothalamic paraventricular nucleus lesions produce overeating and obesity in the rat. Physiology & Behavior. 1981; 27: 1031-1040. DOI: 10.1016/0031-9384(81)90366-8

[12] Schwartz MW, Woods SC, Porte D, Seeley RJ, Baskin, DG. Central nervous system control of food intake. Nature. 2000; 404: 661-671. DOI: 10.1038/35007534

[13] Könner AC, Klöckener T, Brüning JC. Control of energy homeostasis by insulin and leptin: Targeting the arcuate nucleus and beyond. Physiology & Behavior. 2009; 97: 632-638. DOI: 10.1016/j.physbeh.2009.03.027

[14] Zhang Y, Proenca R, Maffei M, Barone M, Leopold L, Friedman J. Positional cloning of the mouse obese gene and its human homologue. Nature. 1994; 372: 425-432. DOI: 10.1038/372425a0

[15] King BM. Amygdaloid lesion-induced obesity: Relation to sexual behavior, olfaction, and the ventromedial hypothalamus. American Journal of Physiology. 2006; 291: R1201-R1214. DOI: 10.1152/ajpregu.00199.2006

[16] King BM, Kass JM, Cadieux NL, Sam H, Neville KL, Arceneaux ER. Hyperphagia and obesity in female rats with temporal lobe lesions. Physiology & Behavior. 1993; 54: 759-765. DOI: 10.1016/0031-9384(93)90088-W

[17] Woods SC. Signals that influence food intake and body weight. Physiology & Behavior. 2005; 86: 709-716. DOI: 10.1016/j.physbeh.2005.08.060

[18] Levin BE. Factors promoting and ameliorating the development of obesity. Physiology & Behavior. 2005; 86: 633-639. DOI: 10.1016/j.physbeh.2005.08.054

[19] de Graaf C, Blom WAM, Smeets PAM, Stafleu A, Hendriks HFJ. Biomarkers of satiation and satiety. American Journal of Clinical Nutrition. 2004; 79: 946-961.

[20] Cabanac M, Rabe EF. Influence of a monotonous food on body weight regulation in humans. Physiology & Behavior. 1976; 17: 675-678. DOI: 10.1016/0031-9384(76)90168-2

[21] Cameron J, Doucet É. Getting to the bottom of feeding behavior: Who's on top? Applied Physiology, Nutrition, and Metabolism. 2007; 32: 177-189. DOI: 10.1139/H06-072

[22] Egger G, Swinburn B. An "ecological" approach to the obesity pandemic. British Medical Journal. 1997; 315: 477. DOI: 10.1136/bmj.315.7106.477

[23] King BM. The modern obesity epidemic, ancestral hunter-gatherers, and the sensory/reward control of food intake. American Psychologist. 2013; 68: 88-96. DOI: 10.1037/a0030684

[24] Levitsky DA. The non-regulation of food intake in humans: Hope for reversing the epidemic of obesity. Physiology & Behavior. 2005; 86: 623-632. DOI: 10.1016/j.physbeh.2005.08.053

[25] Pinel JPJ, Assanand S, Lehman DR. Hunger, eating, and ill health. American Psychologist. 2000; 55: 1105-1116. DOI: 10.1037/0003-066X.55.10.1105

[26] Swinburn BA, Sacks G, Hall KD, McPherson K, Finegood DT, Moodie ML, et al. The global obesity pandemic: Shaped by global drivers and local environments. Lancet. 2011; 378: 804-814. DOI: 10.1016/S0140-6736(11)60813-1

[27] de Castro JM. The control of food intake of free-living humans: Putting the pieces back together. Physiology & Behavior. 2010; 100: 446-453. DOI: 10.1016/j.physbeh.2010.04.028

[28] Ogden CL, Carroll MD, Kit BK, Flegal KM. Prevalence of childhood and adult obesity in the United States, 2011-2012. Journal of the American Medical Association. 2014; 311: 806-814. DOI: 10.1001/jama.2014.732

[29] Finkelstein EA, Khavjou OA, Thompson H, Trogdon JG, Pan L, Sherry B, et al. Obesity and severe obesity forecasts through 2030. American Journal of Preventive Medicine. 2012; 42: 563-570. DOI: 10.1016/j.amepre.2011.10.02

[30] TFAH Release. F as in fat: How obesity threatens America's future 2012. Trust for America's Health and the Robert Wood Johnson Foundation. 2012. Available from: http://www.healthyamericans.org/report/100/ [Accessed: 2016-05-11]

[31] U.S. Public Health Service. Obesity and Health. (Publication No. 1485). Washington, DC: U.S. Department of Health, Education and Welfare. 1966.

[32] Gautier J-F, Chen K, Salbe AD, Bandy D, Pratley RE, Heiman M, et al. Differential brain responses to satiation in obese and lean men. Diabetes. 2000; 49: 838-846. DOI: 10.2337/diabetes.49.5.838

[33] Liu Y, Gao JH, Liu HL, Fox PT. The temporal response of the brain after eating revealed by functional MRI. Nature. 2000; 405: 1058-1062. DOI: 10.1038/35016590

[34] Matsuda M, Liu Y, Mahankali S, Pu Y, Mahankali A, Wang J, et al. Altered hypothalamic function in response to glucose injection in obese humans. Diabetes. 1999; 48: 1801-1806. DOI: 10.2337/diabetes.48.9.1801

[35] Brooks SJ, Cedernaes J, Schiöth HB. Increased prefrontal and parahippocampal activation with reduced dorsolateral prefrontal and insular cortex activation to food images in obesity: A meta-analysis of fMRI studies. Plos One. 2013; 8(4): e60393. DOI: 10.1371/journal.pone.0060393

[36] Carnell S, Gibson C, Benson L, Ochner CN, Geliebter A. Neuroimaging and obesity: Current knowledge and future directions. Obesity Reviews. 2012; 13: 43-56. DOI: 10.1111/j.1467-789X.2011.00927.x

[37] Stice E, Figlewicz DP, Gosnell BA, Levine AS, Pratt WE. The contribution of brain reward circuits to the obesity epidemic. Neuroscience and Biobehavioral Reviews. 2013; 37: 2047-2058. DOI: 10.1016/j.neubiorev.2012.12.001

[38] Stice E, Yokum S, Bohon C, Marti N, Smolen A. Reward circuitry responsivity to food predicts future increases in body mass: Moderating effects of DRD_2 and DRD_4. Neuroimage. 2010; 50: 1618-1625. DOI: 10.1016/j.neuroimage.2010.01.081

[39] Stice E, Yokum S, Burger KS, Epstein LH, Small DM. Youth at risk for obesity show greater activation of striatal and somatosensory regions to food. Journal of Neuroscience. 2011; 31: 4360-4366. DOI: 10.1523/JNEUROSCI.6604-10.2011

[40] DelParigi A, Chen K, Salbe AD, Hill JO, Wing RR, Reiman EM, et al. Persistence of abnormal neural responses to a meal in postobese individuals. International Journal of Obesity and Related Metabolic Disorders. 2004; 28: 370-377. DOI: 10.1038/sj.ijo.0802558

[41] Zhang Y, von Deneen KM, Tian J, Gold MS, Liu Y. Food addiction and neuroimaging. Current Pharmaceutical Design. 2011; 17: 1149-1157. DOI: 10.2174/138161211795656855

[42] Devore I. Diet and hunter-gatherers. Anthroquest. 1984; 30: 3-5.

[43] Lee RB, Devore I. Problems in the study of hunters and gatherers. In: Lee RB, Devore I, editors. Man the Hunter. Chicago, IL: Aldine; 1968. p. 3-12.

[44] Neel JV. Diabetes mellitus: A "thrifty" genotype rendered detrimental by "progress"? American Journal of Human Genetics. 1962; 14: 353-362.

[45] Mattson MP, Allison DB, Fontana L, Harvie M, Longo VD, Malaisse WJ, et al. Meal frequency and timing in health and disease. Proceedings of the National Academy of Sciences. 2014; 111: 16647-16653. DOI: 10.1073/pnas.1413965111

[46] Horne BD, Muhlestein JB, Anderson, JL. Health effects of intermittent fasting: Hormesis or harm? A systematic review. American Journal of Clinical Nutrition. 2015; 102: 464-470. DOI: 10.3945/ajcn.115.109553

[47] Patterson RE, Laughlin GA, LaCroix AZ, Hartman SJ, Natarajan L, Senger CM, et al. Intermittent fasting and human metabolic health. Journal of the Academy of Nutrition and Dietetics. 2015; 115: 1203-1212. DOI: 10.1016/j.jand.2015.02.018

[48] Tinsley GM, La Bounty PM. Effects of intermittent fasting on body composition and clinical health markers in humans. Nutrition Reviews. 2015; 73: 661-674. DOI: 10.1093/nutrit/nuv041

[49] Cohen MN. Introduction: Rethinking the origins of agriculture. Current Anthropology. 2009; 50: 591-595. DOI: 10.1086/603548

[50] Lichtenstein AH. Dietary fat: A history. Nutrition Reviews. 1999; 57: 11-14. DOI: 10.1111/j.1753-4887.1999.tb01770.x

[51] Outram AK. Hunter-gatherers and the first farmers: The evolution of taste in prehistory. In: Freedman P, editor. Food: The History of Taste. Volume 21. Berkeley, CA: University of California Press; 2007. p. 34-61.

[52] Armelagos GJ. The omnivore's dilemma: The evolution of the brain and the determinants of food choice. Journal of Anthropological Research. 2010; 66: 161-186. DOI: 10.3998/jar.0521004.0066.201

[53] Grey MA. The industrial food stream and its alternatives in the United States: An introduction. Human Organization. 2000; 59: 143-150. DOI: 10.17730/humo.59.2.xm3235743p6618j3

[54] Popkin BM, Duffey K, Gordon-Larse P. Environmental influences on food choice, physical activity and energy balance. Physiology & Behavior. 2005; 86: 603-613. DOI: 10.1016/j.physbeh.2005.08.051

[55] Putnam J, Allshouse J, Kantor LS. US per capita food supply trends: More calories, refined carbohydrates, and fats. Food Reviews. 2002; 25: 2-15.

[56] Technomic, Inc. Technomic Foodservice Segment Time Series: Limited Service Restaurants (1975-2005). Chicago, IL: Technomic, Inc.; 2004.

[57] Briefel RR, Johnson CL. Secular trends in dietary intake in the United States. Annual Review of Nutrition. 2004; 24: 401-431. DOI: 10.1146/annurev.nutr.23.011702.073349

[58] Nielsen SJ, Popkin BM. Changes in beverage intake between 1977 and 2001. American Journal of Preventive Medicine. 2004; 27: 205-210. DOI: 10.1016/j.amepre.2004.05.005

[59] Fraser LK, Edwards KL. The association between the geography of fast food outlets and childhood obesity rates in Leeds, UK. Health & Place. 2010; 16: 1124-1128. DOI: 10.1016/j.healthplace.2010.07.003

[60] Inagami S, Cohen DA, Brown AF, Asch SM. Body mass index, neighborhood fast food and restaurant concentration, and car ownership. Journal of Urban Health. 2009; 86: 683-695. DOI: 10.1007/s11524-009-9379-y

[61] Maddock J. The relationship between obesity and the prevalence of fast food restaurants: State-level analysis. American Journal of Health Promotion. 2004; 19: 137-143. DOI: 10.4278/0890-1171-19.2.137

[62] Mehta NK, Chang VW. Weight status and restaurant availability: A multilevel analysis. American Journal of Preventive Medicine. 2008; 34: 127-133. DOI: 10.1016/j.amepre.2007.09.031

[63] Papas MA, Alberg AJ, Ewing R, Helzlsover KJ, Gary TL, Klassen AC. The built environment and obesity. Epidemiologic Reviews. 2007; 29: 129-143. DOI: 10.1093/epirev/mxm009

[64] Spence JC, Cutumisu N, Edwards J, Raine KD, Smoyer-Tomic K. Relation between local food environments and obesity among adults. BMC Public Health. 2009; 9: 192. DOI: 10.1186/1471-2458-9-192

[65] Anderson B, Rafferty AP, Lyon-Callo S, Fussma C, Imes G. Fast-food consumption and obesity among Michigan adults. Preventing Chronic Disease. 2011; 8(4): A71.

[66] Bezerra IN, Curioni C, Sichieri R. Association between eating out of home and body weight. Nutrition Reviews. 2012; 70: 65-79. DOI: 10.1111/j.1753-4887.2011.00459.x

[67] Duffey KJ, Gordon-Larsen P, Jacobs DR, Williams OD, Popkin BM. Differential associations of fast food and restaurant food consumption with 3-y change in body mass index: The coronary artery risk development in young adults study. American Journal of Clinical Nutrition. 2007; 85: 201-208.

[68] Holsten JE. Obesity and the community food environment: A systematic review. Public Health and Nutrition. 2009; 12: 397-405. DOI: 10.1017/S1368980008002267

[69] McCrory MA, Fuss PJ, Hays NP, Vinken AG, Greenberg A, Roberts SB. Overeating in America: Association between restaurant food consumption and body fatness in

healthy adult men and women ages 19 to 80. Obesity Research. 1999; 7: 564-571. DOI: 10.1002/j.1550-8528.1999.tb00715.x

[70] Thompson OM, Ballew C, Resnicow K, Must A, Bandini LG, Cyr H, et al. Food purchased away from home as a predictor of change in BMI z-score among girls. International Journal of Obesity and Related Metabolic Disorders. 2004; 28: 282-289. DOI: 10.1038/sj.ijo.0802538

[71] Lachat C, Nago G, Verstraeten R, Roberfroid D, Van Camp J, Kolsteren P. Eating out of home and its association with dietary intake: A systematic review of the evidence. Obesity Reviews. 2012; 13: 329-346. DOI: 10.1111/j.1467-789X.2011.00953x

[72] de Castro JM, King GA, Duarte-Gardea M, Gonzalez-Ayala S, Kooshian CH. Overweight and obese humans overeat away from home. Appetite. 2012; 59: 204-211. DOI: 10.1016/j.appet.2012.04.020

[73] Goel MS, McCarthy EP, Phillips RS, Wee CC. Obesity among US immigrant subgroups by duration of residence. Journal of the American Medical Association. 2004; 292: 2860-2867. DOI: 10.1001/jama.292.23.2860

[74] Levitsky DA, Halbmaier CA, Mrdjenovic G. The freshman weight gain: A model for the study of the epidemic of obesity. International Journal of Obesity and Related Metabolic Disorders. 2004; 28: 1435-1442. DOI: 10.1038/sj.ijo.0802776

[75] Blundell JE, Stubbs RJ, Golding C, Croden F, Alam R, Whybrow S, et al. Resistance and susceptibility to weight gain: Individual variability in response to a high-fat diet. Physiology & Behavior. 2005; 86: 614-622. DOI: 10.1016/j.physbeh.2005.08.052

[76] Carnell S, Haworth CMA, Plomin R, Wardle J. Genetic influence on appetite in children. International Journal of Obesity. 2008; 32: 1468-1473. DOI: 10.1038/ijo.2008.127

[77] Carnell S, Wardle J. Appetite and adiposity in children: Evidence for a behavioral susceptibility theory of obesity. American Journal of Clinical Nutrition. 2008; 88: 22-29.

[78] Jansen A, Theunissen N, Slechten K, Nederkoorn C, Boon B, Mulkens S, et al. Overweight children overeat after exposure to food cues. Eating Behaviors. 2003; 4: 197-209. DOI: 10.1016/S1471-0153(03)00011-4

[79] Carnell S, Kim Y, Pryor K. Fat brains, greedy genes, and parent power: A biobehavioural risk model of child and adult obesity. International Review of Psychiatry. 2012; 24: 189-199. DOI: 10.3109/09540261.2012.676988

[80] Bonato DP, Boland FJ. Delay of gratification in obese children. Addictive Behaviors. 1983; 8: 71-74. DOI: 10.1016/0306-4603(83)90059-X

[81] Geller SE, Keane TM, Scheirer CJ. Delay of gratification, locus of control, and eating patterns in obese and nonobese children. Addictive Behaviors. 1981; 6: 9-14. DOI: 10.1016/S0306-4603(81)80002-0

[82] Johnson WG, Parry W, Drabman RS. The performance of obese and normal size children on a delay of gratification task. Addictive Behaviors. 1978; 3: 205-208. DOI: 10.1016/0306-4603(78)90020-5

[83] Weller RE, Cook EW, Avsar KB, Cox JE. Obese women show greater delay discounting than healthy-weight women. Appetite. 2008; 51: 563-569. DOI: 10.1016/j.appet.2008.04.010

[84] de Castro JM. The relationship of cognitive restraint to the spontaneous food and fluid intake of free-living humans. Physiology & Behavior. 1995; 57: 287-295. DOI: 10.1016/0031-9384(94)00229-X

[85] de Castro JM, Lilenfeld L. The influence of heredity on dietary restraint, disinhibition, and perceived hunger in humans. Nutrition. 2005; 21: 446-455. DOI: 10.1016/j.nut.2004.07.010

[86] Maffeis C. Aetiology of overweight and obesity in children and adolescents. European Journal of Pediatrics. 2000; 159: S35-S44. DOI: 10.1007/PL00014361

[87] Speliotes EK, Willer CJ, Berndt SI, Monda KL, Thorleifsson G, Jackson AU, et al. Association analyses of 249,796 individuals reveal 18 new loci associated with body mass index. Nature Genetics. 2010; 42: 937-948. DOI: 10.1038/ng.686

[88] Rodgers GP, Collins FS. The next generation of obesity research. No time to waste. Journal of the American Medical Association. 2012; 308: 1095-1096. DOI: 10.1001/2012.jama.11853

[89] Christiansen T, Bruun JM, Madsen EL, Richelsen B. Weight loss maintenance in severely obese adults after an intensive lifestyle intervention: 2- to 4-year follow-up. Obesity. 2007; 15: 413-420. DOI: 10.1038/oby.2007.530

[90] LeBlanc ES, O'Connor E, Whitlock EP, Patnode CD, Kapka T. Effectiveness of primary care-relevant treatments for obesity in adults: A systematic evidence review for the U.S. Preventive Services Task Force. Annals of Internal Medicine. 2011; 155: 434-447. DOI: 10.7326/0003-4819-155-7-201110040-00006

[91] Cornell Conferences on Therapy. The management of obesity. New York State Journal of Medicine. 1958; 58: 79-87.

[92] Heymsfield SB, Greenberg AS, Fujioka K, Dixon RM, Kushner R, Hunt T, et al. Recombinant leptin for weight loss in obese and lean adults: A randomized, controlled, dose-escalation trial. Journal of the American Medical Association. 1999; 282: 1568-1575. DOI: 10.1001/jama.282.16.1568

[93] Li Z, Maglione M, Tu W, Majica W, Arterburn D, Shugarman LR, et al. Meta-analysis: Pharmacologic treatment of obesity. Annals of Internal Medicine. 2005; 142: 532-546. DOI: 10.7326/0003-4819-142-7-200504050-00012

[94] Rucker D, Padwal R, Li SK, Curioni C, Lau DC. Long term pharmacotherapy for obesity and overweight: Updated meta-analysis. British Medical Journal. 2007; 335: 1194-1199. DOI: 10.1136/bmj.39385.413113.25

[95] Yanovski SZ, Yanovski JA. Long-term drug treatment for obesity. A systematic and clinical review. Journal of the American Medical Association. 2014; 311: 74-86. DOI: 10.1001/jama.2013.281361

[96] Bray GA, Tartaglia LA. Medicinal strategies in the treatment of obesity. Nature. 2000; 404: 672-677. DOI: 10.1038/35007544

[97] Cobourn C, Chapman MA, Ali A, Amrhein J. Five-year weight loss experience of outpatients receiving laparoscopic adjustable gastric band surgery. Obesity Surgery. 2013; 23: 903-910. DOI: 10.1007/s11695-013-0881-7

[98] O'Brien PE, MacDonald L, Anderson M, Brennan L, Brown WA. Long-term outcomes after bariatric surgery: Fifteen-year follow-up of adjustable gastric banding and a systematic review of the bariatric surgical literature. Annals of Surgery. 2013; 257: 87-94. DOI: 10.1097/SLA.ob013e31827b6c02

[99] Vest AR, Heneghan HM, Agarwal S, Schaver PR, Young JB. Bariatric surgery and cardiovascular outcomes: A systematic review. Heart. 2012; 98: 1763-1777. DOI: 10.1136/heartjnl-2012-301778

[100] Livhits M, Mercado C, Yermilov I, Parikh JA, Dutson E, Mehran A, et al. Preoperative predictors of weight loss following bariatric surgery: Systematic review. Obesity Surgery. 2012; 22: 70-89. DOI: 10.1007/s11695-011-0472-4

[101] Christou NV, Look D, MacLean LD. Weight gain after short- and long-limb gastric bypass in patients followed for longer than 10 years. Annals of Surgery. 2006; 244: 734-740. DOI: 10.1097/01.sla.0000217592.04061.d5

[102] Institute of Medicine. Accelerating progress in obesity prevention: Solving the weight of the nation. 2012. Available from: http://www.iom.edu/Reports/2012/Accelerating-Progress-in-Obesity-Prevention.aspx [Accessed: 2016-05-11]

[103] Barry CL, Gollust SE, Niederdeppe J. Are Americans ready to solve the weight of the nation? New England Journal of Medicine. 2012; 367: 389-391. DOI: 10.1056/NEJMp1206519

[104] Mitchell NS. Obesity: Overview of an epidemic. Psychiatric Clinics of North America. 2011; 34: 717-732. DOI: 10.1016/j.psc.2011.08.005

[105] Mwanri L, Foley W, Coveney J, Muller R, Verity F, Ward PR, et al. Food supply and the obesity scourge: Is there a relationship? Health. 2012; 4: 1457-1463. DOI: 10.4236/health.2012.412A210

10

Dietary and Hormonal Factors Involved in Healthy or Unhealthy Visceral Adipose Tissue Expansion

María Guillermina Zubiría, Ana Alzamendi,
Luisina Ongaro, Eduardo Spinedi and
Andrés Giovambattista

Abstract

White adipose tissue (WAT) expansion is related to the development of metabolic disorders found in obesity. WAT expansion is the result of generation of new adipose cells by activation of adipogenesis and/or the increase in adipose cell size (hypertrophy). The balance between these two processes determines whether WAT expansion occurs predominantly by hyperplasia, which means the increase in the number of adipocytes, or hypertrophy. Hypertrophic adipocytes are characterized by changes in adipokine secretion pattern, insulin resistance and altered lipid metabolism, which is the reason why WAT-hypertrophic expansion is considered unhealthy. Conversely, the generation of new mature adipocytes by adipogenesis contributes to reduction of the development of hypertrophic adipocytes and therefore maintain normal WAT functions, leading to healthy hyperplastic expansion. The adipogenic capacity of adipose tissue depends on the adipogenic potential and the number of adipocyte precursor cells. Different factors are known to regulate adipogenic process and adipose tissue function, contributing to a healthy or unhealthy expansion that occurs under positive energy balance. This chapter discusses the role of fructose intake and glucocorticoids and testosterone as regulators of adipose tissue function and expansion.

Keywords: fructose-rich diet, glucocorticoid, testosterone, adipogenesis

1. Introduction

Obesity has been defined by the World Health Organization as the excess of adipose tissue (AT) mass that can be harmful or not for the health. The incidence of this disorder has reached epidemic levels during the last few decades. It is associated with a high risk of developing different pathologies such as type 2 diabetes mellitus (T2DM), cardiovascular diseases, dyslipidaemias and cancer, among others. White AT (WAT) dysfunction plays an important role in the development of metabolic disorders associated to obesity. Anatomically, WAT presents a discontinuous distribution in the organism and it is divided into two major depots, visceral and subcutaneous (VAT and SAT, respectively). VAT is mainly located in the abdominal cavity (peri-renal, retroperitoneal (RPAT), mesenteric, omental and gonadal) and SAT is distributed below the dermis (femoral, gluteal, abdominal and gonadal). Studies in humans and animal models indicate that VAT expansion is associated with an increase in metabolic risk and mortality, whereas accumulation of SAT improves insulin sensitivity and reduces the risk of developing T2DM.

WAT increase is the consequence of two processes: the increase in the size (hypertrophy) and/or in the number of adipocytes (hyperplasia). The form in which WAT expands correlates with the presence or absence of WAT-functional alterations. It is well known that hypertrophy of adipose cells is associated with the change in the pattern of adipokine secretion, increasing the release of leptin [1] and pro-inflammatory cytokines [2], and decreasing the release of adiponectin [2]. This profile of adipokine secretion contributes to the development of insulin resistance (IR) observed in hypertrophic adipocytes [3]. Moreover, the increase in cell size is associated with changes in lipid metabolism [4]. Conversely, adipogenesis activation leads to an increase in the number of adipose cells, and therefore prevents the development of hypertrophy thus contributing to normal WAT function.

WAT has been recently reported to express brown AT (BAT) markers, and its exposure to cold or beta-adrenergic receptors stimulation to increase the presence of brown-like-multilocular cells [5]; this process is called WAT 'browning'. Since these cells are different from brown and white adipocytes, they have been called beige or brite adipocytes (from the combination of brown and white). It is known that brown and beige adipocytes originate from different lineages; while brown adipocytes are generated from MYF5$^+$ precursors, beige ones derive from precursors that express platelet-derived growth factor receptor (PDGFR-α^+) and stem cells antigen 1 (Sca1$^+$) or from smooth muscle-like precursors that express myosin heavy-chain 11 (MYH11$^+$) [6, 7]. Previous reports have suggested that beige adipocytes could arise through a less-studied mechanism of transdifferentiation of pre-existent white adipocytes. The most important functional difference between beige and white adipocytes is the expression of the mitochondrial-uncoupling protein 1 (UCP-1), which allows the production of heat via the respiratory-uncoupling reaction. UCP-1 is activated by an increase of free fatty acids (FFAs), product of cold-induced lipolysis [8]. Peroxisome proliferator-activated receptor-γ coactivator-1α (PGC1α) is a transcription co-activator which promotes the expression of thermogenic genes during cold-induced browning of WAT. Thereby, enhancing the number of beige adipocytes results quite relevant because of the consequent increase in energy expenditure that would avoid or reduce unhealthy hypertrophic WAT expansion. This could protect organisms against metabolic disorders associated to obesity.

Adipogenesis is a process that can be divided into two sequential steps: (a) commitment of mesenchymal stem cells into adipocyte precursor cells (APCs), acquiring the adipogenic potential and restricting them to the adipocyte lineage; and (b) the terminal adipocyte differentiation wherein APCs under specific adipogenic stimuli differentiate into mature adipocytes. In the first step, APCs begin to express CD34, a cell surface antigen that distinguishes between adipogenic and non-adipogenic cell subpopulations [9]. It is important to highlight that APCs are not a homogeneous cell population, presenting different ability to differentiate into mature adipocytes. This cell ability has been called APCs competency and is mainly determined by the expression of two transcription factors, zinc finger protein 423 (Zfp423) and peroxisome proliferator-activated receptor (PPAR)-γ2, that are considered competency markers. Initially, APCs express Zfp423 [10], which in turn activates the basal expression of PPAR-γ2, a key pro-adipogenic signal that assures APCs conversion into adipocytes [11]. APCs differentiation capacity is inversely correlated with the expression of anti-adipogenic factors, such as preadipocyte factor 1 (Pref-1) and wingless-type MMTV 10b (mouse mammary tumour virus) (Wnt-10b). Pref-1 is produced by APCs and exerts the most potent inhibitory signal of the adipogenic process, by suppressing CCAAT/enhancer-binding proteins (C/EBPs) gene expression [12]. Pref-1 expression decreases progressively in cells undergoing differentiation, becoming undetectable in mature adipocytes. Also, the increase of Wnt-10b levels inhibits APCs differentiation *in vitro* and *in vivo* [13].

Terminal adipocyte differentiation is under the control of different transcription factors and hormones. PPAR-γ2 is one of the most important factors that induce adipocyte differentiation, and its expression is absolutely required for adipocyte differentiation. C/EBP-α, -β and -δ have been the first transcription factors described as involved in the differentiation of AT cells. The expression of C/EBP-β and -δ increases immediately after induction of adipogenesis and stimulates the expression of C/EBP-α and PPARγ-2. The increase in C/EBP-α occurs at the end of adipogenesis and is more abundant in mature adipocytes, being crucial for the normal sensitivity to insulin in adipocytes.

Several factors influence the biology and adipogenic potential of WAT, which contribute to a healthy or unhealthy expansion that occurs under positive-energy balance. The purpose of this chapter is to discuss the role of three of these factors, such as fructose intake, glucocorticoids (GCs) and testosterone, affecting WAT function and expansion (**Figure 1**).

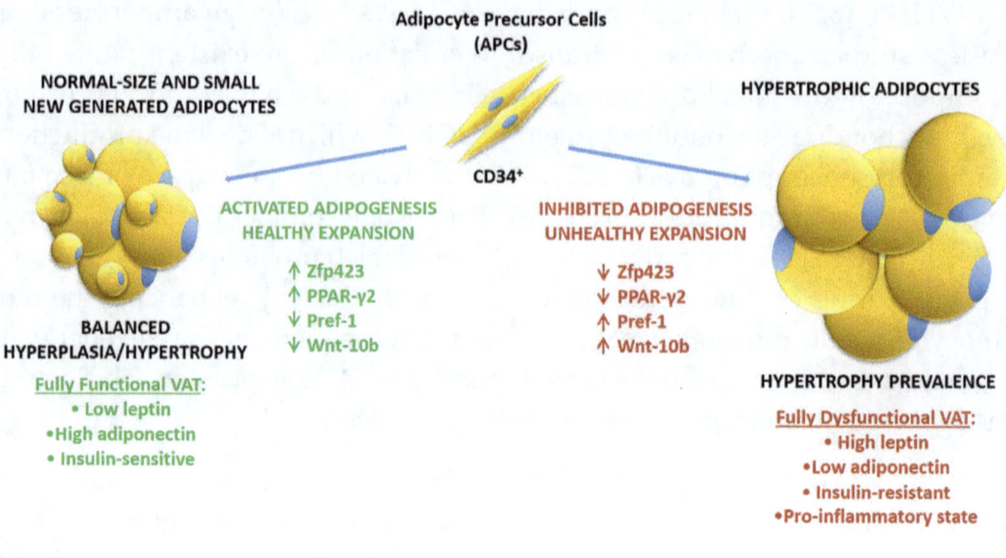

Figure 1. Adipocyte precursor cells (APCs) are committed mesenchymal stem cells that have acquired the adipogenic potential, and are restricted to adipocyte lineage. During healthy adipose tissue (AT) expansion, adipogenesis is active and AT is composed by normal sized and small new generated adipocytes, maintaining normal functions. When AT undergoes an unhealthy expansion, VAT expands mainly by hypertrophy, and becomes dysfunctional, characterized by insulin-resistant adipocytes, with abnormal endocrine function and local pro-inflammatory state.

2. Deleterious effects of high-fructose diet

2.1. Fructose-rich diet intake and fructose metabolism

Fructose is a natural sugar found in fruits and vegetables, also known as levulose and fruit sugar. Although the intake of natural sources of fructose has been relatively stable for the last 40 years, the introduction of high-fructose corn syrups has led to an exponential increase of free fructose in food supply [14].

Fructose is metabolized primarily by the liver, although both the small intestinal mucosa and kidney also contain the enzymes necessary for fructose catabolism [15]. Fructose is transported into cells by two membrane proteins: GLUT5, a specific fructose transporter highly expressed along the small intestine, and GLUT2, a transporter of both glucose and fructose which is expressed in the liver, small intestine and pancreas. Most of ingested fructose passes via the portal circulation to the liver where it is rapidly cleared. Fructose liver metabolism bypasses the main glycolysis metabolic control. Therefore, fructose metabolism will generate pyruvate and acetyl-CoA even during positive-energy balance, and both of them will end in fatty acid synthesis. This phenomenon explains why high-fructose consumption, more than other sugar intake, increases *de novo* lipogenesis, dyslipidaemia and visceral fat deposition, all of them components of the metabolic syndrome (MS).

2.1.1. Fructose impacts on adipose tissue function and adipogenesis

Fructose effects were initially described by observational studies showing the association between cardiometabolic diseases and consumption of fructose-containing sugars, but not with lactose [16]. These considerations were also confirmed by several pre-clinical and clinical studies globally showing that dietary fructose can induce several metabolic alterations closely similar to the MS phenotype.

There is considerable evidence suggesting that the intake of added sugars or sugar-sweetened beverages is associated with increased body weight, presence of unfavourable lipid levels, IR, fatty liver, cardiovascular disease and MS [17], while these alterations are not found using artificial sweeteners [18]. Specifically, fructose-sweetened beverages have been reported to cause body-weight increase and intra-abdominal fat deposition, which would be related to high circulating levels of triglycerides found after fructose-rich diet (FRD) [19]. Indeed, dietary fructose activates de novo lipogenesis in liver and therefore increases AT fatty acid uptake. This powerful lipogenic effect has not been observed after the ingestion of other carbohydrates, since fructose metabolism is driven almost completely to fatty acid synthesis, as mentioned above. Another effect related to fructose consumption is the advanced glycation end products (AGEs) formation. Fructose produces 10 times more AGEs than glucose does and these AGEs indirectly contribute to the inflammation and oxidative stress that characterize the MS phenotype [20].

As in men, fructose ingestion by rats induces body-weight gain, morphological and functional VAT modifications and MS-like phenotype, while this does not occur when glucose or starch is administered to rats [21–23]. Previous studies from our group showed that FRD given to adult rats during 3 and 8 weeks, induced an increase in circulating levels of key adipokines secreted by RPAT, such as leptin, adiponectin and PAI-1. Interestingly, this altered secretion pattern was accompanied by enlarged adipocytes and decreased expression of insulin receptor substrates (IRS-1 and IRS-2) in adipocytes [24–28], suggesting an IR state. On the other hand, Pektas et al. showed that FRD increases gene expression of insulin-signalling pathway components and pro- and anti-inflammatory markers in WAT from male and female rats. Gender-dependent differences in fructose feeding were not significant, suggesting that females were not protected from harmful effects of fructose [29]. In summary, FRD ingestion during short or long periods of time induces deep changes in VAT functionality, predominantly by favouring hypertrophic VAT mass expansion.

The deleterious effect of high-fructose intake on hypertrophic AT mass expansion has been extensively studied; however, the study of fructose effects on adipogenesis is now emerging. It has been observed that rats fed with FRD during short and long periods showed an increase in the adipogenic potential of APCs from RPAT, displaying high levels of competency markers, PPAR-γ2 and Zfp423 [26, 28]. These changes in the cell expression pattern of both competency factors are related to an increased APCs ability to differentiate into mature adipocytes. Indeed, APCs from FRD-fed rats differentiated into adipocytes showed high intracellular lipid content and high expression levels of adipogenic genes indicating that FRD intake generates APCs with a greater ability to become mature adipocytes [26, 28]. Another factor that could influence cell adipogenic potential in AT depots is APCs number. High-fat diet intake increases APCs number in different AT depots [30, 31]. Interestingly, we previously reported that a 3-week FRD intake did not induce any change in RPAT APCs number [26]. However, prolonged FRD intake (8 weeks) increased RPAT APCs number, indicating that this effect is dependent on the time period of fructose consumption; thus, prolonged periods of fructose intake increase RPAT APCs number.

Though literature about the effects of fructose on WAT browning is rather scarce, some authors have shown that dietary factors are related with this phenomenon. It has been observed that high-fat ingestion is associated with an increase in UCP-1 expression in BAT and WAT, in mice [32, 33] and rats [34]. Conversely, other studies show a decrease or no differences in UCP-1 WAT expression [35]. Moreover, changes in the micronutrient composition induce WAT browning in rodents [36]. Nevertheless, dietary effects on beige adipocytes generation and precursors remain to be further studied.

2.1.2. Direct effects of fructose on adipocyte precursor cells

As mentioned above, fructose is extensively extracted and metabolized (50–75%) primarily by the liver; however, a percentage of fructose enters into the systemic circulation and is metabolized by extra-hepatic tissues, such as the AT [37]. In fact, fructose concentration in the portal circulation around VAT can easily reach 5–10 mM [38, 39]. So, it suggests that some of the effects of FRD intake on AT mass expansion could be the result from a direct fructose effect on APCs.

In this regard, there are some available reports describing direct fructose effects on adipogenesis, and most of them have been focused on the terminal differentiation stage of 3T3-L1 preadipocytes [40]. The addition of fructose into the culture medium of 3T3-L1 preadipocytes stimulates the terminal stage of adipogenesis, a mechanism that is GLUT5-dependent [40, 41]. Both 3T3-L1 preadipocytes and adipocytes express GLUT5 [40, 42]. It has been described that GLUT5 gene expression is higher in undifferentiated than in differentiated 3T3-L1 cells, in which it is almost undetectable [40, 43]. This indicates that adipocyte precursors are a better target for fructose action than mature adipocytes. Several effects have been described using fructose in the culture medium. In differentiated 3T3-L1 cells, fructose increased lipolysis and the activity of 11-β hydroxysteroid dehydrogenase-1 [41]. Also, the presence of fructose (55–5500 μM) during adipocyte differentiation induced an increase in several pro-adipogenic factors, and either GLUT5 knockdown or its over-expression reduced or increased this effect, respectively [40].

Previous reports have described direct effects of fructose on cultured RPAT APCs from adult normal male rats when they were cultured in the presence of fructose (5500 μM) in the culture medium. Under this condition, APCs expressed high levels of competency factors, showing greater APCs potential to become adipocytes. Similar results were found when cells were cultured with a comparable concentration of glucose [28]. It has been proposed that the balance between mineralocorticoid (MR)/glucocorticoid (GR) receptors plays a key role in the pro-adipogenic effect of GCs. Fructose decreases GR expression in adipocytes [44], in agreement with these data APCs grown in the presence of fructose, but not in the presence of glucose, displayed higher MR and lower GR mRNA levels. Interestingly, when fructose-exposed APCs were induced to differentiate, they accumulated high lipid content, indicating that the imprinting of fructose in APCs is reflected in the mature adipocytes differentiation capacity [28].

As mentioned before, there are two possible mechanisms by which adipogenic potential of AT can be increased, that is, by enhancing APCs competency and increasing APCs number. Fructose effects on APCs competency have already been presented. Regarding the direct effect of fructose on APCs number, our previous studies showed that fructose directly increased the $CD34^+$ adipogenic cell subpopulation in the WAT stromal vascular fraction (SVF), indicating an increase on APCs [28]. Interestingly, these results were not observed when glucose was used, which confirms a fructose-specific effect. Taken together, these results are similar to those observed in cells from FRD-fed rats, thus it is plausible that some effects observed in RPAT mass expansion from FRD-fed rats can be a consequence of direct fructose effects on APCs.

2.1.3. Fructose-rich diet intake and metabolic imprinting

The concept of 'developmental origins of adult disease' states [45] that environmental factors, including maternal nutrition, experienced *in utero* and during early postnatal life, can elicit permanent metabolic and physiological modifications in individuals, leading to enhanced susceptibility to develop diseases later in life. Limited data are available on the long-term effects of high fructose exposure during gestation, lactation and infancy. Emerging research suggests that fructose consumption by mothers and/or their offspring during early life can lead to persistent neuroendocrine and metabolic dysfunctions.

Our group has studied the effect of fructose exposure during gestation or lactation, on adult male pups. Maternal consumption of FRD during gestation alters offspring development causing impaired insulin sensitivity and RPAT dysfunction, evidenced by hypertrophic adipocytes that secrete larger amounts of leptin *in vitro*, though with decreased AT mass. A paradoxical situation could at least partially be the result of a reduced RPAT APCs number [46]. Adult male offspring born to FRD-fed dams throughout gestation were reported to develop IR, dyslipidaemia, with a distorted pattern of peripheral adipokines and enhanced oxidative stress [47]. Interestingly, later in life, the offspring normalized their metabolic profile [48]. Conversely, another study showed that FRD intake by gestating mothers resulted in pro-

even after following their progress up to 6 months of age [49].

When FRD was administered to lactating dams, the offspring showed increased body weight, hypothalamic leptin resistance, increased food intake, IR and increased VAT mass (due to both fat mass and adipocyte size) [50].

It was reported that offspring born from mothers consuming FRD during pregnancy and lactation displayed decreased body weight, hyperinsulinaemia and hypoglycaemia at weaning [51]. Moreover, rat pups consuming high-carbohydrate milk during lactation did develop obesity at adulthood [52], characterized by increased body weight, hyperinsulinaemia and augmented skeletal muscle fatty acid transport at adult life [53]. Excessive insulin secretion in turn promotes enhanced lipogenesis [54] and adipogenesis [55]. Regarding WAT browning, FRD effects have not been yet studied. Nevertheless, maternal perinatal undernutrition has been reported to increase the appearance of beige adipocytes in gonadal WAT of rats at weaning [56]. There is still much to investigate about this mechanism.

In summary, FRD administration during an individual´s development (gestation or lactation periods) induces a permanent alteration in AT development, increasing its susceptibility to have an unhealthy RPAT expansion, and leading to unfavourable metabolic consequences seen at adult age.

2.2. The role of glucocorticoids in adipose tissue biology

GCs have numerous effects on AT biology and functionality. Among others, they regulate AT endocrine function, AT inflammation in obesity and lipogenic-lipolysis balance [57]. High GC levels in blood or in AT depots would be expected to increase the breakdown of lipids; however, the GC effects on AT metabolism are controversial. Many reports agree that GCs increase lipolysis in mature adipocytes [58, 59], while others state that GCs have an inhibitory effect on lipolysis [59, 60]. Regarding lipogenesis, dexamethasone (DXM), a synthetic GC, has been shown to potentiate the stimulatory effect of insulin on *de novo* lipogenesis in adipocytes [61]. GCs also may cause an increase in VAT lipoprotein lipase (LPL) activity, particularly in men [62]. Consequently, a greater amount of fatty acids would be available for uptake in the VAT, and could help to explain central AT accumulation seen in individuals with high GC levels. The global balance of GC effects on AT lipid metabolism seems to indicate that GCs may favour lipid accumulation in adipocytes, contributing to cell hypertrophy.

Another important effect of GCs on AT is the regulation of fat distribution, promoting VAT deposition [63]. One clear example is Cushing's syndrome (CS) phenotype, mainly characterized by high-serum GC levels and increased VAT rather than SAT mass [64]. CS has several features in common with MS phenotype, such as the presence of VAT-hypertrophic adipocytes, altered lipid metabolism and impaired adipokine secretion [65]. Chronic treatment with GCs induces obesity and MS, impairing AT metabolism. These alterations suggest that GCs have a pivotal role in the pathogenesis of central obesity and the associated alterations

a rat model of CS reverses most of dysfunctions [66].

Although plasmatic levels of GC seem not to be increased in human obesity, increased local production of cortisol within the AT is associated with this disorder [67]. Local cortisol levels are regulated by 11β-hydroxysteroid dehydrogenase type-1 and -2 (HSD1 and HSD2, respectively). Both enzymes are expressed in AT, where they act regulating the interconversion from the inactive to the active forms of GCs and vice versa, respectively. HSD1 is expressed at higher levels than HSD2 in AT, generating higher concentrations of the active form, which may play an important role in GCs-driven AT mass expansion. In animal models, overexpression of HSD1 in mature adipocytes has generated a model for VAT accumulation [68], whereas HSD1 knockout mice are resistant to central obesity [69].

GCs are required for the differentiation of APCs [70] and for the maintenance of adipogenic gene expression in cultured adipocytes and AT [71]. In fact, DXM has been widely used *in vitro* as a component of traditional differentiation cocktails, due to its potent adipogenic stimulus. The main effect of GCs during early stages of adipogenesis results from the inhibition of anti-adipogenic and the activation of pro-adipogenic transcriptional factors, as well as the increase of APCs competency factors. GCs decrease Pref-1 and Wnt-10b expression [72, 73], both factors are highly expressed in preadipocytes, absent in mature adipocytes and responsible for the undifferentiated phenotype maintenance [74, 75]. Experiments in 3T3-L1 preadipocytes showed that Pref-1 is an early target for DXM action and that its expression decreases with high DXM concentrations, at the same time that adipocyte differentiation increases [72]. Similarly, methylprednisolone (another synthetic GCs) or DXM inhibit Wnt/b-catenin-signalling pathway, promoting adipocyte differentiation [73, 76]. In cultured APCs from hypercorticosteronaemic rats, mRNA levels of Pref-1 and Wnt-10b decreased at the time that all differentiation parameters increased, for example, lipid content, expression levels of mature adipocytes genes (Ob, adiponectin, C/EBP-α, PPAR-γ2) and leptin secretion [77]. On the other hand, GCs increased mRNA levels of the pro-adipogenic factors C/EBP-δ and C/EBP-β [78], which subsequently regulated the expression of mature adipocytes genes. Additionally, it has been previously shown that GCs can activate APCs by enhancing the expression of the competency factors, PPAR-γ2 and Zfp423 [77], and consequently increasing their adipogenic potential.

The actions of GC on AT cells can be exerted through their binding to MR and GR [79, 80], although the contribution of MR and GR in mediating GC effects on AT cells has not been fully understood. In 3T3-L1 and in mouse and human preadipocytes, MR rather than GR has been reported to be important in mediating the pro-adipogenic effects of GCs [79, 81, 82].

However, another study by Lee et al. found that human preadipocytes express lower levels of MR than those of GR. Moreover, the blockade of GR but not of MR inhibited adipogenesis activation caused by GCs [80]. Nevertheless, the participation of MR or GR in the biological actions of GCs upon the AT is still a matter for debate, while there is currently no consensus about this.

Most studies on the stimulatory role of GCs on preadipocyte differentiation have been largely limited to the 3T3-L1 cell line [83, 84]. However, the role of GCs *in vivo* should not be assumed on the basis of those studies. Taking into account the potent pro-adipogenic action of GCs, it is difficult to explain the presence of hypertrophic adipocytes under conditions of high GC levels, when they are supposed to favour the generation of new cells and therefore small adipocytes through a continuously activated adipogenesis. In this regard, previous reports show evidence for a dual behaviour of the adipogenesis in a model of high GC levels, characterized by initial activation and a subsequent inhibition of the adipogenic process [66, 77]. This dual behaviour could be in part because of differential expression levels of MR: while MR expression does not change in early stages of hypercorticosteronaemia, it decreases under chronic high GC levels condition. This fact could suggest that MR is involved in the development of a GCs-resistant state in AT and it could explain, at least in part, the inhibition of adipogenesis in a powerful pro-adipogenic environment. However, the contribution of GR to the lack of GCs effect cannot be disregarded, even in the presence of similar GR expression levels.

The recruitment of immune cells, such as macrophages, lymphocytes and natural killer (NK) cells, occurs in VAT during obesity and contributes to the development of a chronic inflammatory state [85]. Furthermore, there is a macrophage polarization towards the M1 pro-inflammatory type in detriment to the M2 anti-inflammatory type [85]. The role of GCs mediating the inflammatory response in AT depends on MR or GR activation, which will determine a pro- or anti-inflammatory response, respectively. While GR activation induces a decrease of pro-inflammatory cytokine secretion, MR activation generates the opposite effect [86]. Nevertheless, in CS patients the establishment of an AT inflammatory state is debated [87, 88]. In our animal model of high GC levels, the RPAT expression of macrophages infiltration markers (TNF-α, IL-6, MCP-1 and F4/80) does not increase [66]. This suggests an anti-inflammatory effect of GCs exerted through GR activation or a lower pro-inflammatory effect due to low MR expression [66].

It has been described that GCs suppress thermogenesis in rodents BAT, by decreasing the expression of UCP-1 [89]. Also, GCs treatment decreases BAT-specific genes expression in a brown adipose cell line [90]. However, available information about GCs action on beige adipocytes generation is contradictory and inconclusive. MR antagonist in high-fat-fed mice has been observed to promote WAT browning, inducing the expression of UCP-1 in VAT and SAT (inguinal) and the generation of brown-like adipocytes [91]. On the other hand, human and mouse adipocytes expressed lower levels of UCP-1 when cultured in the presence of DXM [92]. Additionally, DXM-treated mice showed decreased UCP-1 mRNA levels in both SAT and WAT depots, at the same time that developed glucose intolerance and hypertrophic adipocytes [92]. Further studies are needed to clarify the role of GCs on WAT browning and the potential effects on metabolic disorders.

The molecular basis and a more complete understanding of GCs effects on *in vivo* AT mass expansion remain to be defined. Adipogenesis activation or inhibition, depending on the competency and number of APCs, could be one factor modulating the way in which an AT depot expands. This fact is crucial because the metabolic dysfunctions associated with obesity are dependent on the development of adipocyte hypertrophy. Thus, the possibility to increase APCs adipogenic potential could result in the activation of adipogenesis (hyperplastic AT mass expansion), and probably the compensation of adipocyte hypertrophy, with consequent benefits for AT functionality. The fact that CS patients as well as GCs-treated rodents show enlarged adipocytes [93, 94] suggests that GCs must also stimulate hypertrophy, through either increased lipogenesis or decreased lipolysis, in addition to hyperplasia, through adipogenesis activation, probably in balance where hypertrophy exceeds hyperplasia.

2.3. Testosterone modulates fat store deposition and function

It is well known that AT mass and distribution pattern display a clear dimorphism between genders, which has been observed in humans, non-human primates and laboratory animals. Women have greater percentage of AT and proportionately lower lean mass than men. Furthermore, there is a differential distribution of AT among individuals, while men have greater predisposition to accumulate VAT (android distribution), women accumulate gluteal-femoral AT (gynoid distribution). Since VAT expansion is associated to high risk of T2DM and cardiovascular disease development, the greater predisposition to VAT accumulation in men is one of the reasons for higher male incidence in metabolic disorders development. In physiological range, plasma testosterone levels are inversely correlated with VAT mass and therefore associated with a favourable metabolic profile. The same relation has been shown with plasmatic sex hormone-binding globulin (SHBG) concentration and VAT mass. Dehydroepiandrosterone (DHEA) is an adrenal precursor of the peripheral steroid synthesis and it is considered a weak androgen. Some studies have found an inverse correlation between the DHEA levels and central obesity. However, this relationship is not clear with supra- or sub-physiological testosterone levels. Treatments with testosterone in transsexual individuals are accompanied by an increase in AT mass [95], while in patients with hypo-

cardiovascular diseases was enhanced [95–97].

The relationship between blood androgen levels and AT function in women is more complex. It is accepted that androgen excess is associated with central obesity, although there are studies that are not consistent with this assumption. Women with polycystic ovary syndrome (PCOS) often have hyperandrogenaemia associated with IR and accumulate VAT mass. It has been seen that in humans, testosterone induces IR in adipocytes, in part by decreasing glucose uptake by these cells. Neonatal androgenization, an experimental model of PCOS, clearly showed that transiently testosterone excess altered AT function, increasing VAT mass [98], adipocyte size and plasmatic leptin, PAI-1 and FFA levels. These alterations shifted towards those favouring IR and inflammation in adult life [27]. On the other hand, neonatal treatment with a non-steroidal antagonist of the androgen receptor (AR), flutamide, induced a decrease in the levels of leptin and greater LPS-induced TNF-α secretion [99]. In general, the treatment with testosterone in the first days of life increases the susceptibility to the development of MS [76] and, on the contrary, the treatment with flutamide improves this condition, showing that testosterone effects are specific receptor-dependent (AR) [100].

The effects of androgens on lipid metabolism, insulin sensitivity and adipogenic process are well known. Androgens exert their biological actions through its specific receptor, which is part of the nuclear receptors family that includes GR, MR and PPAR-γ, among others. AR is expressed in both adipose cells and APCs [101]. However, the levels of its expression differ among AT depots. VAT has higher AR expression levels than SAT [101–103], which would explain in part the differential actions of testosterone on these different AT depots.

It is accepted that androgens have stimulating effects on lipolysis. In rats, castration inhibits catecholamines- or cAMP-induced lipolysis [104], while testosterone treatment increases forskolin- and adrenaline-induced lipolysis [105]. Also, DHEA has positive effects on the lipolytic process. It has been found that rats treated with DHEA show an increase in plasma glycerol and FFA, and in the epididymal AT pad it increases the expression levels of adipose triglyceride lipase (ATGL) and hormone-sensitive lipase (HSL) [106]. In humans, androgen effects on lipolysis are dependent of the AT depot being studied. Treatment with testosterone in transsexual individuals has been reported to increase lipolysis in VAT, but not in the SAT. *In vivo* studies also show that testosterone increases catecholamine-induced lipolysis in abdominal AT, but not in the femoral fat pad. There is a correlation between plasma testosterone levels and the degree of post-stimulation lipolysis in omental AT [107].

In vitro studies with preadipocyte cell line 3T3-L1 and multipotent cell lines C3H10T1/2, have shown that androgens (e.g. testosterone, dihydrotestosterone (DHT) and DHEA) inhibit cell proliferation and differentiation into mature adipocytes [108–110]. The same inhibitory effect was observed in human APCs from different AT depots (mesenteric, omental and abdominal subcutaneous). In rats, castration produces a dual effect according to the AT depot studied; while increasing adipogenic potential of APCs from peri-renal AT, a decreased effect was observed in epididymal AT [111]. Part of the anti-adipogenic action of androgens would be exerted through the inhibition of PPAR-γ2 and C/EBP-α. On the other hand, it has been observed that testosterone and DHT also inhibit the commitment of mesenchymal cells into APCs obtained from lean and obese women [112, 113]. The induction of the APCs to differentiate into mature adipocytes increases the expression of the AR [103], although Dieudonne et al. showed that this protein level decreases [101]. It is important to emphasize that most of the literature related to androgen effects on adipogenesis is focused on the terminal phase of this process, but very little is known about the actions on APCs number and competency.

Androgens effects on WAT browning have not been yet explored. However, the thermogenic capacity of BAT is associated with sexual dimorphism, evidenced by differential UCP-1 expression levels between males and females [114, 115]. It has been observed that testosterone inhibited the expression of UCP-1 [116] and PGC1-α in cultured precursors of brown adipocytes [117]. These results coincide with the lowest mitochondrial activity observed in male compared to female rats [118]. These observations show that androgens inhibit thermogenic capacity in brown adipocytes and therefore the same effect could be expected on beige adipocytes.

In obesity, plasmatic testosterone levels are diminished, favouring the increase in VAT mass. At the same time, low levels of testosterone induce inhibition of lipolytic metabolism and stimulate LPL expression favouring lipogenesis [119]. This altered lipolysis/lipogenesis balance contributes to an increase lipid storage in adipose cells and therefore to the development of unhealthy VAT mass expansion. Adipocyte hypertrophy is associated with higher leptin secretion into circulation. Leptin impacts on reproductive axis function by inhibiting testis testosterone production [120]. These feedback effects contribute to generate a vicious cycle between AT dysfunction and androgen.

The development of a pro-inflammatory state is one of the features of unhealthy VAT mass expansion. Androgens have been described as anti-inflammatory factors. In hypogonadism, pro-inflammatory cytokines levels increase, while androgen replacement therapy decreases them [121]. Therefore, the decrease of testosterone levels associated to obesity contributes to the pro-inflammatory state observed. On the other hand, low testosterone levels in circulation would be one of the factors that activate adipogenesis, contributing to the increase of VAT adipocyte number, as observed in obese individuals. However, the effect of low androgen levels on cell hyperplasia is not strong enough to prevent adipocyte hypertrophy development, and therefore VAT depot dysfunction, main characteristics of the hypertrophic obese phenotype.

3. Conclusion

Endocrine-metabolic alterations associated to obesity are related to WAT dysfunction, mainly VAT. However, the increase of VAT mass per se is not an unequivocal indication of VAT dysfunction, whereas the adipocyte size actually is. Therefore, the balance between hypertrophy and hyperplasia will determine the appearance of enlarged adipocytes and, consequently, the development of VAT dysfunction. There are many factors that regulate this balance in WAT expansion. In this chapter, we have addressed three of them: fructose intake, GCs and testosterone. Both, fructose intake and GCs, stimulate adipogenesis by modulating APCs competency and number, and thus terminal differentiation. However, in both cases the chronic exposure to these factors led to hypertrophic adipocytes, and therefore to an unhealthy WAT expansion. Chronic exposure to high GC levels seems to induce a resistance state in APCs that would limit their adipogenic potential, partially by a lower response to GCs stimuli due to MR expression decrease. Conversely, testosterone is an anti-adipogenic factor that favours unhealthy expansion. Obesity is associated with reduced testosterone levels, which would promote adipogenesis; however, much extensive research is needed to determine the role of androgens in APCs adipogenic potential in obesity. Finally, factors inducing adipogenesis could become a therapeutic target against

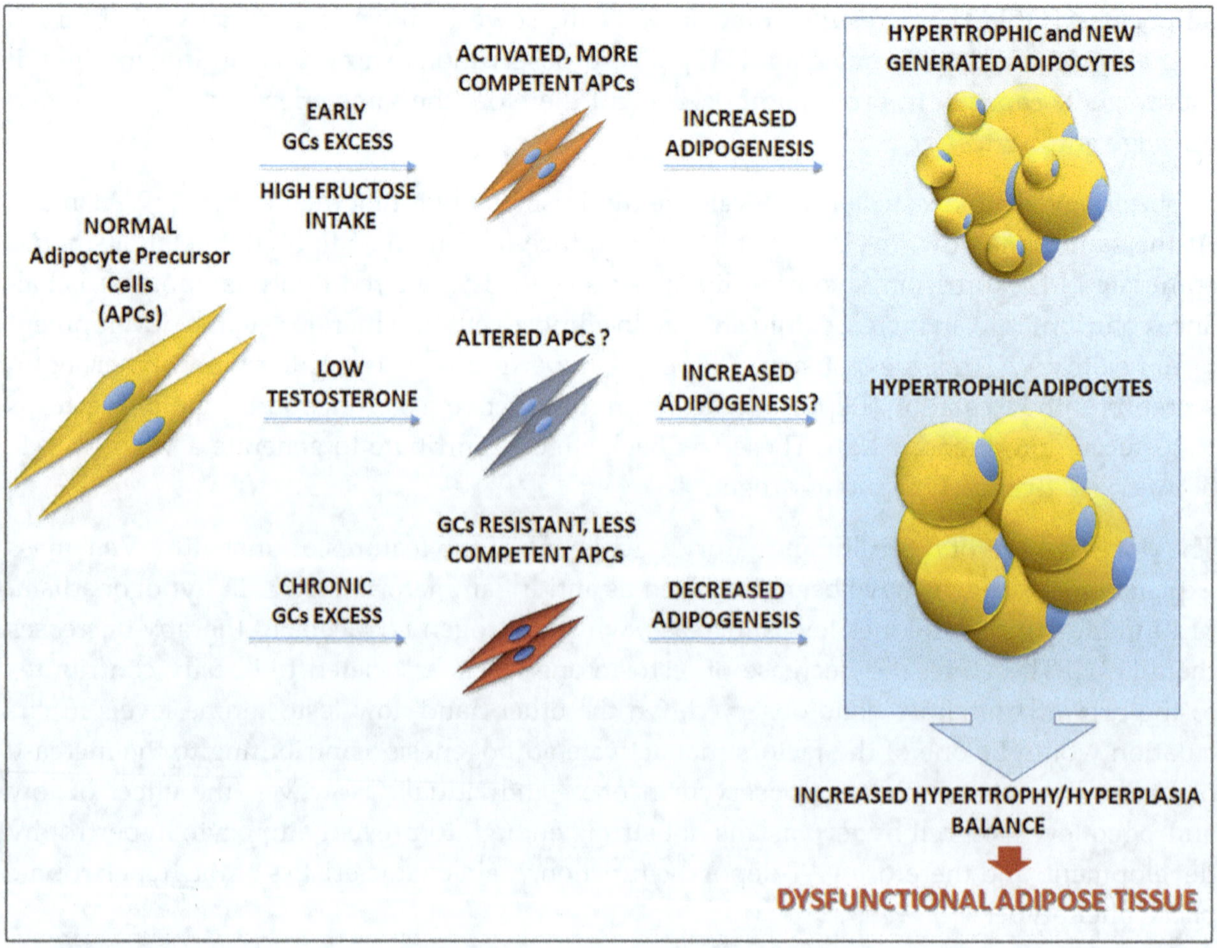

Figure 2. The analysis of three different factors regulating adipogenesis and VAT expansion shows differential effects, depending on the factor analysed. Early GC excess and FRD intake make APCs more competent, this means favouring their ability to differentiate into mature adipocytes, consequently increasing adipogenesis. Nevertheless, this increased adipogenesis occurs in parallel with hypertrophic VAT expansion. GCs chronic excess causes APCs competency to decrease, adipogenesis to fall and VAT expansion mainly by the hypertrophy of pre-existent adipocytes. Effects of low testosterone levels associated to obesity need to be further studied. Nonetheless, it is already known that testosterone is an anti-adipogenic factor involved in unhealthy VAT expansion, favouring adipocyte hypertrophy. In summary, all three factors are involved in increased hypertrophy/hyperplasia balance, generating a dysfunctional VAT.

endocrine-metabolic disorders, favouring WAT healthy expansion and thus mitigating obesity-associated pathologies (**Figure 2**).

Acknowledgements

The authors thank CONICET (PIP 2013-0198), Fondo para la Investigación Científica y Tecnológica (FONCYT, PICT-2013-0930) and Fondation pour la Recherche en Endocrinologie, Diabetologie et Metabolisme (FPREDM 062013). The authors are grateful to Beatriz Tosti for careful manuscript edition/correction.

Author details

María Guillermina Zubiría[1,†], Ana Alzamendi[1,†], Luisina Ongaro[2], Eduardo Spinedi[3] and Andrés Giovambattista[1]*

*Address all correspondence to: agiovamba@imbice.gov.ar

1 Neuroendocrinology Laboratory, Multidisciplinary Institute of Cellular Biology (IMBICE, CICPBA-CONICET-UNLP), La Plata, Argentina

2 Department of Pharmacology and Therapeutics, Centre for Research in Reproduction and Development, McGill University, Montreal, QC, Canada

3 Center of Experimental and Applied Endocrinology (CENEXA, UNLP-CONICET, PAHO/WHO Collaborating Center for Diabetes), La Plata Medical School, National University of La Plata, La Plata, Argentina

† These authors contributed equally to this chapter

References

[1] Wåhlen K, Sjölin E, Löfgren P. Role of fat cell size for plasma leptin in a large population based sample. Exp Clin Endocrinol Diabetes. 2011;119(5):291–4.

[2] Skurk T, Alberti-Huber C, Herder C, Hauner H. Relationship between adipocyte size and adipokine expression and secretion. J Clin Endocrinol Metab. 2007;92(3):1023–33.

[3] Franck N, Stenkula KG, Ost A, Lindström T, Strålfors P, Nystrom FH. Insulin-induced GLUT4 translocation to the plasma membrane is blunted in large compared with small primary fat cells isolated from the same individual. Diabetologia. 2007;50(8):1716–22.

[4] Wueest S, Rapold RA, Rytka JM, Schoenle EJ, Konrad D. Basal lipolysis, not the degree of insulin resistance, differentiates large from small isolated adipocytes in high-fat fed mice. Diabetologia. 2009;52(3):541–6.

[5] Young P, Arch JRS, Ashwell M. Brown adipose tissue in the parametrial fat pad of the mouse. FEBS Lett. 1984;167(1):10–4.

[6] Sanchez-Gurmaches J, Hung C-M, Sparks CA, Tang Y, Li H, Guertin DA. PTEN loss in the Myf5 lineage redistributes body fat and reveals subsets of white adipocytes that arise from Myf5 precursors. Cell Metab. 2012;16(3):348–62.

[7] Wu J, Boström P, Sparks LM, Ye L, Choi JH, Giang A-H, et al. Beige adipocytes are a distinct type of thermogenic fat cell in mouse and human. Cell. 2012;150(2):366–76.

[8] Keipert S, Jastroch M. Brite/beige fat and UCP1 — is it thermogenesis? Biochim Biophys Acta Bioenerg. 2014;1837(7):1075–82.

[9] Sengenès C, Lolmède K, Zakaroff-Girard A, Busse R, Bouloumié A. Preadipocytes in the human subcutaneous adipose tissue display distinct features from the adult mesenchymal and hematopoietic stem cells. J Cell Physiol. 2005;205(1):114–22.

[10] Gupta RK, Arany Z, Seale P, Mepani RJ, Ye L, Conroe HM, et al. Transcriptional control of preadipocyte determination by Zfp423. Nature. 2010;464(7288):619–23.

[11] Tontonoz P, Spiegelman BM. Fat and beyond: the diverse biology of PPARgamma. Annu Rev Biochem. 2008;77:289–312.

[12] Sul HS. Minireview: Pref-1: role in adipogenesis and mesenchymal cell fate. Mol Endocrinol. 2009;23(11):1717–25.

[13] Longo KA, Wright WS, Kang S, Gerin I, Chiang S-H, Lucas PC, et al. Wnt10b inhibits development of white and brown adipose tissues. J Biol Chem. 2004;279(34):35503–9.

[14] Stephan BCM, Wells JCK, Brayne C, Albanese E, Siervo M. Increased fructose intake as a risk factor for dementia. J Gerontol A Biol Sci Med Sci. 2010;65(8):809–14.

[15] Van den Berghe G. Fructose: metabolism and short-term effects on carbohydrate and purine metabolic pathways. Prog Biochem Pharmacol. 1986;21:1–32.

[16] Lallès J-P. Dairy products and the French paradox: could alkaline phosphatases play a role? Med Hypotheses. 2016;92:7–11.

[17] Dhingra R, Sullivan L, Jacques PF, Wang TJ, Fox CS, Meigs JB, et al. Soft drink consumption and risk of developing cardiometabolic risk factors and the metabolic syndrome in middle-aged adults in the community. Circulation. 2007;116(5):480–8.

[18] Raben A, Vasilaras TH, Møller AC, Astrup A. Sucrose compared with artificial sweeteners: different effects on ad libitum food intake and body weight after 10 wk of supplementation in overweight subjects. Am J Clin Nutr. 2002;76(4):721–9.

[19] Stanhope KL, Havel PJ. Fructose consumption: considerations for future research on its effects on adipose distribution, lipid metabolism, and insulin sensitivity in humans. J Nutr. 2009;139(6):1236S–1241S.

[20] Miller A, Adeli K. Dietary fructose and the metabolic syndrome. Curr Opin Gastroenterol. 2008;24(2):204–9.

[21] Nakagawa T, Hu H, Zharikov S, Tuttle KR, Short RA, Glushakova O, et al. A causal role for uric acid in fructose-induced metabolic syndrome. Am J Physiol Renal Physiol. 2006;290(3):F625–31.

[22] Kanarek RB, Orthen-Gambill N. Differential effects of sucrose, fructose and glucose on carbohydrate-induced obesity in rats. J Nutr. 1982;112(8):1546–54.

[23] Crescenzo R, Bianco F, Coppola P, Mazzoli A, Valiante S, Liverini G, et al. Adipose tissue remodeling in rats exhibiting fructose-induced obesity. Eur J Nutr. 2014;53(2):413–9.

[24] Alzamendi A, Giovambattista A, García ME, Rebolledo OR, Gagliardino JJ, Spinedi E. Effect of pioglitazone on the fructose-induced abdominal adipose tissue dysfunction. PPAR Res. 2012;2012:259093.

[25] Alzamendi A, Giovambattista A, Raschia A, Madrid V, Gaillard RC, Rebolledo O, et al. Fructose-rich diet-induced abdominal adipose tissue endocrine dysfunction in normal male rats. Endocrine. 2009;35(2):227–32.

[26] Zubiría MG, Fariña JP, Moreno G, Gagliardino JJ, Spinedi E, Giovambattista A. Excess fructose intake-induced hypertrophic visceral adipose tissue results from unbalanced precursor cell adipogenic signals. FEBS J. 2013;280(22):5864–74.

[27] Alzamendi A, Castrogiovanni D, Ortega HH, Gaillard RC, Giovambattista A, Spinedi E. Parametrial adipose tissue and metabolic dysfunctions induced by fructose-rich diet in normal and neonatal-androgenized adult female rats. Obesity (Silver Spring). 2010;18(3):441–8.

[28] Zubiría MG, Alzamendi A, Moreno G, Rey MA, Spinedi E, Giovambattista A. Long-term fructose intake increases adipogenic potential: evidence of direct effects of fructose on adipocyte precursor cells. Nutrients. 2016;8(4):198.

[29] Pektas MB, Koca HB, Sadi G, Akar F. Dietary fructose activates insulin signaling and inflammation in adipose tissue: modulatory role of resveratrol. Biomed Res Int. 2016;2016:8014252.

[30] Joe AWB, Yi L, Even Y, Vogl AW, Rossi FMV. Depot-specific differences in adipogenic progenitor abundance and proliferative response to high-fat diet. Stem Cells. 2009;27(10):2563–70.

[31] Macotela Y, Emanuelli B, Mori MA, Gesta S, Schulz TJ, Tseng Y-H, et al. Intrinsic differences in adipocyte precursor cells from different white fat depots. Diabetes. 2012;61(7):1691–9.

[32] García-Ruiz E, Reynés B, Díaz-Rúa R, Ceresi E, Oliver P, Palou A. The intake of high-fat diets induces the acquisition of brown adipocyte gene expression features in white adipose tissue. Int J Obes (Lond). 2015;39(11):1619–29.

[33] Wang QA, Tao C, Gupta RK, Scherer PE. Tracking adipogenesis during white adipose tissue development, expansion and regeneration. Nat Med. 2013;19(10):1338–44.

[34] Margareto J, Larrarte E, Marti A, Martinez JA. Up-regulation of a thermogenesis-related gene (UCP1) and down-regulation of PPARγ and aP2 genes in adipose tissue: possible features of the antiobesity effects of a β3-adrenergic agonist. Biochem Pharmacol. 2001;61(12):1471–8.

[35] Fromme T, Klingenspor M, Akagiri S, Naito Y, Ichikawa H, Mizushima K, et al. Uncoupling protein 1 expression and high-fat diets. Am J Physiol Regul Integr Comp Physiol. 2011;300(1):R1–8.

[36] Bonet ML, Oliver P, Palou A. Pharmacological and nutritional agents promoting browning of white adipose tissue. Biochim Biophys Acta Mol Cell Biol Lipids. 2013;1831(5):969–85.

[37] Bray GA. How bad is fructose? Am J Clin Nutr. 2007;86(4):895–6.

[38] Mayes PA. Intermediary metabolism of fructose. Am J Clin Nutr. 1993;58(5 Suppl.): 754S–765S.

[39] Bizeau ME, Pagliassotti MJ. Hepatic adaptations to sucrose and fructose. Metabolism. 2005;54(9):1189–201.

[40] Du L, Heaney AP. Regulation of adipose differentiation by fructose and GluT5. Mol Endocrinol. 2012;26(10):1773–82.

[41] Legeza B, Balázs Z, Odermatt A. Fructose promotes the differentiation of 3T3-L1 adipocytes and accelerates lipid metabolism. FEBS Lett. 2014;588(3):490–6.

[42] Hajduch E, Darakhshan F, Hundal HS. Fructose uptake in rat adipocytes: GLUT5 expression and the effects of streptozotocin-induced diabetes. Diabetologia. 1998; 41(7):821–8.

[43] del Mar Romero M, Sabater D, Fernández-López JA, Remesar X, Alemany M. Glycerol production from glucose and fructose by 3T3-L1 Cells: a mechanism of adipocyte defense from excess substrate. PLoS One. 2015;10(10):e0139502.

[44] Kovačević S, Nestorov J, Matić G, Elaković I. Dietary fructose-related adiposity and glucocorticoid receptor function in visceral adipose tissue of female rats. Eur J Nutr. 2014;53(6):1409–20.

[45] Barker DJP. The origins of the developmental origins theory. J Intern Med. 2007; 261(5):412–7.

[46] Alzamendi A, Zubiría G, Moreno G, Portales A, Spinedi E, Giovambattista A. High risk of metabolic and adipose tissue dysfunctions in adult male progeny, due to prenatal and adulthood malnutrition induced by fructose rich diet. Nutrients. 2016;8(3):178.

[47] Rodríguez L, Otero P, Panadero MI, Rodrigo S, Álvarez-Millán JJ, Bocos C. Maternal fructose intake induces insulin resistance and oxidative stress in male, but not female, offspring. J Nutr Metab. 2015;2015:158091.

[48] Rodríguez L, Panadero MI, Roglans N, Otero P, Rodrigo S, Álvarez-Millán JJ, et al. Fructose only in pregnancy provokes hyperinsulinemia, hypoadiponectinemia, and impaired insulin signaling in adult male, but not female, progeny. Eur J Nutr. 2016;55(2):665–74.

[49] Lineker C, Kerr PM, Nguyen P, Bloor I, Astbury S, Patel N, et al. High fructose consumption in pregnancy alters the perinatal environment without increasing metabolic disease in the offspring. Reprod Fertil Dev. 2015;28:2007–2015.

[50] Alzamendi A, Castrogiovanni D, Gaillard RC, Spinedi E, Giovambattista A. Increased male offspring's risk of metabolic-neuroendocrine dysfunction and overweight after fructose-rich diet intake by the lactating mother. Endocrinology. 2010;151(9):4214–23.

[51] Rawana S, Clark K, Zhong S, Buison A, Chackunkal S, Jen KL. Low dose fructose ingestion during gestation and lactation affects carbohydrate metabolism in rat dams and their offspring. J Nutr. 1993;123(12):2158–65.

[52] Srinivasan M, Dodds C, Ghanim H, Gao T, Ross PJ, Browne RW, et al. Maternal obesity and fetal programming: effects of a high-carbohydrate nutritional modification in the immediate postnatal life of female rats. Am J Physiol Endocrinol Metab. 2008;295(4):E895–903.

[53] Huynh M, Luiken JJJP, Coumans W, Bell RC. Dietary fructose during the suckling period increases body weight and fatty acid uptake into skeletal muscle in adult rats. Obesity (Silver Spring). 2008;16(8):1755–62.

[54] Kreier F, Fliers E, Voshol PJ, Van Eden CG, Havekes LM, Kalsbeek A, et al. Selective parasympathetic innervation of subcutaneous and intra-abdominal fat—functional implications. J Clin Invest. 2002;110(9):1243–50.

[55] Gregoire FM, Smas CM, Sul HS, Adams M, Reginato MJ, Shao D, et al. Understanding adipocyte differentiation. Physiol Rev. 1998;78(3):783–809.

[56] Delahaye F, Lukaszewski M-A, Wattez J-S, Cisse O, Dutriez-Casteloot I, Fajardy I, et al. Maternal perinatal undernutrition programs a "brown-like" phenotype of gonadal white fat in male rat at weaning. Am J Physiol Regul Integr Comp Physiol. 2010;299(1):R101–10.

[57] Lee M-J, Pramyothin P, Karastergiou K, Fried SK. Deconstructing the roles of glucocorticoids in adipose tissue biology and the development of central obesity. Biochim Biophys Act. 2014;1842(3):473–81.

[58] Xu C, He J, Jiang H, Zu L, Zhai W, Pu S, et al. Direct effect of glucocorticoids on lipolysis in adipocytes. Mol Endocrinol. 2009;23(8):1161–70.

[59] Campbell JE, Peckett AJ, D'souza AM, Hawke TJ, Riddell MC. Adipogenic and lipolytic effects of chronic glucocorticoid exposure. Am J Physiol Cell Physiol. 2011; 300(1):C198–209.

[60] Ottosson M, Lönnroth P, Björntorp P, Edén S. Effects of cortisol and growth hormone on lipolysis in human adipose tissue. J Clin Endocrinol Metab. 2000;85(2):799–803.

[61] Wang Y, Jones Voy B, Urs S, Kim S, Soltani-Bejnood M, Quigley N, et al. The human fatty acid synthase gene and de novo lipogenesis are coordinately regulated in human adipose tissue. J Nutr. 2004;134(5):1032–8.

[62] Fried SK, Bunkin DA, Greenberg AS. Omental and subcutaneous adipose tissues of obese subjects release interleukin-6: depot difference and regulation by glucocorticoid. J Clin Endocrinol Metab. 1998;83(3):847–50.

[63] Geer EB, Shen W, Gallagher D, Punyanitya M, Looker HC, Post KD, et al. MRI assessment of lean and adipose tissue distribution in female patients with Cushing's disease. Clin Endocrinol (Oxf). 2010;73(4):469–75.

[64] Mayo-Smith W, Hayes CW, Biller BM, Klibanski A, Rosenthal H, Rosenthal DI. Body fat distribution measured with CT: correlations in healthy subjects, patients with anorexia nervosa, and patients with Cushing syndrome. Radiology. 1989;170(2):515–8.

[65] Chanson P, Salenave S. Metabolic syndrome in Cushing's syndrome. Neuroendocrinology. 2010;92(Suppl. 1):96–101.

[66] Zubiría MG, Vidal-Bravo J, Spinedi E, Giovambattista A. Relationship between impaired adipogenesis of retroperitoneal adipose tissue and hypertrophic obesity: role of endogenous glucocorticoid excess. J Cell Mol Med. 2014;18(8):1549–61.

[67] Engeli S, Böhnke J, Feldpausch M, Gorzelniak K, Heintze U, Janke J, et al. Regulation of 11beta-HSD genes in human adipose tissue: influence of central obesity and weight loss. Obes Res. 2004;12(1):9–17.

[68] Masuzaki H, Paterson J, Shinyama H, Morton NM, Mullins JJ, Seckl JR, et al. A transgenic model of visceral obesity and the metabolic syndrome. Science. 2001; 294(5549):2166–70.

[69] Morton NM, Holmes MC, Fiévet C, Staels B, Tailleux A, Mullins JJ, et al. Improved lipid and lipoprotein profile, hepatic insulin sensitivity, and glucose tolerance in 11beta-hydroxysteroid dehydrogenase type 1 null mice. J Biol Chem. 2001; 276(44):41293–300.

[70] Hauner H, Schmid P, Pfeiffer EF. Glucocorticoids and insulin promote the differentiation of human adipocyte precursor cells into fat cells. J Clin Endocrinol Metab. 1987;64(4):832–5.

[71] Lee M-J, Fried SK. Integration of hormonal and nutrient signals that regulate leptin synthesis and secretion. Am J Physiol Endocrinol Metab. 2009;296(6):E1230–8.

[72] Smas CM, Chen L, Zhao L, Latasa MJ, Sul HS. Transcriptional repression of pref-1 by glucocorticoids promotes 3T3-L1 adipocyte differentiation. J Biol Chem. 1999;274(18):12632–41.

[73] Xiao X, Li H, Yang J, Qi X, Zu X, Yang J, et al. Wnt/β-catenin signaling pathway and lipolysis enzymes participate in methylprednisolone induced fat differential distribution between subcutaneous and visceral adipose tissue. Steroids. 2014;84:30–5.

[74] Christodoulides C, Lagathu C, Sethi JK, Vidal-Puig A. Adipogenesis and WNT signalling. Trends Endocrinol Metab. 2009;20(1):16–24.

[75] Wang Y, Hudak C, Sul HS. Role of preadipocyte factor 1 in adipocyte differentiation. Clin Lipidol. 2010;5(1):109–15.

[76] Pantoja C, Huff JT, Yamamoto KR. Glucocorticoid signaling defines a novel commitment state during adipogenesis in vitro. Mol Biol Cell. 2008;19(10):4032–41.

[77] Zubiría MG, Alzamendi A, Moreno G, Portales A, Castrogiovanni D, Spinedi E, et al. Relationship between the balance of hypertrophic/hyperplastic adipose tissue expansion and the metabolic profile in a high glucocorticoids model. Nutreints. 2016;8(7):410.

[78] Tomlinson JJ, Boudreau A, Wu D, Atlas E, Haché RJG. Modulation of early human preadipocyte differentiation by glucocorticoids. Endocrinology. 2006;147(11):5284–93.

[79] Caprio M, Fève B, Claës A, Viengchareun S, Lombès M, Zennaro M-C. Pivotal role of the mineralocorticoid receptor in corticosteroid-induced adipogenesis. FASEB J Off Publ Fed Am Soc Exp Biol. 2007;21(9):2185–94.

[80] Lee M-J, Fried SK. The glucocorticoid receptor, not the mineralocorticoid receptor, plays the dominant role in adipogenesis and adipokine production in human adipocytes. Int J Obes (Lond). 2014;38(9):1228–33.

[81] Caprio M, Antelmi A, Chetrite G, Muscat A, Mammi C, Marzolla V, et al. Antiadipogenic effects of the mineralocorticoid receptor antagonist drospirenone: potential implications for the treatment of metabolic syndrome. Endocrinology. 2011;152(1):113–25.

[82] Hirata A, Maeda N, Nakatsuji H, Hiuge-Shimizu A, Okada T, Funahashi T, et al. Contribution of glucocorticoid-mineralocorticoid receptor pathway on the obesity-related adipocyte dysfunction. Biochem Biophys Res Commun. 2012;419(2):182–7.

[83] Mandrup S, Loftus TM, MacDougald OA, Kuhajda FP, Lane MD. Obese gene expression at in vivo levels by fat pads derived from s.c. implanted 3T3-F442A preadipocytes. Proc Natl Acad Sci USA. 1997;94(9):4300–5.

[84] Green H, Kehinde O. Spontaneous heritable changes leading to increased adipose conversion in 3T3 cells. Cell. 1976;7(1):105–13.

[85] Choe SS, Huh JY, Hwang IJ, Kim JI, Kim JB. Adipose tissue remodeling: its role in energy metabolism and metabolic disorders. Front Endocrinol (Lausanne). 2016;7:30.

[86] Hoppmann J, Perwitz N, Meier B, Fasshauer M, Hadaschik D, Lehnert H, et al. The balance between gluco- and mineralo-corticoid action critically determines inflammatory adipocyte responses. J Endocrinol. 2010;204(2):153–64.

[87] Barahona M-J, Sucunza N, Resmini E, Fernández-Real J-M, Ricart W, Moreno-Navarrete J-M, et al. Persistent body fat mass and inflammatory marker increases after long-term cure of Cushing's syndrome. J Clin Endocrinol Metab. 2009;94(9):3365–71.

[88] Setola E, Losa M, Lanzi R, Lucotti P, Monti LD, Castrignanò T, et al. Increased insulin-stimulated endothelin-1 release is a distinct vascular phenotype distinguishing Cushing's disease from metabolic syndrome. Clin Endocrinol (Oxf). 2007;66(4):586–92.

[89] Poggioli R, Ueta CB, Drigo RAE, Castillo M, Fonseca TL, Bianco AC. Dexamethasone reduces energy expenditure and increases susceptibility to diet-induced obesity in mice. Obesity (Silver Spring). 2013;21(9):E415–20.

[90] Soumano K, Desbiens S, Rabelo R, Bakopanos E, Camirand A, Silva JE. Glucocorticoids inhibit the transcriptional response of the uncoupling protein-1 gene to adrenergic stimulation in a brown adipose cell line. Mol Cell Endocrinol. 2000;165(1–2):7–15.

[91] Armani A, Cinti F, Marzolla V, Morgan J, Cranston GA, Antelmi A, et al. Mineralocorticoid receptor antagonism induces browning of white adipose tissue through impairment of autophagy and prevents adipocyte dysfunction in high-fat-diet-fed mice. FASEB J. 2014;28(8):3745–57.

[92] Kong X, Yu J, Bi J, Qi H, Di W, Wu L, et al. Glucocorticoids transcriptionally regulate miR-27b expression promoting body fat accumulation via suppressing the browning of white adipose tissue. Diabetes. 2015;64(2):393–404.

[93] Rebuffé-Scrive M, Krotkiewski M, Elfverson J, Björntorp P. Muscle and adipose tissue morphology and metabolism in Cushing's syndrome. J Clin Endocrinol Metab. 1988;67(6):1122–8.

[94] Rebuffé-Scrive M, Walsh UA, McEwen B, Rodin J. Effect of chronic stress and exogenous glucocorticoids on regional fat distribution and metabolism. Physiol Behav. 1992;52(3):583–90.

[95] Elbers JMH, Giltay EJ, Teerlink T, Scheffer PG, Asscheman H, Seidell JC, et al. Effects of sex steroids on components of the insulin resistance syndrome in transsexual subjects. Clin Endocrinol (Oxf). 2003;58(5):562–71.

[96] Boyanov MA, Boneva Z, Christov VG. Testosterone supplementation in men with type 2 diabetes, visceral obesity and partial androgen deficiency. Aging Male. 2003;6(1):1–7.

[97] Blouin K, Després J-P, Couillard C, Tremblay A, Prud'homme D, Bouchard C, et al. Contribution of age and declining androgen levels to features of the metabolic syndrome in men. Metabolism. 2005;54(8):1034–40.

[98] Perelló M, Castrogiovanni D, Moreno G, Gaillard RC, Spinedi E. Neonatal hypothalamic androgenization in the female rat induces changes in peripheral insulin sensitivity and adiposity function at adulthood. Neuro Endocrinol Lett. 2003;24(3–4):241–8.

[99] Ongaro L, Castrogiovanni D, Giovambattista A, Gaillard RC, Spinedi E. Enhanced proinflammatory cytokine response to bacterial lipopolysaccharide in the adult male rat after either neonatal or prepubertal ablation of biological testosterone activity. Neuroimmunomodulation. 2011;18(4):254–60.

[100] Ongaro L, Giovambattista A, Spinedi E. Impact of neonatal manipulation of androgen receptor function on endocrine-metabolic programming in the juvenile female rat. ISRN Endocrinol. 2013;2013:181950.

[101] Dieudonne MN, Pecquery R, Boumediene A, Leneveu MC, Giudicelli Y. Androgen receptors in human preadipocytes and adipocytes: regional specificities and regulation by sex steroids. Am J Physiol. 1998;274(6 Pt 1):C1645–52.

[102] Rodriguez-Cuenca S, Monjo M, Proenza AM, Roca P. Depot differences in steroid receptor expression in adipose tissue: possible role of the local steroid milieu. Am J Physiol Endocrinol Metab. 2005;288(1):E200–7.

[103] Joyner J, Hutley L, Cameron D. Intrinsic regional differences in androgen receptors and dihydrotestosterone metabolism in human preadipocytes. Horm Metab Res. 2002;34(5):223–8.

[104] Elbers JMH, Giltay EJ, Teerlink T, Scheffer PG, Asscheman H, Seidell JC, et al. Effects of sex steroids on components of the insulin resistance syndrome in transsexual subjects. Clin Endocrinol (Oxf). 2003;58(5):562–71.

[105] Xu XF, De Pergola G, Björntorp P. Testosterone increases lipolysis and the number of beta-adrenoceptors in male rat adipocytes. Endocrinology. 1991;128(1):379–82.

[106] Mårin P, Lönn L, Andersson B, Odén B, Olbe L, Bengtsson BA, et al. Assimilation of triglycerides in subcutaneous and intraabdominal adipose tissues in vivo in men: effects of testosterone. J Clin Endocrinol Metab. 1996;81(3):1018–22.

[107] Mårin P, Andersson B, Ottosson M, Olbe L, Chowdhury B, Kvist H, et al. The morphology and metabolism of intraabdominal adipose tissue in men. Metabolism. 1992;41(11):1242–8.

[108] Singh R, Artaza JN, Taylor WE, Braga M, Yuan X, Gonzalez-Cadavid NF, et al. Testosterone inhibits adipogenic differentiation in 3T3-L1 cells: nuclear translocation of androgen receptor complex with beta-catenin and T-cell factor 4 may bypass canonical Wnt signaling to down-regulate adipogenic transcription factors. Endocrinology. 2006;147(1):141–54.

[109] McIntosh M, Hausman D, Martin R, Hausman G. Dehydroepiandrosterone attenuates preadipocyte growth in primary cultures of stromal-vascular cells. Am J Physiol. 1998;275(2 Pt 1):E285–93.

[110] Singh R, Artaza JN, Taylor WE, Gonzalez-Cadavid NF, Bhasin S. Androgens stimulate myogenic differentiation and inhibit adipogenesis in C3H 10T1/2 pluripotent cells through an androgen receptor-mediated pathway. Endocrinology. 2003;144(11):5081–8.

[111] Lacasa D, Agli B, Moynard D, Giudicelli Y. Evidence for a regional-specific control of rat preadipocyte proliferation and differentiation by the androgenic status. Endocrine. 1995;3(11):789–93.

[112] Gupta V, Bhasin S, Guo W, Singh R, Miki R, Chauhan P, et al. Effects of dihydrotestosterone on differentiation and proliferation of human mesenchymal stem cells and preadipocytes. Mol Cell Endocrinol. 2008;296(1):32–40.

[113] Chazenbalk G, Singh P, Irge D, Shah A, Abbott DH, Dumesic DA. Androgens inhibit adipogenesis during human adipose stem cell commitment to preadipocyte formation. Steroids. 2013;78(9):920–6.

[114] Quevedo S, Roca P, Picó C, Palou A. Sex-associated differences in cold-induced UCP1 synthesis in rodent brown adipose tissue. Pflügers Arch Eur J Physiol. 1998;436(5):689–95.

[115] Roca P, Rodriguez AM, Oliver P, Bonet ML, Quevedo S, Picó C, et al. Brown adipose tissue response to cafeteria diet-feeding involves induction of the UCP2 gene and is impaired in female rats as compared to males. Pflügers Arch Eur J Physiol. 1999;438(5):628–34.

[116] Rodriguez AM, Monjo M, Roca P, Palou A. Opposite actions of testosterone and progesterone on UCP1 mRNA expression in cultured brown adipocytes. Cell Mol Life Sci. 2002;59(10):1714–23.

[117] Rodríguez-Cuenca S, Monjo M, Gianotti M, Proenza AM, Roca P. Expression of mitochondrial biogenesis-signaling factors in brown adipocytes is influenced specifically by 17beta-estradiol, testosterone, and progesterone. Am J Physiol Endocrinol Metab. 2007;292(1):E340–6.

[118] Amengual-Cladera E, Lladó I, Gianotti M, Proenza AM, Conde J, Scotece M, et al. Sex differences in the effect of high-fat diet feeding on rat white adipose tissue mitochondrial function and insulin sensitivity. Metabolism. 2012;61(8):1108–17.

[119] Björntorp P. Growth hormone, insulin-like growth factor-I and lipid metabolism: interactions with sex steroids. Horm Res. 1996;46(4–5):188–91.

[120] Herrid M, Xia Y, O'Shea T, McFarlane JR. Leptin inhibits basal but not gonadotrophin-stimulated testosterone production in the immature mouse and sheep testis. Reprod Fertil Dev. 2008;20(4):519–28.

[121] Dhindsa S, Ghanim H, Batra M, Kuhadiya ND, Abuaysheh S, Sandhu S, et al. Insulin resistance and inflammation in hypogonadotropic hypogonadism and their reduction after testosterone replacement in men with type 2 diabetes. Diabetes Care. 2016;39(1):82–91.

11

Childhood Obesity

Laura Mihaela Trandafir, Ileana Ioniuc and
Ingrith Miron

Abstract

Currently, the prevalence of obesity among children and adolescents and related complications is considered one of the most important nutritional problems globally. The prevalence of childhood obesity in Europe is 10 times higher now than it was in the 1970s. Initial assessments of these patients should include taking a careful history (investigating comorbidities, family history and potentially modifiable behaviors) and physical examination. The degree of investigation is dependent on the patient's age and severity of obesity, the findings on history and physical examination and associated familial risk factors. Childhood obesity treatment is based on sustained lifestyle changes with family involvement. Management intervention strategies include nutrition, physical activity, behavior and lifestyle changes, medication and surgical considerations.

Keywords: obesity, childhood, adolescents

1. Introduction

Obesity is a chronic disorder of the state of nutrition characterized by an increase in body weight due to excessive adipose tissue, which occurs when the calorie intake exceeds the caloric needs of a body with low energy expenditure. Obesity is currently a significant public health problem, as we have witnessed a dramatic increase in the number of obese and overweight children worldwide in the last years. Children's risk of obesity varies by age and sex groups, ethnic/racial groups, socioeconomic status, geographic and rural/urban regions. The obesity etiology is complex, involving genetic, environmental, psycho-socio-cultural, neuroendocrine and metabolic factors. Complications of pediatric obesity occur during childhood and adolescence and increase the risk for morbidity and mortality in adulthood.

2. Nosologic framework of obesity in children and adolescent

2.1. Definition

Obesity is an important pediatric public health problem associated with risk of complications in childhood and increased morbidity and mortality throughout life. Overweight and obesity predispose people to noncommunicable diseases such as heart disease, diabetes mellitus, musculoskeletal and psychological disorders and certain types of cancer [1].

Without intervention, obese infants and young children will likely continue to be obese during childhood, adolescence and adulthood [1–3].

The methodological problem of inconsistency between criteria of childhood obesity classification is a major obstacle in studying global trends for younger age group. The body mass index [BMI: weight (kg)/height $(m)^2$] is the parameter used for the screening of overweight and obesity in childhood because it is easy to determine, it tends to correlate well with body fat, and it has been widely used in adults to define obesity. It decreases until the period called "adiposity rebound" when body fat is at the lowest level (between 3 and 7 years) and after then BMI increases again until the adulthood [4, 5].

The child's BMI must be plotted on nationally recommended BMI—for age charts. The classification of overweight and obesity varies among guidelines, such as those from Centre for Disease Control (CDC), International Obesity Task Force (IOTF) and World Health Organization (WHO).

For example, in UK (IOTF BMI values) the cut off points for and are the BMI >91st and >98th percentile, respectively.

The definition of overweight and obesity using BMI percentiles in the USA: children aged 2 years and older with a BMI between the 85th and 95th percentile is overweight, and those with a BMI greater than the 95th percentile for a specific age and sex subgroup are obese [4–6].

According to WHO, for children aged between 5 and 19 years, overweight is >2 standard deviations and obesity is defined as a BMI-for-age >1 standard deviation, above the WHO growth reference median [1].

The IOTF BMI values represent standard international references that allow the screening of adiposity in children and adolescents worldwide under the same criterion, without variations depending on geographic, social and secular trends [5].

2.2. Epidemiological data

Currently, the prevalence of obesity among children and adolescents and related complications is considered one of the most important nutritional problem globally. The obesity epidemic among children is the result of excess energy intake and inadequate energy expenditure [2]. The prevalence of childhood overweight and obesity has increased worldwide in recent decades, and the numbers of those affected continue to rise at an alarming rate [6].

In recent years, the epidemiology of overweight and obesity is well described in many European countries and the data showed the increasing trends in the prevalence of childhood obesity. The current prevalence of childhood obesity is ten times higher than it was in the 1970s [5].

The incidence of overweight and obesity increased progressively from infancy through adolescence [5, 6]. High prevalence of obesity in 0- to 6-year-old children is warning signs and risk for increased rates of obesity in adolescence and adulthood reported.

North America and some countries in Europe have shown consistent year-on-year increases in prevalence of overweight (20–30%) and obesity (5–15%), although recent surveys indicate that the rising trends are easing, with a plateau in prevalence levels shown since around 2005 [6].

Children's risk of obesity varies by age and sex groups, ethnic/racial groups, socioeconomic status, geographic and rural/urban regions. The key reason for the variations is due to the considerable socioeconomic and lifestyle differences and the differences in differing criteria for obesity and overweight definition [4, 7].

Several countries of Southern Europe appear to be showing high prevalence of childhood obesity (20–35%) in the Italy, Greece, Malta, Portugal and Spain. The highest levels of overweight and obesity were in Southern Italy (30.1 and 33.1% in preschool boys and, respectively, girls) and in various regions of Spain (29.4% in both sexes, increasing to 32.6% among children aged 7- to 10-year old), followed by Greece (19.1 and 23.6% in boys and, respectively, girls) [7–9]. Children and adolescents residing in countries surrounding the Mediterranean Sea show the highest rates ranging from 20 to 40%, too [7]. Studies concerning obesity with regard to its prevalence in Portugal reported a rate of overweight in children under the age of 6 years, 13.6% in boys and 20.4% in girls, and, obesity varied between 6.5% in boys and 6.9%, respectively, in girls [10]. The very high prevalence of childhood obesity in Mediterranean countries could be secondary to lifestyle changes (switching from a healthy Mediterranean diet to a fast food type of diet and lower physical activity levels) [7].

In children and adolescents residing the Scandinavian countries and Central Western European countries, the prevalence of overweight and obesity is far lower (10–20%). Scandinavian countries have the lowest prevalence of obesity in all age groups, except Finland which reported the prevalence of overweight and obesity in school children of 23.6 and 19.1% for boys and, respectively, girls [7, 11]. It is important to note that among preschool children, the highest prevalence rates of overweight and obesity were in Ireland (26 and 29% in boys and, respectively, girls), United Kingdom (24.1 and 21.4% in boys and, respectively, girls). In school children, the prevalence of overweight and obesity has increased to 32.7% and, respectively, 29.2% in 2007 the United Kingdom [7]. In developed countries, an increasing number of studies suggest that children of lower-income families are vulnerable to becoming obese, possibly due to poor dietary habits and limited opportunities for physical activity [7, 12]. In the UK, the prevalence of overweight and obesity in 11- to 12-year-old children was 25%, with higher rates in girls (29%) and students from lower socioeconomic backgrounds (31%), and the highest rates was observed in black girls (38%) [13].

Data from Eastern European countries indicate the prevalence rate is smaller (15%), but rising. In Lithuania, the Russian Federation, Slovakia and Poland, the overweight and obesity prevalence ranges from 8.46 to 15.8% in children aged 6–12 years. It is likely that the huge economic burden and the associated poverty following the political transition in the 1990s may have contributed to the relatively low obesity prevalence in Eastern Europe [7].

3. The etiology of obesity and the risk factors

Obesity is a multifactorial disease with a complex etiology being involved genetic, environmental, psycho-socio-cultural, neuroendocrine and metabolic factors, intestinal microbiota. The factors involved in its etiology included the 'obesogenic' environment, and the unhealthy dietary behaviors and patterns of physical activity [14].

There is growing interest in the role of experience in early life in the risk of becoming overweight or obese. In children, prenatal life may be a critical period when the long-term regulation of energy balance is permanently 'programmed'. The perinatal parameters and factors implicated in the etiology of obesity include maternal obesity, excessive weight gain in pregnancy, gestational diabetes, and maternal smoking, duration of breastfeeding, rapid infancy weight gain and other cultural or familial factors associated with childhood eating patterns and activity levels [14, 15].

Maternal obesity is a strong predictor of overweight and obesity in children. Obesity in pregnant women was found to be associated to high newborn weight and also causing obesity and metabolic syndrome risk in later life of the individual. Intrauterine growth restriction is associated with the development of central adiposity and adult-onset cardiovascular risk [4, 14].

Child's exposure to passive smoking, since the product conception stage, predisposes to the development of obesity and obesity related diseases as a result [14, 16, 17].

Breastfeeding could help infants to better recognize satiety signals and hence to better self-regulate energy intake. The prevalence and duration of breastfeeding is higher in countries with relatively lower prevalence of childhood obesity such as Sweden, Finland and Austria, in comparison to countries such as Italy, Greece and the UK, where is less [7, 14, 15].

Ethnicity is associated with differences in eating behaviors, preferences, and cultural influences may contribute to obesity among children and youth in minority populations.

The environmental factors are represented by: over-nutrition (high fat, high sugar diets), sedentary lifestyle, short sleep duration, abuse of drugs (antibiotics, corticosteroids, anti-epileptics drugs), smoking and alcohol. Almost all obesity in children is strongly influenced by environmental factors, caused by a sedentary lifestyle or a caloric intake that is greater than needs. However, this explains only a part of obesity risk, but is important targets for treatment such they can be modifiable.

Sugar-sweetened beverages—the literature evidence suggests that consumption of sugar-sweetened beverages is an important factor in the development of obesity in some individuals.

In the United States, sugar-sweetened beverages supplied an average of 270 kcal/day, representing 10–15% of total caloric intake. In a separate randomized trial on children aged 5–12 (primarily normal weight), consuming one serving of a sugar-free beverage daily was associated with less weight gain and fat accumulation than consuming one serving of a sugar-sweetened beverage. Other studies have found that dietary salt intake is associated with increased intake of sugar-sweetened beverages, perhaps because of increased thirst [18, 19].

Television viewing is an environmental influence on the development of obesity in children. Contact of a child with television begins in the newborn stage and tends to increase continuously. In the first year of life, children react to the screen characters with mimics and voice. Toddlers spend approximately 1 h a day watching television, and from the 4th year of life the exposure to other type of media expands and rises significantly to reach 7 out of 24 h per day. The presence of a television in a child's bedroom and any time spent in watching television are directly related to the prevalence of obesity in children and adolescents. A significant association between advert exposure and childhood obesity has been demonstrated in a cross-cultural study which included data from the USA, Australia and eight European countries [18, 20–22].

Video games—the use of PC or console games has been associated with obesity in children. Half of American children have either a DVD, video or game console in their bedroom and, third, a computer with access to Internet [22, 23].

Sleep—there is a reported association between shortened sleep duration and obesity. A causal association arises from a short-term experimental study in which sleep deprivation for 1 week was associated with increased food intake, weight gain and higher leptin levels as compared to the child's usual sleep. Moreover, sleep may have an association with insulin resistance, independent of its association with obesity. The mechanism between sleep duration and obesity has not been well-known, but may comprise dysfunction in serum leptin and/or ghrelin levels, both are involved in the regulation of appetite [4, 18]. A meta-analysis found that sleep is positively associated with fat mass in toddlers. A positive association between nighttime sleep and BMI *z*-scores were observed in the study reported by Kuzik and Carson [24].

Medications that may cause weight gain in children include cortisol and other glucocorticoids, sulfonylureas, tricyclic antidepressants (TCAs), monoamine oxidase inhibitors, such as phenelzine, oral contraceptives, insulin (in excessive doses), thiazolidinediones, risperidone, clozapine [25].

Other environmental factors that have been proposed as possible contributors to obesity include the influences of gut microbiota, toxins and viruses. Due to the influence of gut microbiota, it has been suggested that there exists a relationship between the resident intestinal bacteria and the potential for weight gain. Effect of microbiota may be partially responsible for increased rate of obesity in children born via cesarean section. Intestinal bacteria seem to influence several factors leading to development of obesity complications such us nonalcoholic steatohepatitis, cardiovascular disease and insulin resistance in humans [26]. It has been suggested that obesity can be triggered or worsened by exposure to a virus. Adenovirus 36 increases body fat in several animal models [18].

Other epidemiologic studies highlight the possibility that obesity could be triggered or exacerbated by exposure to environmental endocrine disrupting chemicals (dichlorodiphenyltrichloroethane—DDT and bisphenol A—BPA). Some studies in adults and children establish an association between urinary BPA levels and obesity or obesity related diseases, as well as diabetes and cardiovascular disease [18].

Endocrine disruptors can disturb every level of the endocrine system. They can interrupt the action of enzymes involved in steroidogenesis. The endocrine disruptors inducing obesity are called obesogens and have been revealed to target transcription regulators that function to control intracellular lipid homeostasis as well as proliferation and differentiation of adipocytes. The main group of regulators that are targeted represent a group of nuclear hormone receptors recognized as peroxisome proliferator-activated receptors (PPARα, δ and γ). PPARγ is considered to be the master regulator of adipogenesis and plays key roles in nearly all aspects of adipocyte biology. Other endocrine disruptors are known to promote adipogenesis, but probably do not act through PPARγ, these include BPA, organophosphate pesticides and monosodium glutamate [27].

Hormonal disorders associated with childhood obesity include growth hormone deficiency, growth hormone resistance, hypothyroidism, leptin deficiency or resistance to leptin action, glucocorticoid excess (Cushing syndrome), precocious puberty, polycystic ovary syndrome (PCOS), prolactin-secreting tumors. Furthermore, in obese individuals, dysfunction in the gut-brain hypothalamic axis and ghrelin/leptin hormonal pathway has been proposed to have a role in excess energy intake and abnormal appetite control [28].

3.1. Genetic factors

Specific syndromes and single gene defects that are linked to obesity in children have been identified. These are very rarely causes of obesity, Generally, monogenic forms of childhood obesity are very rare, accounting for <1% in children. Mutations in only a few genes are known to cause the development of severe obesity in early childhood. Single gene disorders that can cause obesity include deficiency in leptin or its receptor, mutation in leptin gene, deficiency of proopiomelanocortin (POMC), haploinsufficiency receptor 4 and accessory protein receptor 2 of melanocortin, also disorders of protein convertase 1 [4, 18]. The leptin/leptin receptor system regulate food intake through reduce feeding and increased energy expenditure. Some forms of monogenic obesity like congenital leptin deficiency benefits from leptin substitution therapy that leads to significant decrease in weight [29].

Moreover, children with genetic syndromes associated with obesity typically have early onset obesity and characteristic signs on physical examination, including dysmorphic features, developmental delay, short stature or intellectual disability, retinal changes or deafness. The Prader Willi syndrome is the most common among obesity syndromes and is characterized by hypotonia and feeding difficulties during infancy, hyperphagia and obesity developing during early childhood and developmental delay. Other syndromes associated with childhood obesity are Pseudohypoparathyroidism, Laurence Moon Biedl (Bardet Biedl) syndrome, Cohen syndrome, Down syndrome and Turner syndrome [30].

4. Pathophysiology of comorbidities of pediatric obesity

Complications of pediatric obesity occur during childhood and adolescence and increased the risk for morbidity and mortality into adulthood.

Obesity, particularly abdominal, has been shown to be an important risk factor for a number of chronic diseases in adults. Associated with obesity in childhood is a wide range of health serious complications and increased risk of premature onset year of illnesses. The most important organic complications are dyslipidemia, arterial hypertension, type 2 diabetes mellitus, nonalcoholic fatty liver disease, polycystic ovaries syndrome, orthopedic and respiratory complications. The metabolic syndrome (central obesity, hypertension, glucose intolerance and hyperlipidemia) increases risk for cardiovascular morbidity and mortality. The most frequent psychological complications are disorders concerning body image, eating habits and depression [4, 19].

Insulin resistance is defined as a decreased response of tissue to the action of insulin, and due to lowering of the capacity of insulin to stimulate glucose utilization by muscle cells and fat cells and to suppress hepatic glucose production, and insulin resistance in the protein and lipid metabolism. The association of obesity with insulin resistance is well-known: the factors and the mechanism by which the insulin resistance compensation is produced by beta islet cells and those that lead to the "failure" of the pancreatic beta cells in obese patients. It seems that microvascular changes associated with diabetes begin early stages still hyperinsulinemia with normal glycaemia or impaired oral glucose tolerance test. A central role in regulating central nervous system appears to have fat in the body's glucose metabolism by integrating information neural hormonal and nutritional. Insulin via the insulin receptor in the central nervous system regulates food intake and energy homeostasis. Adipose tissue seems to play a role in insulin resistance by metabolites, hormones and adipocytokines influencing different stages of insulin action. Fat distribution is an important determinant of insulin resistance, abdominal fat tissue lipolysis is easier and is less sensitive to insulin anti-lipolysis than subcutaneous adipose tissue. Total fat in children correlates well with the visceral and the relationship of visceral adipose tissue and the cardiovascular risk factors demonstrated in adults appears to differ [4, 31].

4.1. Dyslipidemia

Research on elucidating the relationship between obesity and atherogenic dyslipidemia appears to show a close relationship with insulin resistance. Three major events are based on atherogenic dyslipidemia of obesity with insulin resistance: excessive production of very low density lipoprotein-cholesterol, lipoprotein catabolism and defective catabolism of high density lipoprotein-cholesterol. Visceral fat is associated with impaired insulin-glucose homeostasis, the plasma lipoprotein, in particular increased triglycerides and decreased high density lipoprotein-cholesterol [4].

Arterial hypertension is recognized as an important component of metabolic syndrome in adults, but in children, its role is not very clear. While some studies hypertension is considered the direct effect of obesity, insulin resistance in others, it is considered a predictor of hypertension, independent of BMI. Arterial hypertension in the pathogenesis of obesity and insulin resistance may play a role in which leptin resistance physiological actions of insulin that leptin central nervous system vessels and kidneys should be changed. Studies suggest the involvement of oxidative stress in the pathogenesis and hypertension by stimulating reactive oxygen species by the renin–angiotensin–aldosterone system [32].

5. Clinical assessment of obesity

Obesity is more complicated to diagnose in children than in adults because children increase in height, weight and body fat naturally as they grow. The criteria for defining obesity in children are the fat mass assessment, the distribution of the body fat measure by age and sex and a centile cut off to define the point in the body fat measure distribution corresponding to obesity [33].

Initial assessments of these patients should include taking a careful history (investigating comorbidities, family history and potentially modifiable behaviors) and physical examination with BMI plotted on a BMI-for-age chart.

The careful history includes as follows: elements of perinatal life (gestational diabetes, maternal obesity, birth weight, infant feeding, medications—glucocorticoids, some antiepileptics, antipsychotics), weight history (onset of parental and child obesity, current eating behaviors, management interventions), complications (psychological, sleeping disorders, gastrointestinal and orthopedic complications, menstrual disturbances in girls), family history (ethnicity, history of obesity, type 2 diabetes, cardiovascular disease, dyslipidemia, obstructive sleep apnea, polycystic ovary syndrome, bariatric, surgery, eating disorders) and lifestyle history (detailed exploration of family eating, nutritional, and activity patterns, sleep) [34].

Physical examination should include the following: anthropometric data (weight, height, BMI, abdominal circumference), adiposity distribution (central versus generalized), assess blood pressure, markers of comorbidities and physical stigmata of a genetic syndrome, endocrine disorders, congenital or acquired hypothalamic alterations (fewer than 5% of cases) [4, 34].

The child's BMI must be plotted on nationally recommended BMI—for age charts. Children and adolescents with a BMI ≥99th percentile are even more likely to have comorbidities [4].

Abdominal circumference (AC) is also used for assessing excess fatty tissue is an indirect method for assessing abdominal fat tissue. Given the strong association between body fat distribution and risk of metabolic complications, it is helpful to calculate in all children with excess weight from the age of 5 years and upwards the relationship between waist circumference and height.

Other methods of measuring fat, such as bioelectrical impedance, and total body water measurement are used in research, but not in clinical evaluation [4].

Careful screening for hypertension using an appropriately sized blood pressure cuff is important (e.g., hypertension is diagnosed if systolic or diastolic blood pressure falls over 95th percentile for age, gender and height in at least three occasions) [35, 36].

Endocrine problems must be considered carefully on signs suggesting hypothyroidism (goiter), insulin resistance (acanthosis nigricans), polycystic ovary syndrome (hirsutism, excessive acne) and Cushing syndrome (violaceous striae, moon face) [36].

Symptoms of polyuria, nocturia or polydipsia may be the result of type 2 diabetes mellitus. Depending on their durations, overweight and obesity are important potential risk factors for respiratory complications (asthma, sleep apnea), abdominal pain or hepatomegaly (gastroesophagial reflux, nonalcoholic fatty liver), musculoskeletal problems (hip or knee pain, genu valgum, slipped capital femoral epiphysis, Blount disease) and psychological disorders (depression, body dissatisfaction, bulimia nervosa impaired social relationships and decreased health-related quality of life depression) [4, 37–39].

Reproductive system and Tanner stage disturbance can reveal premature puberty, apparent micropenis (but normal penis may be hidden in fat), undescended testis/micropenis (Prader Willi syndrome) and must be evaluated [4].

The degree of investigation is dependent on the patient's age and severity of obesity, the findings on history and physical examination, and associated familial risk factors.

First-line investigations recommended in cases of childhood obesity include fasting plasma glucose, triglycerides, low-density lipoprotein and high-density lipoprotein cholesterol, liver function tests and, possibly, insulinemia [4, 34, 35].

The investigations for overweight children include the fasting lipid screening test. If this children present risk factors represented by hypertension, dyslipidemia and family history of diabetes, it is necessary to evaluated the serum levels of fasting glucose, alanine aminotransferase (ALT) and aspartate aminotransferase (AST) to every 2 years (increased value of ALT and AST is associated with possible non-alcoholic fatty liver disease) [36].

In obese, children is necessary to evaluated serum levels of fasting lipids, glucose, ALT and AST every 2 years, and insulinemia [4, 34, 35].

Second-line investigations may include liver ultrasound, an oral glucose tolerance test, more detailed endocrine assessment and polysomnography [4, 34].

Patients with fasting blood glucose >100 mg/dL or overweight children (BMI 85th to 95th percentile) who have a family history of diabetes mellitus or signs of insulin resistance (acanthosis nigricans), polycystic ovary syndrome, or metabolic syndrome should also be evaluated with an oral glucose tolerance test [4, 34, 35]. If the result of oral glucose tolerance test is more than 126 mg/dL, counseling and repeating test is necessary because pediatric obesity can lead to impaired glucose tolerance. The value of HbA1c of 40 mmol/mol (5.8%) is an appropriate screening tool for diagnosing impaired glucose tolerance [40, 41].

Liver ultrasound is recommended for all obese children and adolescents. In children with confirmed ALT >40 IU/L or palpable liver, more thorough diagnostic tests are advisable with gamma-GT and differential diagnosis of hepatitis [41].

Other laboratory tests such as thyroid function tests (if there is a faster increase in weight than height), pelvic ultrasound and hormonal doses in cases of suspected polycystic ovary syndrome have been recommended [4, 41].

Psychological and psychiatric evaluations are essential to identify psychological disturbances including depression, loss-of-control eating, unhealthy and extreme weight control behaviors, and decreased health-related quality of life which are warning signs of bulimia nervosa and binge-eating disorder [39].

In patients with hypertension more diagnostic tests should be done: cardiac exam: ECG and echocardiogram, standard urinalysis, microalbuminuria, creatinine and potassium levels [4, 41].

We should realize screening for diagnosis of metabolic syndrome in the presence of at least three of the following situations: BMI indicate obesity or waist circumference/height ratio >0.5, systolic and/or diastolic blood pressure >95th percentile, fasting blood glucose >100 mg/dL, serum level of triglycerides >95th percentile, serum level of HDL cholesterol [4, 41].

According to International Diabetes Federation (IDF), the consensus definition of metabolic syndrome in children (older than 6 years) and adolescents are as follows:

- for children aged 6–10 years:

- obesity mean a waist circumference >90th percentile

- in case of metabolic syndrome that cannot be diagnosed, the measurements should be made if there is a family history of metabolic syndrome, type 2 diabetes mellitus, dyslipidemia, cardiovascular disease, hypertension or obesity.

- IDF suggests for weight reduction to use an appropriate message in patients with abdominal obesity.

- for children aged 10–16 years:

- obesity mean a waist circumference >90th percentile (or adult cut-off if lower).

- serum triglycerides level >1.7 mmol/l

- serum HDL cholesterol level <1.03 mmol/l

- systolic blood pressure >130 mmHg or diastolic blood pressure >85 mmHg

- blood glucose >5.6 mmol/l (oral glucose tolerance test recommended) or medical history of type 2 diabetes mellitus

- for children >16 years:

- should use the IDF criteria for adults. According to the recent IDF definition, a person with metabolic syndrome must have central obesity (defined as waist circumference using ethnicity-specific values) and any two of the following four factors:

- serum triglyceride levels >150 mg/dl (1.7 mmol/l) or specific treatment recommended for this abnormality

- reduced serum HDL cholesterol level <40 mg/dl (1.03 mmol/l) in males and <50 mg/dl (1.29 mmol/l) in females, or specific treatment for this lipid abnormality

- raised blood pressure: systolic blood pressure >130 mmHg or diastolic blood pressure of 85 mmHg or treatment for previously diagnosed hypertension

- raised fasting plasma glucose >100 mg/dl (5.6 mmol/l) or previously diagnosed type 2 diabetes (if above 5.6 mmol/l or 100 mg/dl, the oral glucose tolerance test is strongly recommended but is not necessary to define the presence of this syndrome) [32, 42].

Vitamin D deficiency is common in obese children and is associated with risk factors for type 2 diabetes in obese children, but they are not still recommended by national clinical practice guidelines as routine measures [43].

6. Management of child obesity

Prevention is the best cost/benefit approach for the management of obesity in children and, in the future, of adulthood. Childhood obesity is a multifaceted problem embedded in physiological, behavioral, genetic, socioeconomic, environmental and political contexts, and the actions to prevent childhood obesity must therefore be taken in multiple settings. Public awareness campaigns, social marketing and behavior-change communication related to nutrition and physical activity implemented in countries together are very important strategies regarding childhood obesity prevention. The critical periods of pediatric obesity characterized by important changes in adiposity growth velocity or obesity related behavior are represented by the first year of life, the preschool ("adiposity rebound") and adolescence years. The transition period from childhood to adolescence is characterized by important behavioral changes and decreased physical activity [44]. The obesity primary prevention begins in pregnancy period (healthy food diet), continuing with promoting the breastfeeding in the first 2 years of life, and then with support for healthy eating habits (low sugar consumption, eat breakfast every day, eat at home with family, avoid fast—food meals, avoid television in the first years of life and limit television to less than 2 h per day after then, etc. [4, 41, 45, 46].

Management of obesity should be based on risk factors, including age, severity of overweight and obesity and comorbidities, as well as family history and support. Management intervention strategies are available and include nutrition, physical activity, behavior and lifestyle changes, medication and surgical considerations. Treatment largely focuses on sustained lifestyle changes with family involvement. There are several broad principles of conventional management: management of comorbidities, family involvement, taking a developmentally appropriate approach, the use of a range of behavior change techniques, long-term dietary change, increased physical activity and decreased sedentary behaviors. The primary goal for all children with uncomplicated obesity is the long-term improvement of physical health through healthy lifestyles. In obese children with a secondary complication, specific treatment of the complication is an important goal. Effective weight reduction is one of the key elements in the treatment of comorbidities. In morbid obesity, bariatric surgery and laparoscopic sleeve gastrectomy have been used in adolescence [4, 34, 41].

In order to plan a developmentally appropriate approach, it is essential to consider the developmental age of the patient and the resultant level of parental engagement that will be required. Most successful interventions have been family based and take into account the child's developmental age. In preadolescent children, a parent-based program, without direct engagement of the child, might be more appropriate than a child centered approach.

Depending on the age of the child, the present of parents must be or not compulsory. For example, if we talk about adolescents, the present of parents in not recommended. However, the parents must participate at counseling session that are designed for them.

Because obesity is multifactorial, not all children and adolescents will respond to the same approach. Behavior therapy, healthy diet and increasing physical activity are the great sections of obesity treatment. Referral to multidisciplinary, comprehensive pediatric weight—management programs is ideal for obese children whenever possible [4, 34].

Behavior modification strategy has a large effect on weight reduction. The set of techniques employed to change thought processes and actions associated with eating, physical activity and sedentary are components of behavior strategies. For the obese adolescent, there are several ways to help him acquiring a healthy lifestyle: to log daily his physical effort and food intake; to participate to motivational interview; to receive permanent psychological support for positive lifestyle changes [34, 41, 46].

Dietary interventions are usually part of a broader lifestyle change program can be effective in achieving relative weight loss in children and adolescents. Dietary interventions should follow national nutrition guidelines which have an emphasis on:

- at least five meals over the day (three meals + two snacks)

- restrict/replace specific high calorie foods with others less rich in calories

- the protein content: it is suggested the 14 meals per week: meat, three to four times a week; fish, three to four times a week; legumes, three to four times a week; cheese and eggs, once a week.

- carbohydrates should account for at least 50% of total calories, preferring low glycemic index foods: cereals such as pasta, barley and whole wheat products—twice a day; legumes; fruit and vegetables (not canned or pureed) five servings a day) and by limiting foods that combine a high glycemic index to a high glycemic load (bread, rice, potatoes, sweets, sugar, fruit juices, sweet drinks).

- the total fat in the diet should account for no more than 30% of total calories.

- the adequate intake of fiber in grams/day: five servings a day of fruits and vegetables in season, not canned or pureed, and legumes four times a week are recommended.

- decreased portion sizes.

- drinking water as the main beverage and reduction in sugary drink intake.

- involvement of the entire family in making sustainable dietary changes [34, 41].

Increasing physical activity can decrease risk for cardiovascular disease, improve well-being and contribute to weight loss:

- walking or cycling for transport,

- undertaking household chores and playing,

- organized exercise programs,

- limiting television and other small screen recreation to less than 2 h per day is particularly strategic, but may be challenging,

- is recommended at least 60 min of moderate exercise.

Parental involvement is vital and may include monitoring and limiting television use, role modeling of healthy behaviors and providing access to recreation areas or recreational equipment.

Existing recommendations on management of pediatric obesity suggest that drug therapy can be used in the treatment of severely obese adolescents. Orlistat can be useful as an adjunct to lifestyle changes in severely obese adolescents and metformin can be used in older children and adolescents with clinical insulin resistance [4, 34, 41].

Bariatric surgery should be considered in adolescents with complete or near-complete skeletal maturity, who are severely obese with a body mass index of more than 40 kg/m^2 or weight exceeding 100% of ideal body, and a medical complication resulting from obesity, after they have failed 6 months of a multidisciplinary weight management program. Preoperative care and counselling is very important if we want to have good long-term results for bariatric surgery patients. This care must be provided by specialist in various medical fields: endocrinology, gastroenterology, cardiovascular, pneumology, etc. All this effort must by sustained with nutritional and psychological support [4, 34, 41,47, 48].

Childhood obesity treatment is based on sustained lifestyle changes with family involvement. Behavior therapy, healthy diet and increasing physical activity are the great sections of obesity treatment.

7. Conclusions

Childhood and adolescent obesity is a major health problem. The prevalence of childhood obesity in Europe is ten times higher than it was in the 1970s. The increasing occurrence in children of disorders, such as type 2 diabetes, is a consequence of this obesity epidemic. Initial assessments of these patients should include taking a careful history (investigating comorbidities, family history and potentially modifiable behaviors) and physical examination. The degree of investigation is dependent on the patient's age and severity of obesity, the findings on history and physical examination, and associated familial risk factors. The increased prevalence of obesity in childhood and adolescence highlights the need for effective treatment approaches. There are several broad principles of conventional management: management of comorbidities, family involvement, the use of a range of behavior change techniques, long-term dietary change, increased physical activity and decreased sedentary behaviors. Pediatric patients and their families should be counselled on nutritional interventions including limiting sugar-sweetened beverages, eating nutrient-dense breakfasts, limiting eating out at fast food restaurants, families eating together, increased exercise and decreased time in front of computer and TV screens. For adolescents with severe obesity, lifestyle changes are mandatory. This change must be supported with medical therapy (the only drugs approved by the health organizations are Orlistat and Metformin; these treatments do not exclude metabolic surgery). Finally, given the high prevalence and chronic nature of obesity, coordinated models of care for health service delivery for the management of pediatric obesity are needed.

Author details

Laura Mihaela Trandafir*, Ileana Ioniuc and Ingrith Miron

*Address all correspondence to: trandafirlaura@yahoo.com

Pediatric Department, University of Medicine and Pharmacy "Grigore T. Popa", Iasi, Romania

References

[1] World Health Organization. Obesity and Overweight [Internet]. 2015 [Updated: 2016]. Available from: http://www.who.int/mediacentre/factsheets/fs311/en/

[2] Hill Jo: Understanding and addressing the epidemic of obesity: an energy balance perspective. Endocrine Reviews. 2006;27:750–761. doi:10.1210/er.2006-0032

[3] World Health Organization. Global Status Report on Non-communicable Diseases [Internet]. 2014. Available from: http://www.who.int/nmh/publications/ncd-status-report-2014/en/ [Accessed: 2016]

[4] Gahagan S. Overweight and Obesity. In: Kliegman RM, Stanton BF, St. Geme JWIII, Schor NF, editors. Nelson Textbook of Pediatrics. 20th ed. Philadelphia: Elsevier Saunders; 2016. p. 307–316. doi:978-1-4557-7566-8, 2823-2831

[5] Rodríguez G, Pietrobelli A, Wang Y, Moreno LA. Methodological Aspects for Childhood and Adolescence Obesity Epidemiology. In: Moreno AL, Pigeot I, Ahrens W, editors.

Epidemiology of Obesity in Children and Adolescents—Prevalence and Etiology. New York: Springer; 2011. p. 21–40. doi:10.1007/978-1-4419-6039-9

[6] Lobstein T. Prevalence and Trends Across the World. In: M.L. Frelut, editor. The ECOG's eBook on Child and Adolescent Obesity. ebook.ecog-obesity.eu:2015.

[7] Manios Y, Costarelli V. Childhood Obesity in the WHO European Region. In: Moreno AL, Pigeot I, Ahrens W, editors. Epidemiology of Obesity in Children and Adolescents—Prevalence and Etiology. New York: Springer; 2011. p. 43–68. doi:10.1007/978-1-4419-6039-9

[8] Larranaga, N., Amiano, P., Arrizabalaga, J., Bidaurrazaga, J.J., Gorostiza E. Prevalence of obesity in 4-18-year-old population in the Basque Country, Spain. Obesity Reviews. 2007;**8**(4):281–287. doi:10.1111/j.1467-789X.2006.00306

[9] Kontogianni, M.D., Vidra, N., Farmaki, A.E., Koinaki, S., Belogianni, K., Sofrona, S., Magkanari, F., Yannakouli M. Adherence rates to the mediterranean diet are low in a representative sample of Greek children and adolescents. Journal of Nutrition. 2008; **138**:1951–1956.

[10] Moreira P. Overweight and obesity in Portuguese children and adolescents. Journal of Public Health. 2007;**15**(3):155–161. doi:10.1007/s10389-007-0109-1

[11] Hakanen, M., Lagstrom, H., Kaitosaari, T., Niinikoski, H., Nanto-Salonen K., Jokinen, E., Sillanmaki, L., Viikari, J., Ronnemaa, T., Simell, O. Development of overweight in an atherosclerosis prevention trial starting in early childhood. The STRIP study. International Journal of Obesity.2006;**30**:618–626.

[12] Kumanyika S.K. Environmental influences on childhood obesity: ethnic and cultural influences in context. Physiology & Behaviour. 2008;**94**(1):61–70. doi:10.1016/j.physbeh.2007.11.019

[13] Wardle J., Brodersen N.H., Cole T.J., Jarvis M.J., Boniface D.R. Development of adiposity in adolescence: five-year longitudinal study of an ethnically and socioeconomically diverse sample of young people in Britain. British Medical Journal. 2006;**332**:1130–1135. doi:10.1136/bmj.38807.594792.AE

[14] Hollis J, Robinson S. Prenatal Experience and Childhood Obesity. In: M.L. Frelut, editor. The ECOG's eBook on Child and Adolescent Obesity. ebook.ecog-obesity.eu 2015.

[15] Socha P. Metabolic Programming, Breastfeeding and Later Risk of Obesity. In: In M.L. Frelut, editor. The ECOG's eBook on Child and Adolescent Obesity. Retrieved from ebook.ecog-obesity.eu. 2015.

[16] Oken E., Levitan E., Giillman M. Maternal smoking during pregnancy and child overweight systematic review and meta-analysis. International Journal of Obesity. 2008;**32**(2):201–210. doi:10.1038/sj.ijo.0803760

[17] Riedel C., Schönberger K., Yang S., Koshy G., Chen Y.C., Gopinath B., Ziebarth S., von Kries R. Parental smoking and childhood obesity: higher effect estimates for maternal smoking in pregnancy compared with paternal smoking—a meta-analysis. International Journal of Epidemiology. 2014;**43**(5):1593–1606. doi:10.1093/ije/dyu150

[18] Klish W.J. Definition; epidemiology; and etiology of obesity in children and adolescents, http://www.uptodate.com/contents/definition-epidemiology-and-etiology-of-obesity-in-children-and-adolescents [Internet].

[19] Klish W.J. Comorbidities and Complications of Obesity in Children and Adolescents. http://www.uptodate.com/contents/comorbidities-and-complications-of-obesityin-children-and-adolescents [Internet].

[20] Tu A.W., Mâsse L.C., Lear S.A., Gotay C.C., Richardson C.G. Exploring the mediating roles of physical activity and television time on the relationship between the neighbourhood environment and childhood obesity. Canadian Journal of Public Health. 2016;**107**(2):168–175. doi:10.17269/cjph.107. 5268

[21] Lobstein T., Dibb S. Evidence of a possible link between obesogenic food advertising and child overweight. Obesity Reviews. 2005;**6**(3):203–208. doi:10.1111/j.1467-789X.2005. 00191.x

[22] Mazur A., Radziewicz-Winnicki I. Obesity and Media. In: In M.L. Frelut, editor. The ECOG's eBook on Child and Adolescent Obesity. Retrieved from ebook.ecog-obesity.eu. 2015. The ECOG's eBook

[23] Bhadoria A.S., Kapil U., Kaur S. Association of duration of time spent on television, computer and video games with obesity amongst children in National Capital Territory of Delhi. Journal of Preventive Medicine. 2015;**6**(1):80. doi:10.4103/2008-7802.164090

[24] Kuzik N., Carson V. The association between physical activity, sedentary behavior, sleep, and body mass index z-scores in different settings among toddlers and preschoolers. ***BMC Pediatrics. 2016;**16**. doi:10.1186/s12887-016-0642-6

[25] emedicine. http://emedicine.medscape.com/article/985333-overview#a5 [Internet]

[26] Telega G. Intestinal Microbiome. In Obesity. In: In M.L. Frelut, editor. The ECOG's eBook on Child and Adolescent Obesity. Retrieved from ebook.ecog-obesity.eu. 2015.

[27] Yang O., Kim H.L., Weon J.I., Seo Y.R. Endocrine-disrupting Chemicals: Review of Toxicological Mechanisms Using Molecular Pathway Analysis. Journal of Cancer Prevention. 2015;**20**(1):12–24. doi:10.15430/JCP.2015.20.1.12

[28] http://emedicine.medscape.com/article/985333-overview#a5 [Internet].

[29] Funcke J.B., Schnurbein J., Lennerz B., Lahr G., Debatin K.M., Fischer-Posovszky P., Wabitsch M. Monogenic Forms of Childhood Obesity due to Mutations in the Leptin Gene [Internet]. 2014 . Available from: http://molcellped.springeropen.com/articles/10.1186/s40348-014-0003-1

[30] http://emedicine.medscape.com/article/985333-overview [Internet].

[31] Cinti S. The Adipose Organ: Implications for Prevention and Treatment of Obesity. In: In M.L. Frelut, editor. The ECOG's eBook on Child and Adolescent Obesity. Retrieved from ebook.ecogobesity. 2015.

[32] Wabitsch M, Körner A. Definitions. In: Kiess W, Wabitsch M, Maffeis C, Sharma AM, editors. Metabolic Syndrome and Obesity in Childhood and Adolescence. Pediatr Adolesc Med. Basel, Karger; 2015. p. 1–12. doi:10.1159/000368101

[33] Tim J Cole. How to Measure Obesity in Children [Internet]. 2014. Available from: https://thewinnower.com/discussions/14-how-to-measure-obesity-in-children

[34] Baur LA. Management of Child and Adolescent Obesity. In: Berthold Koletzko, editors. Pediatric Nutrition in Practice. 2nd ed. Basel: Karger; 2015. p. 161–167. (1660–2242)

[35] Balow SE. Expert committee recommendations regarding the prevention, assessment, and treatment of child and adolescent overweight and obesity: summary report. Pediatrics. 2007;**120**(Suppl 4):164–192.

[36] Zahra Alizadeh, Shahrzad Khosravi,Sima Borna/Iraninan Journal of Pediatrics. Obese and Overweight Children and Adolescents: An Algorithmic Clinical Approach [Internet]. 2013. Available from: http://www.ncbi.nlm.nih.gov/pmc/articles/PMC4025117/

[37] Ruiz Extremera A., Carazo A., Salmerón A., León J., Casado J., Goicoechea A., Fernandez J.M., Garofano M., Ocete E., Martín A.B., Pavón E., Salmerón J. Factors associated with hepatic steatosis in obese children and adolescents. Journal of Pediatric Gastroenterology and Nutrition. 2011;**53**(2):1962–1901. doi:10.1097/MPG. 0b013e3182185ac4

[38] Thielemann F., Guenther K.P., Stiehler M. Orthopaedic Aspects of Obesity in Children and Adults. In: Kiess W, Wabitsch M, Maffeis C, Sharma AM, editors. Metabolic Syndrome and Obesity in Childhood and Adolescence. Pediatr Adolesc Med. Basel, Karger; 2015. p. 84–98. doi:10.1159/000368101

[39] Vander Wal J.S., Mitchell E.R. Psychological complications of pediatric obesity. Pediatric Clinics of North America.2011;**58**(6):1393–1401. doi:10.1016/j.pcl.2011.09.008

[40] Lee HS, Park HK, Hwang JS. HbA1c and glucose intolerance in obese children and adolescents. Diabetic Medicine.2012;**29**(7):102–105.

[41] Maffeis C., Licenziati M.R., Vania A., Garofalo P., Di Mauro G., Caroli M., Morino G., Siani P., Chiamenti G. Childhood Obesity. In: P. Sbraccia, editor. Clinical Management of Overweight and Obesity: Recommendations of the Italian Society of Obesity (SIO). Switzerland: Springer International Publishing; 2016. p. 131–147. doi:10.1007/978-3-319-24532-4_10

[42] International Diabetes Federation. Metabolic Syndrome in Children and Adolescents [Internet]. 2007. Available from: http://www.idf.org/webdata/docs/Mets_definition_children.pdf

[43] Olson M.L., Maalouf N.M., Oden J.D., White P.C., Hutchison M.R. Vitamin D deficiency in obese children and its relationship to glucose homeostasis. Journal of Clinical Endocrinology & Metabolism. 2012;**97**(1):279–285. doi:10.1210/jc.2011-1507

[44] Joan C. Han, Debbie A. Lawlor, Sue Y.S. Kimm. Childhood Obesity –2010: Progress and Challenges [Internet]. 2011. Available from: http://www.ncbi.nlm.nih.gov/pmc/articles/PMC3073855/

[45] Kugelberg S., Jewell J., Breda J. Prevention Across Europe. In: M.L. Frelut, editor. The ECOG's eBook on Child and Adolescent Obesity. Retrieved from ebook.ecog-obesity.eu. 2015.

[46] Han J.C., Lawlor D.A, Kimm S.Y.S. Childhood obesity–2010: Progress and challenges. Lancet. 2010;**15**:1737–1748. doi:10.1016/S0140-6736(10)60171-7

[47] Baur L.A., Hazelton B., Shrewsbury V.A. Assessment and management of obesity in childhood and adolescence. Nature Reviews Gastroenterology and Hepatology. 2011;**8**:635–645doi:10.1038/nrgastro.2011.165

[48] Barlow S.E. Expert committee: Expert committee recommendations regarding the prevention, assessment, and treatment and obesity: Summary report. Pediatrics. 2007;**120** (suppl 4):S164–S192.

12

Lay Theories of Obesity: Causes and Consequences

Paul H. Thibodeau and Stephen J. Flusberg

Abstract

Both the scientific community and the general public have come to recognize the increasing prevalence of obesity as a significant public health crisis. To help address this issue, recent research has begun to explore *lay theories* of obesity—the mental models that structure how non-experts think about the causes and consequences of the condition. In this chapter, we develop an integrative review of the literature on lay theories of obesity, drawing on research in public health, communications, and psychology to illuminate the factors that shape beliefs and attitudes toward the condition, as well as the consequences of specific lay theories for cognition and behavior. At the individual level, we discuss how certain ways of thinking about obesity facilitate obesity treatment and prevention. At the societal level, we discuss how certain ways of thinking about obesity lead people to support (and oppose) specific types of obesity-related policy interventions. We pay special attention to the role of narrative framing and individual demographics in the etiology of lay beliefs and explore how particular psychological mechanisms (e.g., empathy) can affect attributions and attitudes.

Keywords: obesity, framing, narrative, communication, lay theories, causal attribution

1. Introduction

It is now common knowledge that obesity is unhealthy and poses a significant risk to millions of adults and children worldwide [1]. Being overweight predisposes people to a variety of serious medical conditions [2, 3] and is associated with a lower quality of life and expected life span [4–6]. But despite widespread appreciation of the dangers of being extremely overweight, incidence rates have been steadily climbing for years, resulting in what many doctors and public health officials view as an urgent public health crisis [2, 3]. In the past 50 years, obesity rates have risen rapidly all over the world, at all levels of age, race, and sex [7].

As our scientific understanding of the causes and consequences of obesity grows, it is especially important to track how the general public thinks about the condition. People have "lay theories" [8] about the causes and consequences of obesity that can differ markedly from the comparatively complex and nuanced scientific perspectives on obesity that have developed in recent years. For example, although public health officials have identified a range of complex social, physiological, and psychological factors that contribute to being obese [9], many people still think that individuals alone are responsible for maintaining a healthy weight [10, 11] (but see [12]). Such a disconnect represents an important obstacle for policy makers who seek to design and implement interventions that would address causes of obesity outside a person's control—since many people deny that obesity results from anything other than poor lifestyle decisions made at the individual level. In a democracy, public perceptions can be just as important for addressing complex issues as scientific theories and breakthroughs, since policy interventions are more likely to be accepted when they are consistent with the general public's understanding of an issue such as obesity [13, 14].

By investigating lay theories of obesity, therefore, researchers may gain a better understanding of why obesity rates are on the rise while at the same time they may be able to identify effective ways to address this public health crisis [15–17]. For example, it is important to know whether people think that self-regulatory behaviors such as diet and exercise can help maintain a healthy weight or whether people think that their weight is primarily determined by factors outside of their control. Several recent, but controversial, scientific studies have questioned the efficacy of diet and exercise for the prevention and treatment of obesity [18, 19]. This work has received substantial attention in the popular press, which is often distilled to pithy headlines such as, "Why you can't lose weight on a diet" [20]. How do people interpret these claims in light of what they know about obesity—and what do people know about obesity in the first place? Can messaging strategies be developed to promote support for the kinds of interventions that public health officials have argued will provide better treatments for obesity and reduce the prevalence of an issue that poses significant costs to individuals and society?

In this chapter, we develop an integrative review of the literature on lay theories of obesity, drawing on research in public health, communications, and psychology to illuminate the factors that shape beliefs and attitudes toward the condition, as well as the consequences of specific lay theories for cognition and behavior. We pay special attention to the role of narrative framing and individual demographics in the etiology of lay beliefs, and explore how particular psychological mechanisms (e.g., empathy) can affect how people think and reason about obesity.

2. Trait theories

People often think about obesity in the same way they think about other physical or psychological traits: as a basic attribute that individuals possess to varying degrees. Dweck et al. [21, 22] have identified two opposing lay theories that characterize how people think and reason about a variety of traits, which are distinguished by the degree to which the trait is viewed as malleable [21, 22]. People who hold an "entity theory" of intelligence (also known as "fixed mindset"), for example, think about the intellect as something hard-wired and stable, while those who hold an "incremental theory" (also known as a "growth mindset") believe their intellectual abilities can grow through effort and hard work. Holding one of these theories is associated with a great deal of downstream behavior and cognition. For instance, incremental theorists are more committed to their learning goals and are more persistent in the face of adversity than people who think their intellectual abilities are fixed.

A recent study of dieters [23] found that people who hold incremental theories of obesity adopt qualitatively different strategies for losing weight compared to those who hold an entity theory of obesity. Consistent with prior research, incremental theorists were much more open to changing their lifestyle—to embrace a new diet, implement a novel exercise routine, or attend group meetings—in the service of achieving their weight-loss goal.

3. Causal theories

Another class of lay theories considers the causal origins of obesity, which may or may not have implications for beliefs about malleability. Research suggests that people often rely on narrative structures that include extended metaphors and analogies to think about complex issues like obesity [17, 24–27], and one recent study identified seven common narratives for obesity that capture different causal beliefs about the condition (see **Table 1**; [10]). Importantly, these narratives are also associated with different ways of thinking about how to address the problem of obesity—both at an individual and at a societal level [10, 16, 17].

A critical dimension that differentiates these lay causal theories is the degree to which they attribute personal responsibility or blame to obese individuals for being overweight. At one extreme is the view that individuals are entirely responsible for maintaining a healthy weight —the idea that addiction is a "sinful behavior." At the other extreme are views that suggest obesity is entirely the result of factors outside a person's control, such as a "toxic food environment" or "industry manipulation."

gluttony [28] and places responsibility for maintaining a healthy weight squarely on the everyday decisions that individuals make about diet and exercise. Psychiatrist and media personality Keith Ablow embodies this perspective when he explains that obesity "is largely caused by poor decisions—like binging on food or eating lots of candy, ice cream or Cheetos" ([29], p. 1). On this view, rising rates of obesity are the result of more people making worse decisions about their health; addressing obesity, within this framework, is a challenge for individuals to eat healthier and exercise more.

Barry et al. [10] found that more than half of the participants in their survey of over 1000 people thought that "sinful behavior" was an important cause of obesity. Participants who endorsed this view tended to oppose policy interventions that public health officials argue would have a large impact on obesity [30]: by, for example, requiring restaurants and food producers to list nutritional information on menus and food packaging, to increase the availability of healthy food and opportunities for exercise, and to broaden the reach of laws designed to protect people with disabilities.

Narrative	Theme	Important explanation
Sinful behavior	People are unwilling to work hard to control their impulses. People who are overweight are not even trying to get healthier	50.5%
Addiction	People get hooked on certain things and just cannot quit. When people get hooked on sugary, fatty foods, some cannot keep themselves from eating more and more	71.2%
Time crunch	Work has gotten in the way of important things. Obesity is a symptom of a society that emphasizes work at the expense of well-being	58.0%
Eating disorder	Society sends the wrong messages about what it means to be attractive which leads people to go on fad diets that make them fatter	65.2%
Disability	We blame the victim for things they cannot control. People who are overweight are treated badly even though their weight problems come from their parents	51.3%
Industry manipulation	Commercial interests dictate our choices and values. Advertising distorts how we value food. We used to eat to live, now we live to eat	54.1%
Toxic food environment	We are surrounded by choices that cheap but not good for us. Healthy foods are lost in a sea of unhealthy alternatives	77.5%

Participants identified which ones they thought provided an "important explanation" for why Americans are overweight. The narratives are ordered in terms of how much blame they ascribe to the individual: from highest to lowest.

Table 1. Seven narratives identified by Barry et al. [10] for explaining the obesity epidemic.

In a follow-up study, Thibodeau et al. [17] found that certain demographic characteristics of individuals are associated with thinking that being obese is blameworthy (i.e., to endorse the view that obesity is the result of "sinful behavior"; see [31] to get a sense for how these associations have and have not changed in the past few decades). Specifically, males, conservatives, and people who had a lower body mass index (BMI) or who had not personally suffered from an eating disorder were more likely to endorse the view that obesity is caused by poor decisions about diet and exercise (see also [32, 33], for related evidence that individuals with and without eating disorders have differing views of these conditions). This study replicated Barry et al.'s correlational finding [10]—showing that people who think obesity is blameworthy oppose societal-level interventions designed to prevent people from becoming overweight. In addition, Thibodeau et al. [17] found that these participants were more likely to support policy interventions that would increase individual accountability for maintaining a healthy weight (e.g., policies that would allow health insurers to charge higher premiums to people who are overweight). These results are illustrated in **Figure 1**.

Thibodeau et al. [17] also conducted an experiment to test whether reading a narrative about obesity could causally influence people's beliefs about the condition as well as their support for public policy interventions. Some participants read a narrative that emphasized personal accountability (using a variant of the "sinful behavior" account), while others read a narrative that highlighted factors outside a person's control (combining elements of the "industry manipulation" and "toxic food environment" themes) before being asked about their support for a variety of obesity-related public policies. The results suggested that describing obesity as blameworthy (sinful behavior) decreased support for protective policy interventions (i.e., interventions that would emphasize education, regulation of food-related advertising and manufacturing, and increase legal protections for obese individuals) and increased support for punitive actions (e.g., by allowing health insurers to charge higher premiums to obese individuals). On the other hand, people who were exposed to a narrative that deemphasized individual blameworthiness were less likely to support punitive actions. However, they were no more likely to support societal-level policy interventions. Instead, support for societal-level policy interventions was most strongly predicted by participants' political ideology: left-leaning, politically liberal participants tended to support societal-level policy interventions more than right-leaning, politically conservative individuals.

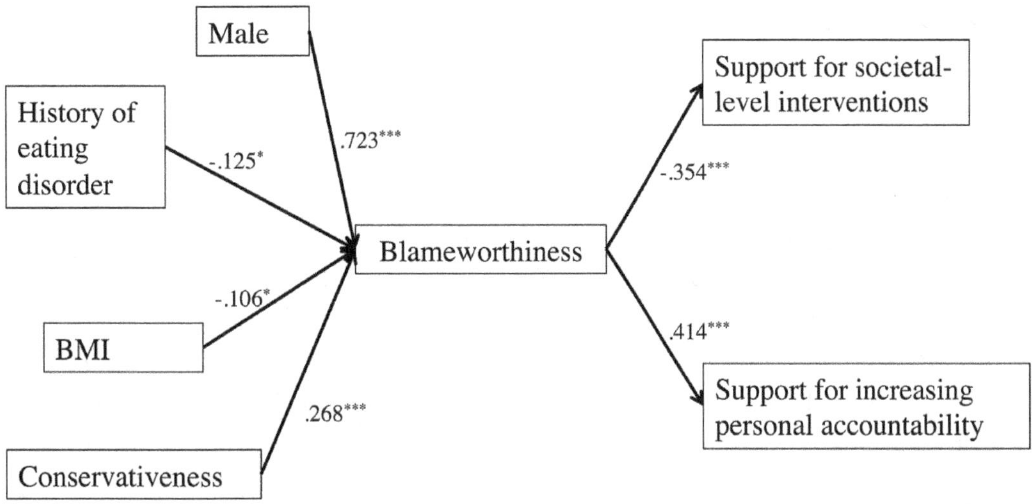

Figure 1. Relationships between demographic characteristics, beliefs about the blameworthiness of obesity (as measured by participants' agreement with narratives for obesity that varied in how they attributed blame for being overweight), and support for different types of interventions designed to address rising rates of obesity found in a study by Thibodeau et al. [17]. Values reflect path coefficients in a structural equation model ($^*p < 0.05$, $^{***}p < 0.001$).

Together, this work suggests that there are several common narratives about the underlying causes of obesity and that these narratives provide a foundation for thinking about different ways of addressing the complex health issue. Specifically, the view that obesity is caused by a lack of personal motivation represents one common lay theory about obesity. The defining characteristic of this view is that it blames obese individuals for being overweight. This blame creates a stigma against obesity and represents a major obstacle to societal-level policy interventions that seek to address causes of obesity that are outside of a person's control (e.g., corporate manipulation and the availability of healthy food). Interestingly, this view can be further broken down into whether people believe it is a lack of exercise or an unhealthy diet that is the central causal factor in obesity, with predictable consequences for behavior: people who believe that lack of exercise plays a larger role in obesity than diet are more likely to consume more food and be overweight [11].

At the other end of the extreme, there are a variety of lay theories about the causes of obesity that blame factors outside of a person's control by highlighting a "toxic food environment" or "corporate manipulation" as culprits in the obesity crisis. Many participants in Barry et al.'s study [10] endorsed these narratives as capturing important causes of the obesity epidemic, and this judgment was correlated with support for more protective policy interventions. However, an experiment designed to test whether reading such narratives would increase support for the protective policy interventions failed to find support for a critical prediction: people who read a narrative that minimized the blame attributed to obese individuals for being overweight were no more likely to support societal-level policy interventions that would address causes of obesity outside a person's control [17]. Below, we discuss a popular alternative causal model of obesity—that it is a "disease"—which may be better suited to eliciting such support.

4. Disease theories

In recent years, doctors and public health officials have sought to reduce the stigma of obesity and increase support for obesity-related research and policy interventions by officially classifying obesity as a "disease" [34–36]. Like narratives that highlight the role of environmental factors in obesity (e.g., "toxic food environment," "corporate manipulation"), describing obesity as a "disease" seems to reduce the personal responsibility associated with the condition. However, rather than appealing to external factors—the social and physical environments in which people live—thinking of obesity as a "disease" makes the condition less blameworthy by appealing to underlying physiological factors as the primary causes of weight gain [36].

Recent research suggests that this biomedical view of obesity has gone from a minority viewpoint just three decades ago to perhaps *the* dominant perspective today [37] (but see [11]). This shift represents an important achievement for public health communications. At a high level, the increased public recognition of obesity as a "disease" in recent years suggests that the way health officials talk about obesity has significant downstream effects on how the general public thinks about the condition. At a more practical level, one of the specific goals of the messaging campaign seems to have been achieved, as a majority of the US population recently reported that thinking of obesity as a disease would facilitate treatment of the condition [37].

However, researchers have also identified drawbacks to the disease model of obesity. The belief that weight is somewhat fixed by biological factors may negatively impact dieting goals and exercise intentions, especially among people who are overweight [15, 38]. In other words, reducing the blameworthiness of being obese is a double-edged sword: it not only mitigates the stigma associated with being overweight but also fosters an entity theory of obesity, reducing an important source of motivation for maintaining healthy habits that can help people lose weight (or gain it in the first place). In one study, for example, overweight participants who read a *New York Times* article describing obesity as a disease displayed lower body-image dissatisfaction compared to those who read an article arguing against the disease construal, but they also expressed less concern for healthy dieting and were more like to make unhealthy food choices when given the chance [15].

There are, certainly, many different types of diseases, and thinking about obesity in terms of one particular type of disease or another may have unique consequences for reasoning and behavior. For instance, conceptualizing obesity as a genetic disorder (i.e., caused by an underlying genetic predisposition) seems to be especially associated with the belief that people have no control over their weight [38]. In comparison to those who read a report that provided a psychosocial explanation for obesity, one study found that people exposed to a genetic explanation for the condition ate more cookies in a follow-up task [38]. On the other hand, conceptualizing obesity as a form of addiction disorder seems to have more inconsistent effects on eating behavior. One experiment revealed that while reading a message stating that food addiction is "real" (as opposed to a "myth") *does* lead people to be more likely to self-identify as a "food addict," these individuals did not consume a greater quantity of indulgent food in a subsequent "taste-test" task (though they did eat a wider variety of items [39]). However, another study found that participants who were told they had high food addiction tendencies (as opposed to low food addiction tendencies) consumed *fewer* calories in a follow-up taste test, a result which was mediated by increased concern for their diet [40].

Taken together, these findings help reveal the nuances underlying the "disease" model of obesity, and the complex, sometimes negative, consequences of messaging campaigns that tap into this way of framing the issue. Recent research suggests that some of the limitations associated with standard messaging strategies may be addressed by exposing people to personal testimonials that describe successful weight loss (rather than basic causal explanations [41, 42]). We discuss this work in the following section, which also hints at a psychological mechanism—empathy—that can be leveraged to increase support for societal-level obesity policy interventions.

5. The role of personal narratives

So far, we have discussed the nature and consequences of several prominent lay theories of obesity. For years, the dominant way of thinking about obesity was that it resulted from poor lifestyle decisions—that it was the result of "sinful behavior." This model represents a challenge to public health officials because it fails to recognize the causes of obesity that are outside a person's control. Alternative lay theories—that highlight "environmental" contributions to obesity or appeal to a person's underlying physiology by classifying the condition as a "disease"—seem to reduce the stigma associated with obesity. However, there are important drawbacks to both. Namely, simply highlighting environmental contributions to obesity does not seem to increase support for important interventions that would reduce the prevalence of obesity (although evidence suggests that reading about the negative consequences of childhood obesity might; see [43]), and simply describing obesity as a disease can make weight gain feel inevitable and weight loss feel impossible.

Recent research suggests that reading personal testimonials about successful weight loss may help people construct a more positive mental model of obesity [41, 43–46]. Stories about individuals struggling (and succeeding or failing) to lose weight are ubiquitous, engaging, and provide a structured framework for thinking about the causes of and solutions to obesity [16, 17, 47]. Consider, for example, the popular reality television program "The Biggest Loser," in which morbidly obese contestants compete, through hard work and dedication, to lose the most weight over the course of the season. Although the show has been criticized for a variety of reasons—for promoting an unhealthy and unrealistic approach to weight loss [48] and because contestants have been found to regain lost weight after the show ends [18]—there is some evidence that it increases viewers' sense that they have control over their weight [49]. This suggests that exposing people to personal testimonials in which a protagonist succeeds at achieving a weight-loss goal—through healthy and realistic diet and exercise—may foster an incremental theory of the condition, making them more optimistic about obesity treatment in general [50].

In other words, it may be more effective to adopt a "bottom-up," rather than "top-down," approach to changing the way people think about obesity. Describing the underlying causes and consequences of obesity at a high level—by classifying the condition as the product of one's "environment" or the result of an underlying "disease"—represents a "top-down" strategy: seeking to change the stigma associated with obesity and increase support for public policy interventions by situating the condition in a particular causal framework (e.g., [51–53]). The drawback of this approach, as noted in the previous section, is that the candidate causal structures seem to encourage some inferences that are at odds with the goals of public health officials.

An alternative "bottom-up" approach would describe specific instances of people successfully losing weight, which could provide the foundation for people to induce the "right" lay theory of obesity: one that acknowledges causes of obesity that are within *and* outside a person's control, which motivates individuals to maintain a healthy lifestyle *and* promotes support for interventions that would address the social and environmental context that has given rise to the current public health crisis.

One specific feature of personal testimonials is that they provide the reader an opportunity to feel empathy for an individual struggling to lose weight [54]. In this context, empathy reflects the process of identifying with someone else's struggle with obesity—taking their perspective and sympathizing with their condition [55]. A natural byproduct of such a feeling is an increased awareness of factors that cause obesity that are outside a person's control [41, 42, 56]. Thus, exposing people to personal narratives that describe successful weight loss may be particularly effective tools for public health officials. Such testimonials may lead people to support policy interventions that would address the social and environmental contexts that have given rise to obesity without completely mitigating the sense of personal responsibility that is needed to maintain healthy habits.

A recent series of studies have tested and found support for this possibility [41, 42]. In one experiment, participants read a personal narrative about a protagonist who had successfully lost weight (or not) and who attributed this outcome to their own personal motivation or to environmental reforms that enabled healthier eating and exercise [42]. One critical finding was that reading about successful weight loss elicited significant empathy from participants—both in the case of a protagonist who attributed successful weight loss to their own motivation and in the case of a protagonist who attributed successful weight loss to environmental reforms. These feelings of empathy were, in turn, highly predictive of support for obesity-related policy interventions.

This line of work suggests that personal testimonials about obesity may facilitate a more responsible and productive mental model of obesity. By describing a specific individual who works hard to lose weight, a personal narrative highlights the role of healthy self-regulation to prevent and reduce obesity. Such a description also seems to elicit empathy from readers, which leads them to recognize causes of obesity that are outside a person's control—and, in turn, to support important policy interventions. In other words, personal narratives seem to achieve the goals that have motivated recent work in the field of public health communications (e.g., by classifying obesity as a disease), and may have fewer or less serious unintended consequences (e.g., such an approach does not seem to undermine the importance of healthy eating and exercise).

6. Conclusions and future directions

In recent years, the general public has come to agree with public health officials who view obesity as a critical global concern. A 2012 survey found that 81% of the American public believes that obesity is an "extremely" or "very serious" problem [1]. However, recent research has found important differences between scientific and lay theories of obesity. While scientists and public health officials recognize an array of social, psychological, and physiological factors that contribute to obesity, non-experts often view the issue through a less sophisticated lens. In this chapter, we have described a variety of lay theories of obesity—focusing on trait-level beliefs, on causal models of obesity, and on personal narratives—that have important implications for the public health crisis.

At the trait level, some people think about psychological and physical attributes as relatively fixed, whereas others think of such attributes as relatively malleable. Empirical research has found that it is important for people to think of weight as malleable in order for obesity-related treatments to work. Talking about obesity as a disease, a strategy that public health officials have adopted in recent years to mitigate the stigma associated with being overweight, may, unfortunately, encourage people to think of weight as being caused by underlying physiological factors that are outside of one's control. Instead, focusing on the individual level—by describing a person who successfully loses weight through diet and exercise—may represent a more effective strategy for public health communications related to obesity. Personal narratives elicit more empathy than causal narratives. As a result, they may be able to mitigate the widespread stigma against obesity and increase support for societal-level policy interventions designed to address causes of weight gain that are outside a person's control, while at the same time encouraging people to adopt an incremental trait theory of the condition.

There are a number of opportunities for future research based on this perspective. One goal of future work should be to consider how personal narratives for obesity affect causal and trait theories of the condition in more detail. For instance, how does a personal narrative about successful weight loss affect people who think of obesity as a disease? What is the most effective way to characterize a causal model of obesity that balances the complex suite of factors that have contributed to the rise of obesity? Another goal will be to figure out how to integrate theoretical and experimental research into scalable public health-messaging campaigns, putting what we now understand about lay theories of obesity—and how to change them—into practice.

Author details

Paul H. Thibodeau[1*] and Stephen J. Flusberg[2]

*Address all correspondence to: paul.thibodeau@oberlin.edu

1 Department of Psychology, Oberlin College, Oberlin, OH, USA

2 Department of Psychology, Purchase College, SUNY, Purchase, NY, USA

References

[1] Mendes, E. (2012). Americans' Concerns about Obesity Soar, Surpass Smoking. http://www.gallup.com/poll/155762/americans-concerns-obesity-soar-surpasssmoking.aspx

[2] Bray, G. A. (2004). Medical consequences of obesity. *The Journal of Clinical Endocrinology & Metabolism, 89,* 2583–2589.

[3] NIH. (2012). Overweight and obesity statistics. Retrieved Aug 22, 2016: https://www.niddk.nih.gov/health-information/health-statistics/Pages/overweight-obesity-statistics.aspx

[4] Fontaine K. R., & Barofsky I. (2001). Obesity and health-related quality of life. *Obesity Review, 2,* 173–182.

[5] Jensen, G. L. (2005). Obesity and functional decline: epidemiology and geriatric consequences. *Clinics in Geriatric Medicine, 21,* 677–687.

[6] Withrow, D., & Alter, D. A. (2011). The economic burden of obesity worldwide: a systematic review of the direct costs of obesity. *Obesity Reviews, 12,* 131–141.

[7] Wang, Y., & Beydoun, M. A. (2007). The obesity epidemic in the Unites States – gender, age, socioeconomic, racial/ethnic, and geographic characteristics; a systematic review and meta-regression analysis. *Epidemiological Review, 29,* 6–28.

[8] Furnham, A., & Manning, R. (1997). Young people's theories of anorexia nervosa and obesity. *Counselling Psychology Quarterly, 10*(4), 389–414.

[9] Allison, D. B., Downey, M., Atkinson, R. L., Billington, C. J., Bray, G. A., Eckel, R. H., Finkelstein, E. A., Jensen, M. D., & Tremblay, A. (2008). Obesity as a disease: A white paper on evidence and arguments commissioned by the Council of the Obesity Society. *Obesity, 16,* 1161–1177.

[10] Barry, C. L., Brescoll, V. L., Brownell, K. D., & Schlesinger, M. (2009). Obesity metaphors: How beliefs about the causes of obesity affect support for public policy. *Milbank Quarterly, 87*(1), 7–47.

[11] McFerran, B., & Mukhopadhyay, A. (2013). Lay theories of obesity predict actual body mass. *Psychological Science, 24,* 1428–1436.

[12] Kwan, S. (2012). Lay perspectives on the biomedical paradigm on 'obesity': Theorizing weight, health and happiness. *Social Theory & Health, 10,* 61–77.

[13] Jansen, M. W., Van Oers, H. A., Kok, G., & De Vries, N. K. (2010). Public health: Disconnections between policy, practice and research. *Health Research Policy and Systems, 8*(1):37.

[14] Rowe, G., & Frewer, L. J. (2000). Public participation methods: A framework for evaluation. *Science, Technology & Human Values, 25,* 3–29.

[15] Hoyt, C. L., Burnette, J. L., & Auster-Gussman, L. (2014). "Obesity is a disease" examining the self-regulatory impact of this public-health message. *Psychological Science, 25,* 997–1002.

[16] Niederdeppe, J., Shapiro, M. A., Kim, H. K., Bartolo, D., & Porticella, N. (2014). Narrative persuasion, causality, complex integration, and support for obesity policy. *Health Communication, 29*(5), 431–444.

[17] Thibodeau, P. H., Perko, V. L., & Flusberg, S. J. (2015). The relationship between narrative classification of obesity and support for public policy interventions. *Social Science & Medicine, 141,* 27–35.

[18] Fothergill E. et al. (2016). Persistent metabolic adaptation 6 years after "The biggest loser competition. *Obesity, 24,* 1612–1619.

[19] Mann, T. (2015). *Secrets from the eating lab: The science of weight loss, the myth of willpower, and why you should never diet again.* New York: Harper Collins Publishers.

[20] Aamodt, S. (May 6, 2016). Why you can't lose weight on a diet. *New York Times.* Retrieved Aug 20, 2016: http://www.nytimes.com/2016/05/08/opinion/sunday/why-you-cant-lose-weight-on-a-diet.html?_r=0

[21] Dweck CS. 2000. *Self Theories: Their Role in Motivation, Personality, and Development.* New York, NY: Psychology Press.

[22] Dweck, C. (2006). *Mindset: The New Psychology of Success.* New York, NY: Random House.

[23] Beruchashvili, M., Moisio, R., & Heisley, D. D. (2014). What are you dieting for? The role of lay theories in dieters' goal setting. *Journal of Consumer Behaviour, 13*(1), 50–59.

[24] Lakoff, G. (2002). *Moral Politics: How Conservatives and Liberals Think.* Chicago: University of Chicago Press.

[25] Niederdeppe, J., Shapiro, M. A., & Porticella, N. (2011). Attributions of responsibility for obesity: Narrative communication reduces reactive counterarguing among liberals. *Human Communication Research, 37*(3), 295-323.

[26] Neumark-Sztainer, D., Story, M., & Harris, T. (1999). Beliefs and attitudes about obesity among teachers and school health care providers working with adolescents. *Journal of Nutrition Education, 31,* 3–9.

[27] Stone, D. (1988). *Policy Paradox and Political Reason.* Glenview, IL: Scott Foresman.

[28] Kersh, R., & Morone, J. (2002). The politics of obesity: seven steps to government action. *Health Affairs, 21,* 142–153.

[29] Ablow, K. (2013). Obesity is not a disease -- and neither is alcoholism. Fox News. Available at: http://www.foxnews.com/health/2013/06/20/dr-keith-ablow-obesity-is-not-disease-and-neither-is-alcoholism/

[30] Brescoll, V. L., Kersh, R., & Brownell, K. D. (2008). Assessing the feasibility and impact of federal childhood obesity policies. *The Annals of the American Academy of Political and Social Science, 615,* 178–194.

[31] Harris, M. B., & Smith, S. D. (1982). Beliefs about obesity: Effects of age, ethnicity, sex and weight. *Psychological Reports, 51,* 1047–1055.

[32] Furnham, A. (1988). *Lay Theories: Everyday Understanding of Problems in the Social Sciences.* Oxford: Pergamon Press.

[33] Salafia, E. H. B., Jones, M. E., Haugen, E. C., & Schaefer, M. K. (2015). Perceptions of the causes of eating disorders: A comparison of individuals with and without eating disorders. *Journal of Eating Disorders, 3,* 1–10.

[34] AMA press release. (2013). Available at: http://www.ama- assn.org/ama/pub/news/news/2013/2013-06-18-new-ama-policies-annual-meeting.page

[35] Jung, R. T. (1997). Obesity as a disease. *British Medical Bulletin, 53*(2), 307–321.

[36] Via, M. A. & Mechanick, J. I. (2014). Obesity as a disease. *Current Obesity Reports, 3*(291), 291–297. doi: 10.1007/s13679-014-0108-9.

[37] Puhl, R. M., & Liu, S. (2015). A national survey of public views about the classification of obesity as a disease. *Obesity, 23*(6), 1288–1295.

[38] Dar-Nimrod, I., Cheung, B. Y., Ruby, M. B., & Heine, S. J. (2014). Can merely learning about obesity genes affect eating behavior? *Appetite, 81*, 269–276.

[39] Hardman, C. A., Rogers, P. J., Dallas, R., Scott, J., Ruddock, H. K., & Robinson, E. (2015). "Food addiction is real." The effects of exposure to this message on self-diagnosed food addiction and eating behaviour. *Appetite, 91*, 179–184.

[40] Ruddock, H. K., Christiansen, P., Jones, A., Robinson, E., Field, M., & Hardman, C. A. (2016). Believing in food addiction: Helpful or counterproductive for eating behavior? *Obesity, 24*(6), 1238–1243.

[41] Niederdeppe, J., Roh, S., & Shapiro, M.A. (2015). Acknowledging individual responsibility while emphasizing social determinants in narratives to promote obesity-reducing public policy: A randomized experiment. *PLoS One, 10*, e0117565.

[42] Thibodeau, P. H., Thompson, B., Uri, R., & Flusberg, S. J. (Under review). Narratives for obesity: Effects of weight loss and attribution on empathy and policy support.

[43] Gollust, S. E., Niederdeppe, J., & Barry, C. L. (2013). Framing the consequences of childhood obesity to increase public support for obesity prevention policy. *American Journal of Public Health, 103*(11), e96–e102.

[44] Braverman, J. (2008). Testimonials versus informational persuasive messages: The moderating effect of delivery mode and personal involvement. *Communication Research, 35*, 666–694.

[45] Busselle, R., & Bilandzic, H. (2008). Fictionality and perceived realism in experiencing stories: A model of narrative comprehension and engagement. *Communication Theory, 18*(2), 255–280.

[46] Slater, M. D., & Rouner, D. (2002). Entertainment—education and elaboration likelihood: Understanding the processing of narrative persuasion. *Communication Theory, 12*, 173–191.

[47] Brochu, P. M., & Esses, V. M. (2009). Weight prejudice and medical policy: support for an ambiguously discriminatory policy is influenced by prejudice-colored glasses. *Analyses of Social Issues and Public Policy, 9*(1), 117–133.

[48] Thomas, S., Hyde, J., & Komesaroff, P. (2007). "Cheapening the struggle:" Obese people's attitudes towards The Biggest Loser. *Obesity Management, 3*, 210-215.

[49] Yoo, J. H. (2013). No clear winner: Effects of The Biggest Loser on the stigmatization of obese persons. *Health Communication, 28*(3), 294–303.

[50] Tomiyama, A.J., & Mann, T. (2013). If shaming reduced obesity, there would be no fat people. *Hastings Center Report, 43*, 4–5.

[51] Carey, S. (1985). *Conceptual Change in Childhood.* Cambridge, MA: Massachusetts Institute of Technology Press.

[52] Gelman, S. A. (1988). The development of induction within natural kind and artifact categories. *Cognitive Psychology, 20,* 65–95.

[53] Medin, D. L. (1989). Concepts and conceptual structure. *American Psychologist, 44*(12), 1469–1481.

[54] Kogut, T., & Ritov, I. (2005). The "identified victim" effect: An identified group, or just a single individual? *Journal of Behavioral Decision Making, 18,* 157–167.

[55] Batson, C. D., Dyck, J. L., Brandt, J. R., Batson, J. G., Powell, A. L., McMaster, M. R., & Griffitt, C. (1988). Five studies testing two new egoistic alternatives to the empathy-altruism hypothesis. *Journal of Personality and Social Psychology, 55*(1), 52–77.

[56] Regan, D. T., & Totten, J. (1975). Empathy and attribution: Turning observers into actors. *Journal of Personality and Social Psychology, 32,* 850–856.

13

Obesity and Anesthesia Management

Ismail Demirel, Esef Bolat and Aysun Yıldız Altun

Abstract

The prevalence of obesity is rapidly increasing throughout the world. Correspondingly, anesthetic procedures in obese patients are also increasing due to both treatment of obesity and other surgical problems of obese patients. Anesthesia-related complications are also seen in obese patients than in normal-weighted population. The importance of anesthetic applications in obese patients originates from physiological and pharmacokinetic alterations. Inhalation of these patients via mask or intubation during general anesthesia may be difficult or even impossible. Determination of extubation time after awakening from anesthesia is also a critical decision. Sleep apnea syndrome and postoperative atelectasis are more common in obese patients than in normal-weighted population. Another vital complication that should be emphasized is thromboembolism, whose incidence and severity may be decreased by pharmacological and functional preventive modalities. This patient population has elevated risk of perioperative mortality and morbidity. Prior to any elective surgical procedure, an obese patient should be thoroughly evaluated to check medical conditions that may increase perioperative mortality risk. Since anesthesiologists will gradually encounter more obese patients, they need a better comprehending of the difficulties of obesity during anesthetic procedures and taking more preventive measures for their patients to avoid complications, or rendering them less traumatic, if any.

Keywords: obesity, airway management, drug dosages, perioperative management, postoperative analgesia

1. Introduction

Though obesity is not a newly emerging problem with its epidemic character at both public and individual levels, there has been recent increase in the number of successful surgical interventions with low likelihood of serious morbidity. Body weight of more than 50% of adults in the United States (US) is 20% more than the body weight regarded optimum for the height. The percentage of such adults has increased from 30 to 50% just in 18 years [1].

Overweight has been defined as an excess of total or expected "normal" body weight, including all tissue components (muscle, bone, water, and fat) of body composition. In practice, the terms obesity and overweight are often used interchangeably to refer to excess body fat, but ideally an index of obesity should reflect only excess adipose tissue and be independent of height, body fluids, and muscle, and skeletal mass.

Body mass index (BMI) is now the standard measure for describing different categories of obesity. It must always be remembered that BMI is an indirect measure of obesity since it only considers height and weight, irrespective of the source of any additional weight. BMI is calculated by dividing patient weight (kilograms, kg) by the square of their height (meters, m); BMI = kg/m^2. An increased BMI can be present from any cause of excess weight (body building, ascites, and very large tumor) even in the absence of additional fat. The United States and many countries classify obesity according to BMI, as shown in **Table 1** [2].

BMI	
<20 kg/m²	Underweight
20–25 kg/m²	Normal
26–29 kg/m²	Overweight
30–39 kg/m²	Obese
≥40 kg/m²	Morbid obese
≥50 kg/m²	Super-obese
≥60 kg/m²	Super-super obese
World Health Organization (WHO) classification: BMI	
30–34.9 kg/m²	Class I
35–39.9 kg/m²	Class II
>40 kg/m²	Class III

Body mass index (BMI) = weight (kilograms, kg) divided by the square of height (meters, m); BMI = Wt (kg)/Ht (m^2).

Table 1. Classification of obesity by body mass index (BMI).

While many obesity complications that pose threat to perioperative period (e.g., airway difficulties or joint problems) may be observed by physical inspection, other complications such as sleep apnea, systemic and pulmonary hypertension, and diabetes mellitus should be comprehensively assessed by careful anamnesis, physical examination, and laboratory tests. Obesity itself, its complications and treatment, is also important for the anesthesiologist. An individual who has 30% excessive weight has a 40% increased mortality risk due to heart disease and a 50% increased mortality risk due to stroke. Hospital costs are also higher in obesity, with increased risk of perioperative morbidity and mortality [3].

Preoperative assessments make perioperative period more efficient, decrease anxiety of both healthcare providers and cared patients, and make patients have realistic expectations which increase satisfaction from pain management and entire perioperative experience. Obesity is a health problem associated with many medical conditions (**Table 2**). Preoperative assessment allows for detection of possible interindividual differences in terms of physiology of airways, pulmonary system, cardiovascular system, metabolic system, and nervous system. Another benefit is the important contribution of anesthesiologists to surgeons in terms of patient's psychological attitude and preparation [4].

Organ system	
Respiratory	Restrictive lung disease, asthma, obstructive sleep apnea (OSA), obesity hyperventilation syndrome (OHS)
Cardiovascular	Hypertension, cardiomyopathy, congestive heart failure, coronary artery disease, peripheral vascular disease, thromboembolism, sudden death
Endocrine/metabolic	Type 2 diabetes mellitus, Cushing's syndrome, hypothyroidism, hyperlipidemia, vitamin deficiencies
Gastrointestinal	Hiatal hernia, inguinal and umbilical hernia, fatty liver, gallbladder stones
Musculoskeletal	Osteoarthritis on weight-bearing joints, low-back pain
Malignancy	Breast, prostate, cervix, uterus, colorectal
Psychiatric	Depression, low self-esteem

Table 2. Obesity-related medical conditions.

2. Preoperative assessment

It is essential to provide a clinical setting that makes obese patients feel comfortable with respect to physical conditions. Outpatient setting or room should be designed according to overweight/obese patients. Primary physicians or surgeons of the patients should not believe mistakenly that they have adequate knowledge about their patients' medical situation. Comorbidities or other accompanying diseases may not frequently be well-documented. Preoperative assessment by anesthesiologist should include the presence of hyperglycemia or type 2 diabetes mellitus, hyperlipidemia, hypertension, coronary artery disease, respiratory problems, liver disease, and obstructive sleep apnea (OSA). As per indicated surgical procedure, impacts of osteoarthritis should be considered regarding positioning of patient especially during elective surgery [5].

An often overlooked, albeit important issue is the evaluation of medical reasons for obesity. Incidence of endocrine disease other than type 2 diabetes mellitus was reported as 47.4% among morbidly obese patients considered for bariatric surgery. Prevalence of hypothyroidism, pituitary diseases, and Cushing's syndrome is shown to be 18.1, 1.9, and 16.3%, respectively. Newly established endocrine diseases are present in 16.3% of all patients [6].

Psychological tests of morbidly obese patients frequently revealed depression, social impairment, and loss of interest in interindividual behaviors. Physicians should be aware of the likelihood of the presence of psychosocial problems in obese patients during the perioperative period [7].

Routine laboratory tests indicated for obese patients are summarized in **Table 3**. If the obese patient had history of bariatric surgery such as gastric bypass or other which represents a potential for malabsorption, a significant protein, vitamin, iron, or calcium deficiency may be present. Therefore, further additional tests are required in such patients to assess metabolic alterations (**Table 4**) [8].

Anesthesiologist should question all current medication of the patient, including over-the-counter and prescribed appetite-stimulating and weight-lowering drugs since most of these agents are associated with serious heart and lung problems and important morbidity and mortality (**Table 5**) [8].

Fasting plasma glucose
Lipid profile
Electrolytes including sodium, potassium, calcium, and phosphorus
Liver function tests including AST, ALT, total, and direct bilirubin
Renal function tests including creatinine level
Complete blood cell count
Ferritin
Vitamin B12
Thyroid stimulating hormone (TSH)
25-Hydroxy vitamin D level
Testosterone level
Electrocardiogram (ECG)
Especially in >55-year-old women and >45-year-old men who has established or suspected heart disease or at higher risk for heart disease
P-A chest X-ray
Especially in >60-year-old patients with established or suspected lung or heart disease
Polysomnography
Other clinically indicated additional tests, such as echocardiography

Table 3. Routine preoperative tests for obese patients.

2.1. Assessment and optimization of airways and pulmonary system

Factors increasing perioperative risks in obese patients in terms of airways and pulmonary system include airway anatomy, rapid desaturation developed during anesthesia induction secondary to reduced functional residual capacity (FRC), tendency to desaturation in supine position, need for induction and recovery in vertical position, tendency to sleep apnea, chronic respiratory insufficiency, pulmonary hypertension, predisposition to deep venous thrombosis and its consequences, and need for active participation to encourage for postoperative mobilization [9].

Test	Month 6	Month 12	Month 18	Month 24	Afterwards
Complete blood count	√	√	√	√	√
Biochemistry profile	√	√	√	√	√
Iron	√	√	√	√	√
Magnesium	√	√	√	√	√
Albumin	√	√		√	√
Vitamin B12	√	√	√	√	√
Vitamin D		√	√	√	√
Other lipid soluble vitamins		√		√	√
Parathyroid hormone	√		√		√
Folate		√		√	√
Bone density		√		√	√
Lipid panel		√			
Uric acid		√			
Vitamin K		√			

Table 4. Preoperative laboratory tests recommended for patients with history of bariatric surgery.

Obesity is a common and important risk factor for obstructive sleep apnea (OSA). A near two-unit increment in BMI raises the probability of OSA by fourfold. While the prevalence of OSA in general population is 2 and 4% in women and men, respectively, it ranges from 3 to 25% and 40 to 78% in morbidly obese women and men, respectively. Sleep apnea in obese patients has usually obstructive character and originated from airway stenosis secondary to excessive amount of peripharyngeal adipose tissue and from reduction of upper airway muscle tonus during rapid eye movement (REM) sleep. BMI, neck diameter, lung function tests (LFT), arterial blood gas measurement during daytime room air, and sleep-related complaints could not adequately predict the presence and severity of OSA in obese patients [10].

Definitive diagnosis of OSA is established by polysomnography, where following criteria should be fulfilled: occurrence of ≥5 apneic events (≥10 s interruption of air flow despite attempting to breath) or ≥15 hypopneic events (>50% reduction of air flow for ≥10 s) per hour during 7-h sleep test. Apneic/hypopneic index (AHI) shows the total number of apneic and/or hypopneic events per slept hour. The severity of OSA is directly correlated with the increase in AHI [11].

The determination of OSA in obese patients has two important implications. First, patients with OSA are more prone to the suppressive effects of hypnotics and opioids on airway muscle tonus and respiration [12]. Postoperative parenteral or neuraxial opioid use may lead to respiratory complications that may result in death or potentially fatal events [13, 14]. Second, OSA complicates laryngoscopy and mask ventilation [15]. Moreover, oxygen stores are decreased due to reduced expiratory reserve volume (ERV) in obese patients [16]. Combination of these factors predispose to serious problems in airways.

Drug	Implications for anesthetic procedures (reported adverse effects)
Diethylpropion	Pulmonary hypertension and psychosis.
Dexfenfluramine	Associated with pulmonary hypertension and cardiac valve disease.
Fenfluramine	Associated with pulmonary hypertension and cardiac valve disease.
Fluoxetine	Selective serotonin reuptake inhibitor. Associated with diarrhea, nausea, headache, and dry mouth. Bradycardia, hemorrhage, convulsion, hyponatremia, hepatotoxicity, and extrapyramidal effects were reported.
Mazindol	Pulmonary hypertension, atrial fibrillation, and syncope episodes were reported.
Metformin	No adverse effect was reported.
Orlistat	Diarrhea and reduced levels of lipid-soluble vitamins were reported.
Phentermine	Association with cardiopulmonary problems could not be excluded.
Phenylpropanolamine	Increases risk of hemorrhagic stroke.
Sibutramine	May lead to mild increases in blood pressure and heart rate. Associated with arrhythmia and hypertension, which is likely to be related to cardiac arrest and stroke.
Diuretics	Hypovolemia, hypokalemia.
Herbal products	
Chitosan	No adverse effect was reported.
Chromium	No adverse effect was reported.
Ephedra	Hypertension, psychiatric symptoms, autonomic dysfunction, gastrointestinal symptoms.
Hydroxycitric acid	No adverse effect was reported.
Pyruvate	Death was reported in a patient with restrictive cardiomyopathy.

Table 5. Weight lowering drugs.

Anamnesis is the easiest way of evaluation of OSA in the preoperative period in patients who did not undergo polysomnography before. Such useful data could be obtained from patient's roommate or sleep partner. Anamnestic data about snoring, interruption of breathing during sleeping (a short-time attempt to inspire after apneic episodes and wheezy breathing or resuscitative nasal breathing), decreased daytime performance, morning headache, and irritability suggest sleep apnea. Systemic hypertension and increased neck diameter (>40–42 cm at cricoid cartilage level) is consistent with probable OSA diagnosis [11, 17]. Other abnormalities of OSA detected during physical examination include somnolence and mask airway and/or intubation difficulties (e.g., Mallampati class III or IV hypognathia, short thyromental distance) [12, 14, 15].

Some obese patients develop chronic daytime hypoventilation, called as obesity-hypoventilation syndrome (OHS) [18]. These patients also have chronic daytime hypoxemia ($PO_2 < 65$ mmHg), which could be easily detected by pulse oximetry at room air. Permanent hypercapnia (($PCO_2 > 45$ mmHg) in the absence of serious obstructive pulmonary disease is pathognomonic for this syndrome in obese patients. These patients usually have advanced obesity (BMI > 40 kg/m^2) and risk of OHS is markedly increased with increasing BMI [19]. Majority of patients with OHS has also OSA; however OHS is not common in OSA patients. Those patients being at the "severe" end of OHS spectrum with cor pulmonale signs and symptoms are called "Pickwickian" [10, 18].

Careful determination of concomitance of obesity and OHS or COPD is important since this combination often leads to chronic daytime hypoxemia, which in turn causes pulmonary hypertension, right ventricular hypertrophy, and/or right ventricular failure. Perioperative morbidity and mortality rates are high in these disorders (Pickwickian), where patients need to undergo many tests to guide for perioperative medical optimization and postoperative care [10, 12, 20].

In perioperative setting, oxygenation is further diminished by reduction in muscular tonus of chest wall and diaphragm following general anesthesia induction and skeletal muscle relaxation. The net effect of this on obesity is the decrease of ERV and FRC by more than 50% and consequent decrease in the number of alveoli making efficient gas exchange, compared to the preinduction phase [21]. In addition, reduction in ERV and FRC increases predisposition to postoperative atelectasis and may inhibit effective clearance of secretions.

Main source of oxygen reserve during apnea is ERV. Therefore, preoxygenation is less effective in obese patients and the time required for hemoglobin desaturation to be reduced to below 90% after apnea is shortened [22]. Obese patients in relaxed condition under anesthesia have increased likelihood of hypoxemic complication due to "reduction in apneic oxygenation reserve" and difficulty of performing positive pressured mask ventilation [15]. In patients considered for bariatric surgery, elective awake tracheal intubation may be the safest approach if there are signs for difficult intubation (e.g., insufficient visualization of posterior pharyngeal wall). Before the induction, after placing a cylinder under the scapula and a support to the occipital region of the patient and asking for full extension at atlanto-occipital joint from the patient may ease awake or conventional laryngoscopy and intubation [23].

A study showed that laryngoscopy was more difficult to perform in obese patients (BMI > 30 kg/m^2) compared to patients with normal BMI [24]. However, authors in another study did not observe any correlation between difficult intubation and BMI, though they found an association between difficult intubation and increased neck diameter (>40–42 cm) or Mallampati score of III or IV [25]. This may be explained by higher probability of incidence of both increased neck diameter and increased Mallampati class in obese patients. Moreover, since obese patients have elevated gastric secretion volume and acidity in the preoperative period, premedication is applied by administration of cimetidine, ranitidine, citric acid, sodium citrate, or metoclopramide. Some investigators suggest this as an indication for awake intubation [26].

2.2. Cardiac assessment

2.2.1. Assessment and prevention of venostasis and thromboembolism

Evaluation of venous system should be prioritized in cardiovascular assessment as implied by mortality data. Venous emboli entered into pulmonary circulation are important causes of pulmonary dysfunction with a 30-day mortality of 1–2%. Majority of 30-day perioperative mortality after bariatric surgery originates from pulmonary embolism (the number of mortality for this reason is ≥ 3 times more than the number of mortality due to anastomosis leakage and consequent sepsis) [27]. Although several agents have been used to diminish the tendency to thrombosis, no consensus has been established. Since low-molecular-weight heparin may limit options for postoperative pain management, preoperative aspirin, and following warfarin (INR 2.0–3.0) may be considered as a reasonable choice. Use of warfarin, a vitamin K antagonist, may elicit some problems during the postoperative period as many patients develop malabsorption of lipids and lipid-soluble substances, including vitamin K after Roux-en-Y gastrojejunostomy (RNYG). Optimizing warfarin dosage may become difficult due to this malabsorption, where daily adjustments are required for at least a couple of weeks [28]. Preoperative exercise, prophylaxis through antithrombotic agents and variceal socks, hematocrit count below the level of polycythemia, increased cardiac output, and early ambulation decrease the risk in this patient group. Therefore, evaluation and prophylaxis including exercise status, pharmacological treatment, absence of symptoms and signs of venous disease and absence of evidence of venous disease, optimal hydration as well as early ambulation should be targeted [29].

2.2.2. Cardiovascular assessment

Cardiac output is expected to increase by 0.01/min for every kilogram of adipose tissue. Consequently, obese patients develop hypertension and associated cardiomegaly and left ventricular failure. To measure blood pressure accurately, an appropriate-sized cuff should be selected, which may not be as easy as it seems. Obesity not only leads to parenteral access difficulty, but also complicates noninvasive blood pressure monitoring. Direct arterial monitoring may be needed for accurate and continuous tracing of blood pressure and frequent arterial blood sampling, based on the extent of cardiopulmonary reserve [30].

Cardiac reserve may be limited in obese patients, where tolerance to hypotension, hypertension, tachycardia, or volume loading-induced stress in preoperative period may be diminished. Most of patients with Pickwickian syndrome also have right-sided heart failure. For this reason, routine preoperative assessment should also include electrocardiogram (ECG) in addition to anamnesis and physical examination featuring drug treatment and cardiopulmonary problems (especially in terms of left or right ventricular hypertrophy, ischemia, and conduction defects). In cases where biventricular failure is severe and not compensated with ≥2 month lasting exercises, measurement of central vascular volume when a large volume of blood loss is expected related to surgery or coagulation status. Physical examination of peripheral venous line may also allow for planning of the possible need for central venous catheter. Some physicians prefer transesophageal echocardiography to assess central volume instead of central venous pressure (CVP) measurement [31]. There are six risk factors to predict perioperative cardiovascular morbidity:

(i) High-risk surgery (e.g., emergent, major thoracic, abdominal, and vascular surgery)

(ii) History of coronary artery disease

(iii) History of congestive heart failure

(iv) History of cerebrovascular disease

(v) Preoperative insulin treatment

(vi) Preoperative plasma creatinine level >2 mg/dL

No additional cardiac tests are required for the elective surgery of patients where these risk factors are absent [32].

2.3. Metabolic assessment

2.3.1. Diabetes mellitus

Although 15% of patients with type I diabetes mellitus has also other comorbid autoimmune diseases such as Graves' disease, Hashimoto's thyroiditis, Addison's disease, and myasthenia gravis, no such an association has been reported in terms of obesity-related diabetes [33].

Current treatment of type II diabetics is initiated with exercise and dietary changes usually. A 5–10 kg weight loss, achieved by a 20% decrease in caloric intake and elevation of daily physical activity to 30 min for a total of 8 weeks often normalize fasting blood glucose levels. Nevertheless, this step is very difficult to achieve for most of patients, and patients will eventually switch to oral hypoglycemic agents, which stimulate secretion of insulin from pancreatic β-cells and improve insulin response of tissues by reversing postbinding defect [34]. Frequently used oral agents include tolazamide, tolbutamide, glyburide, and glipizide, the two latter being sulfonylurea class. Sulfonylureas have more long-lasting glucose-lowering effects (≥24 h) and lower drug-drug interaction potential [35].

By accelerating nonenzymatic glycosylation reactions, higher glucose concentrations lead to the formation of abnormal proteins which decrease flexibility and stretching resistance in wound healing, thereby causing toxic effects. Diminished flexibility may result in stiff joint syndrome and atlanto-occipital joint fixation which could hamper intubation [36].

Anastomosis-related infections are responsible for two-thirds of postoperative complications and about 20% of perioperative mortality in patients undergoing bariatric surgery and constitute number one risk in this patient group. Experimental data show that multiple factors may increase predisposition to infection in patients with glucose intolerance. Many alterations observed in leukocyte functions of hyperglycemic diabetic patients include decreased chemotaxis, impaired phagocytic activity of granulocytes as well as diminished intracellular destruction of pneumococci and staphylococci [37]. Phagocytic functions of granulocytes improve and intracellular killing capacity become near-normal if diabetic patients are aggressively treated, ensuring a blood glucose level <250 mg/dL [38].

2.3.2. Hypocalcemia

Inadequate calcium intake is both associated with obesity and hypertension; indeed, normalization of calcium intake could improve both hypertension and eating crises that lead to obesity [39].

2.3.3. Hyperlipidemia and hypolipidemia

Dietary control is an important treatment modality in all hyperlipidemia types [40]. Clofibrate and gemfibrozil, which are used for the management of hypertriglyceridemia, may cause myopathy especially in patients with hepatic or renal disease. Clofibrate may also increase the formation of gallbladder stones. Apart from bile acids, cholestyramine also binds to oral anticoagulants, digitalis class agents, and thyroid hormones. Nicotinic acid leads to peripheral vasodilatation, which should be likely to discontinue on the day of surgery. Probucol decreases synthesis of apoprotein A1. Rare malodorous perspiration and/or QT interval prolongation are seen during probucol usage, and sudden death in animals [41].

Hypolipidemia, albeit a rare condition, is associated with neuropathy, anemia, and renal failure. Although anesthesia experience is limited in patients with hypolipidemia, following may be recommended: maintenance of caloric intake and perioperative use of intravenous protein hydrolysates and glucose [42].

2.4. Psychological assessment and psychiatric considerations

Psychological assessment is very important for a successful outcome. Not just a week, but even a whole year following the surgery is not an easy period. Each patient needs to have increased awareness and strong-minded with a dedicated attitude of diarizing his/her diet [7]. Evaluations of anesthesiologist may provide important clues. Patient should be emotionally stable. Anesthesiologist may identify several factors about failure, which include drug abuse, untreated major psychiatric disorders, compulsive eating behavior, fibromyalgia, and chronic fatigue syndrome. Investigation, detection, and sharing of any of these may prevent potential frustration of surgical team and avoid patient getting stressed [43].

2.5. Musculoskeletal system assessment and other considerations for patient positioning

Several other considerations about obesity are also important for anesthesiologist in a prognostic and perioperative manner. Appropriate positioning of the patient, binding of monitoring devices, and performing intravenous access become complicated due to excessive and extensive subcutaneous fat tissue and enlarged extremities. Furthermore, assessment of blood pressure is also more difficult compared to normal-weighted patients (difficulty of selecting appropriate cuff) [44].

Assessment of positioning of obese patients prior to the surgery may abolish some postoperative problems. In a retrospective study, incidence of postoperative ulnar neuropathy was reported to be 29% in patients with BMI > 38 kg/m^2, compared to 1% of the control group [45]. Upper brachial plexus injury may also occur secondary to excessive rotation of the head and cervical vertebra to the contralateral side. Hyperabduction of the arm on the affected side may also lead to lower nerve root injury [46].

2.6. Risk classification

According to ASA Physical Status Classification System; patients with 30 < BMI < 40 are classified as ASA II, patients with a BMI ≥40 are classified as ASA III [47]. Also, for these patients, in 2007, DeMaria et al. suggested a risk stratification tool for bariatric patients. The Obesity Surgery-Mortality Risk Score (OS-MRS) assigns one point to each of five preoperative variables: BMI ≥ 50 kg m^2, male gender, hypertension, pulmonary embolic risk factors, and age ≥45 years. A score of 0–1 is classified as "A," 2–3 as "B," and 4–5 as "C" with associated mortality risks of 0.2, 1.1, and 2.4%, respectively [30]. This system was later validated by a multicenter study of more than 4000 patients [48].

3. Intraoperative management

3.1. Positioning in morbidly obese patients

Prevalence of obesity continues to increase rapidly throughout the world [49]. Therefore, all anesthesiologists should be familiar with this issue not only for obesity surgery, but also for other types of surgery [50]. Inappropriate surgical position may lead to serious physiological problems, and even physical injuries [51, 52]. On the other hand, appropriate position may ease procedures, including especially endotracheal intubation, reduce physiological problems, and minimize neural and soft tissue injury [53].

Operation tables having a carrying capacity of near 400 kg should be used for safe anesthetic and surgical procedures in obese patients. If no special operation table is present, two standard ones having a weight-bearing capacity of 200 kg may be adjoined. Patients should be tightly bound to the table, ensuring supporting of areas prone to pressure by gels and pads. These patients may develop renal failure and potentially fatal complications at even supine positions [54, 55]. In a study, Bostanjian et al. [54] described six patients undergoing bariatric surgery, rhabdomyolysis secondary to gluteal muscle necrosis developed after supine position, where the outcomes were fatal in three of cases.

Head-elevated laryngoscopy position, which is described as the position of head and shoulders above the level of the chest, i.e., above an imaginary horizontal line joining sternal notch and external auditory canal, makes laryngoscopy and intubation easy [56]. The position where the head is lifted 25° and reverse Trendelenburg in induction anesthesia were shown to prolong apnea in obese patients without desaturation [57]. Functional residual capacity (FRC) is severely diminished in the supine position after induction of anesthesia. If the reduction in FRC exceeds closure volume, small airways become also closed, ensuing a ventilation perfusion disturbance [58].

Supine position: Switching from the sitting position to the supine position causes an increase in venous load of the heart in some patients. Reduced diaphragmatic movement by abdominal organs leads to increased respiration work, relative hypoxemia, and marked reduction in lung volumes [59]. Lung volume is further decreased in general anesthesia procedures where muscles are completely paralyzed [60]. Compared to normal-weighed patients, FRC and pulmonary compliance are reduced in the supine position in obese patients, eventually increasing ventilation/perfusion mismatch [59]. All these alterations increase as the body mass index (BMI) is elevated. Induction of the anesthesia is recommended to be performed in the lateral decubitus position to overcome these difficulties [61]. Positive end-expiratory pressure (PEEP) may improve lung functions in mechanically ventilated patients [62]. Prolonged supine position should be avoided in patients with reduced cardiac reserve since venous return to the heart is diminished by increased compression onto the inferior vena cava secondary to abdominal pressure and weight. In such cases, operation table or the patient may be turned to the side so as to decrease aortocaval compression [53, 63].

Trendelenburg position: Patient's head is below the horizontal plane in Trendelenburg position, which may increase operative exposure and decrease bleeding in selected cases. It is less tolerated than that in the supine position. In obese patients who already have limited cardiac reserves, blood in lower extremities is added into central and pulmonary circulation by Trendelenburg position, making it hard to tolerate this position [64]. It should be especially avoided in morbidly obese patients. Further diminished residual capacity and pulmonary compliance in this position also lead to atelectasis and hypoxemia. In addition, endotracheal tube may be displaced depending on the position. In brief, this position is often not preferred in obese patients due to all these factors [53, 63].

Head-upward position: Upper torso of morbidly obese patients should be nearly 35–40° in the sitting position or reverse Trendelenburg position in a way where the operation table allows for adequate ventilation. Such position simplifies mask ventilation and conditions of tracheal intubation.

The combined effect of reverse Trendelenburg position and pneumoperitoneum during laparoscopic gastric bypass surgery decreases femoral blood flow and increases venous stasis, thereby increasing risk of pulmonary embolism. Therefore, prolonged applications of this position should be avoided with altering positions occasional breaks during surgery [65].

Prone position: Prone position was shown to increase oxygenation in normal-weighed patients under anesthesia than that in supine position [66]. As long as the chest and pelvis are supported such adequately that allows for abdominal movements, prone position is usually well-tolerated by obese patients. Cardiovascular functions are preserved when appropriate position and supports are provided. Otherwise, cardiac venous return is diminished by compression onto the inferior vena cava and femoral veins, which in turn leads to decreased volume in the left ventricle, causing hypotension. Prone position in obese patients under anesthesia improves pulmonary functions and increase FRC, pulmonary compliance, and oxygenation [53, 67].

Lateral decubitus position: This position is often tolerated well by obese patients. A decrease in the abdominal fat mass' compression on the abdomen diminishes intraabdominal pressure, which eases diaphragmatic movements during mechanical ventilation. However, maintenance of the same position for a long while may lead to vascular congestion and resulting in hypoventilation in underlying lung [68].

Lithotomy position: This position causes increased venous return and cardiac output, and high risk of thromboembolism secondary to venous stasis after prolonged surgery. Another complication of this position may be the development of compartment syndrome when the lower extremities are inappropriately positioned [53, 69].

3.2. Airway management

Obesity leads to many anatomic alterations in airways. Upper thoracic and lower cervical fat pillows result in a limited range of motion in atlantoaxial joints and cervical vertebra. Excessive tissue folds in the pharynx, short and thickened neck, suprasternal, presternal, and posterior cervical fat tissue, and thick submental fat tissue are formed. All these alterations contribute to potentially difficult airway management, which has been reported as 10.3–20.2% in obese patients compared to 1.5–3.2% of general population [70]. Despite all these anatomical and pathological changes, extent of BMI did not appear to influence difficulty of laryngoscopy. This type of difficulty is rather associated with advanced age, male sex, temporomandibular joint pathology, Mallampati class III and IV, history of obstructive sleep apnea, and abnormal upper teeth [71]. Neck diameter has been defined as the best determinant for intubation difficulty in morbidly obese patients. While the probability of problematic intubation was 5% in patients with a neck diameter of 40 cm, this was found to be 35% in patients with a neck diameter of 60 cm [72]. Increased adipose tissue on pharyngeal walls in obese patients complicates mask ventilation and intubation by leading to alterations in upper airway anatomy. The presence of obstructive sleep apnea is an additional pathology that increases the risk for difficult intubation, hence warranting careful consideration in this patient population [73].

The prevalence of aspiration is low in obese patients, though risk of aspiration-related pulmonary complication is known to be increased in this group [74]. Gastroesophageal reflux that may cause aspiration is common in obese patients. Attention should be paid in patients with history of gastric band application especially in terms of aspiration [64].

Intraoperative ideal ventilation strategies are still contradictory in morbidly obese patients, where diminished lung and thorax compliance is particularly important. The increased amount of thoracic fat tissue is associated with decreased FRC that may be increased by elevation of upper torso though this may not provide an increment as effective as in normal-weighed people [75]. While lung volume is not altered, respiratory load, oxygen consumption, and carbon dioxide synthesis are increased following diminution of lung and thorax compliance, which in turn leads to decreased tolerance to respiratory stress. By causing cyclic alveolar collapse, low FRC and unchanged closure volume induce alveolar injury associated with mechanical ventilation [29]. These patients have predisposition for postoperative atelectasis. An association between the extent of atelectasis and the incidence of postoperative ARDS was also demonstrated [76]. An adequate PEEP administration is important to decrease probability of atelectasis during mechanical ventilation. In obese patients, PEEP provides beneficial effects both on PaO_2 and alveolar-arterial oxygen difference, even these benefits were shown to be more prominent as compared to normal-weighed people [15].

Studies showed that applications of PEEP of 10–15 cm H_2O, lung-protective low tidal volume of 6–8 ml/kg, and pressure limit below 30 cm H_2O proved to be beneficial to obese patients [77]. Combined use of recruitment maneuvers and PEEP revealed better effects on intraoperative oxygenation and compliance compared with PEEP use alone during obesity surgery or in surgical obese patients. A meta-analysis reported that pressure-controlled ventilation and volume-controlled ventilation did not differ in terms of outcomes [78].

3.3. Induction and maintenance

All agents used in anesthesia may also be used in obese patients. However, obesity alters pharmacokinetic parameters depending on the lipid solubility and tissue distribution of the administered anesthetic agent. Nonadipose mass is also increased in obese patients. Drug dosages should be adjusted by considering volume of distribution for loading dose and by considering clearance for maintenance dose. Obese people may highly metabolize lipophilic agents compared to underweight people. Pharmacokinetic studies show that weakly or intermediately lipophilic drugs (e.g., vecuronium) are mainly distributed into nonadipose tissues and the dose needs to be calculated according to the ideal body weight. If the clearance is equal to or less than nonobese patients, the ideal body weight should be taken into account for maintenance dose. If the clearance is increased with obesity, then the total body weight should be considered for maintenance dose.

The ideal body weight is calculated as the sum of 49.9 and 0.89 kg for each cm above the height of 152.4 cm in men, and as the sum of 45.4 and 0.89 kg for each cm above the height of 152.4 cm in women. Agents partially distributed into the adipose tissue have variable pharmacokinetic characteristics; they usually have prolonged and unpredictable effects due to altered volume of distribution and clearance rates, respectively [79].

3.4. Induction agents

3.4.1. Thiopental sodium

Thiopental sodium, a frequently used agent for the induction of general anesthesia, is rapidly distributed to highly perfused organs such as brain, liver, lung, intestines, kidneys, heart, and pancreas after bolus administration into the plasma. Reduced plasma concentration and consequent loss of its effect after a short while depends on its rapid distribution to peripheral tissues. High lipophilicity of thiopental increases its volume of distribution and elimination half-life in obese patients. Due to uptake by fatty tissues, its plasma levels decrease within 10 min after induction and the agent is eliminated via liver. A clearance rate of the drug increases twofold in obese patients compared to patients with normal weight. It is reported that administration of the drug according to nonfat body weight is more reasonable for the purposes of induction anesthesia. Nevertheless, increased cardiac output leads to more rapid distribution of thiopental from its effective compartment into the plasma, hence causing an accelerated awaking in procedures where it is administered as single-dose bolus [5, 11].

3.4.2. Propofol

Although propofol has a high lipophilicity, dose adjustment should be performed according to the total body weight due to its high clearance [80]. Its high lipophilicity and rapid distribution from plasma into peripheral tissue render it as the currently most commonly used induction agent in morbidly obese patients. It could be used safely as total intravenous anesthetic drug. Its short-acting nature after single-dose bolus administration is explained by its redistribution from the compartment it acts on, into the plasma and peripheral tissues. As in thiopental sodium, cardiac output is also an important marker in achieving peak plasma concentrations of this agent. When administered as continuous infusion in obese patients, both its volume of distribution and clearance increases along with increased total body weight [53, 59].

3.4.3. Etomidate

Use of etomidate should be considered in patients with hemodynamic instability. Its use is contradictory due to increased incidence of end-organ dysfunction and in-hospital mortality secondary to adrenal suppressive effects in patients administered etomidate for anesthesia induction. Its induction dose should be adjusted by nonfat body weight due to similar pharmacokinetic and pharmacodynamic properties to propofol and thiopental [53, 59].

3.4.4. Opioids

Opioids were quite commonly used to control sympathetic response to tracheal intubation and surgical stress during induction and maintenance of the anesthesia. These agents effectively block the response to nociceptive stimulation in the perioperative period. Increased cardiac output and alteration in body composition (increased fatty tissue and nonfat body weight) in obese patients may change pharmacokinetic properties of the opioids. Administration of opioids leads to upper airway obstruction, central sleep apnea, obstructive sleep apnea, ataxic respiration, and hypoxemia [53, 59].

Fentanyl, one of the most frequently used opioids in anesthesia, has a significantly higher clearance in obese patients, which exhibits a nonlinear increase with the total body weight [53, 59]. As fentanyl, the onset of action of sufentanyl is 3–5 min. Although it has similar plasma clearance, its volume of distribution and elimination half-life is increased in obese patients compared to normal-weighed patients [53, 59, 81].

Alfentanyl, a derivative of fentanyl, has one-tenth of the potency than that of fentanyl. It is more lipophilic and has lower volume of distribution than that in fentanyl. Increased cardiac output decreases concentration of plasma alfentanyl during early distribution phase [53, 59, 81].

Remifentanyl is an ester opioid, which is rapidly metabolized by tissue and plasma esterases. Its administration by continuous infusion is widely adopted. Effects will terminate within 5–10 min after cessation of the infusion, which should be given adjusted to the ideal body weight. Administration of remifentanyl based on the total body weight in obese patients may cause some adverse effects such as bradycardia, hypotension, and muscle rigidity due to supratherapeutic plasma concentrations [53, 59, 81].

3.5. Inhalation agents

Release of inhalation agents is increased due to high solubility in lipids and excessive fat tissue. Furthermore, obese patients were reported to have slow recovery from anesthesia because of extended release of the inhalation agent from adipose tissue [81, 82]. In fact, this slow recovery not only originates from accumulation in adipose tissue but also from increased sensitivity in central nervous system secondary to decreased blood flow in adipose tissue. On the other hand, duration of recovery after procedures of 2–4 h was reported to be similar between obese and nonobese patients [83]. Recovery time after desflurane and sevoflurane, which have low lipid solubility, is also rapid in obese patients [84]. Torri et al. [85] compared obese and nonobese patients and reported that alveolar and inspiratory sevoflurane concentrations were not much changed, yet exhaling of sevoflurane from alveoli was slower in obese patients.

3.5.1. Isoflurane

Isoflurane is more lipophilic than sevoflurane and desflurane, therefore not commonly used in obese patients. Blood flow is decreased as long as the body weight increases. In clinical practice, impact of body mass index on uptake of isoflurane is not clinically relevant [59, 81].

3.5.2. Sevoflurane

Having low lipophilicity and solubility, sevoflurane is rapidly absorbed and eliminated compared to isoflurane [59, 81].

3.5.3. Desflurane

Desflurane, due to its limited distribution in adipose tissue and least lipophilicity and solubility among available inhalation agents, is recommended in obese patients. Nevertheless, the effect of BMI on the absorption of desflurane is not significant. Recovery and wakening from desflurane than that from isoflurane occur more rapidly in both obese and nonobese patients [59, 81].

3.6. Neuromuscular blockers

Neuromuscular blockers are polar and hydrophilic agents, so they have limited distribution in adipose tissue [86]. Except succinylcholine, administrating doses of neuromuscular blockers are usually calculated according to ideal body weight.

3.6.1. Succinylcholine

This neuromuscular blocker is a short-acting agent with a rapid onset of action. It may be preferred in obese patients in order to provide quick tracheal intubation. Pseudocholinesterase levels and extracellular fluid are elevated in obese patients, which determine the duration of action of succinylcholine and thereby warrant the need for dose adjustment with respect to the total body weight [87].

3.6.2. *Vecuronium*

Vecuronium has a nondepolarizing aminosteroid structure and is mainly eliminated via the liver and gallbladder. Since its duration of action may be prolonged when its dose is calculated according to the total body weight, the dose should be adjusted according to the ideal body weight [88].

3.6.3. *Rocuronium*

Being a weakly lipophilic and quaternary ammonium neuromuscular blocker, it is highly ionized with a limited extracellular distribution. Induction dose of 1.2 mg/kg calculated according to the ideal body weight provides excellent intubation settings within 60 s. Administration dose should be adjusted according to the ideal body weight in order to avoid prolonged drug metabolism [59, 87].

3.7. Reversal of neuromuscular blocking agents

Obese patients have increased risk due to upper airway collapse and use of neuromuscular blockers. Therefore, neuromuscular block should be completely reversed before tracheal intubation. Doses of agents reversing neuromuscular blockers should be calculated according to the total body weight. Rapid and thorough reversal of neuromuscular block is particularly important for early restoration of lung functions during early postoperative period [89].

3.7.1. *Neostigmine*

A delayed time to antagonize neuromuscular block by neostigmine has been reported in obese patients. In the study of Suzuki et al. [90], the time elapsed to make train-of-four ratio as 0.9 increased fourfold than normal to antagonize vecuronium. Block should not be reversed by neostigmine under deep neuromuscular block. Recommended dose for neostigmine is 0.04–0.08 mg/kg, whose total dose should not exceed 5 mg [89, 90].

3.7.2. *Sugammadex*

A modified and most potent derivative of cyclodextrin, sugammadex binds to steroidal muscle relaxants with high affinity. Muscle relaxants are encapsulated within lipophilic cavity. Resultant inclusion complex is excreted through kidneys. Affinity of sugammadex to rocuronium is higher than to either pancuronium or vecuronium. It has no effect on acetylcholine, endogenous steroids, or other muscle relaxing agents. It is not recommended for use in severe renal impairment. In intermediate and deep block, dose calculation is inadequate if done according to the ideal body weight; therefore, the dose needs to be adjusted by the total body weight or ideal body weight plus 40% [89, 91].

3.8. Regional anesthesia

Regional anesthesia may be preferred to avoid potentially difficult airway control or postoperative respiratory complications. Detection of landmarks for central blocks or peripheral nerve blocks is especially very compelling in morbidly obese patients. Seventh cervical vertebra or gluteal fissure may be used to identify midline for central blocks. Distribution of the local anesthetics is hard to estimate due to lipid infiltration into epidural space and increased intraabdominal pressure, in which case 75–80% of normal local anesthetic dose may suffice. Regional block practices are regarded as more difficult in obese patients. In a study of 2020 supraclavicular block applications, success rate in obese patients was 94.3% compared with 97.3% in nonobese patients, which was significantly different [92]. The prospective study by Nielsen et al. [93] with over 9000 regional block procedures showed that the failure rate was 1.62 times higher in obese patients than in nonobese patients. Block procedures may be safely performed under the guidance of ultrasonography in obese patients [93, 94].

4. Postoperative care

Obesity is associated with some problems also during postoperative period. The steps of postoperative care of an obese patient should be carefully assessed before the surgery. Postoperative care should aim to prevent from respiratory dysfunction, hypothermia, hemodynamic instability, thromboembolism, nausea, vomiting, and pain [95, 96].

Monitoring should be continued in the recovery unit, while the patient is in sitting position or the head is upward at 45°. Oxygen support should be maintained until arterial oxygen saturation values return to preoperative levels or the patient becomes completely mobilized. In order to be discharged into the ward, the patient should meet routine criteria for leaving wakening room, no hypopnea or apnea period should occur, and preoperative arterial oxygen saturation values should be reached [96].

The prevalence of myocardial infarction is higher in this group compared to nonobese population. In addition, a new onset of atrial fibrillation may be seen during postoperative period. Close monitoring of these patients should be continued also after the surgery [97, 98].

Although being rare, rhabdomyolysis is a fatal complication in this patient population. Predisposing factors include hypotension, dehydration, immobility, and prolonged surgical interventions. In particular, pain in deep tissues of gluteal region should signal rhabdomyolysis. Creatine kinase levels are elevated in such patients [99].

Obesity is a risk factor for thromboembolism, where prophylaxis is recommended in all surgical interventions, except minor surgery. While oral agents such as rivaroxaban and dabigatran are not recommended for obese patients, low-molecular-weight heparin is recommended for prophylactic purposes [96, 100].

The incidence of postoperative nausea-vomiting is not increased in obese patients, albeit a contradictory issue [101].

An effective postoperative pain management is important to prevent pulmonary complications and provides sufficient respiratory depth. Pain management through intramuscular route is not recommended in obese patients. Opioid-induced upper airway obstruction and respiratory depression are more likely to be seen in obese patients with obstructive sleep apnea. When deciding postoperative analgesia in obese patients, selecting a multimodal analgesia method rather than a unimodal method will provide more effective pain control and avoidance of potential complications [95, 96, 102].

4.1. Intensive care

Obesity was found to be associated with increased need for mechanical ventilation and longer duration of stay with tracheostomy and at intensive care unit. No increase in mortality was shown.

For mechanical ventilation, 5–7 ml/kg of tidal volume calculated according to the ideal body weight is recommended as well as maintaining a peak inspiratory pressure below 35 cm/H_2O [76, 103].

If the obese patient is hemodynamically stable and gastrointestinal system is functional, enteral route is preferred over parenteral route for nutrition. Guideline of Society of Critical Care Medicine and American Society for Parental and Enteral Nutrition reports that hypocaloric nutrition support preserves nitrogen balance and decreases morbidity in obese patients [104].

"Obesity paradox" is defined as the better prognosis of obese patients after acute cardiovascular decompensation despite the established role of the obesity for developing of cardiovascular diseases. Nevertheless, the effects of obesity on critical illness, death, or long-term outcomes are conflicting [105].

Author details

Ismail Demirel*, Esef Bolat and Aysun Yıldız Altun

*Address all correspondence to: ismaildemirel23@gmail.com

Department of Anesthesiology and Reanimation, School of Medicine, Fırat University Elazığ, Turkey

References

[1] Ogden CL, Carroll MD, Kit BK, Flegal KM. Prevalence of childhood and adult obesity in the United States, 2011-2012. JAMA 2014; 311(8): 806–814. doi: 10.1001/jama.2014.732

[2] Buchwald H. Bariatric surgery for morbid obesity: health implications for patients, health professionals, and third party payers. J Am Coll Surg. 2005; 200 (4): 593–604.

[3] Buchwald H. The evolution of metabolic/bariatric surgery. Obes Surg. 2014; 24(8): 1126–1135. doi: 10.1007/s11695-014-1354-3.

[4] Leykin Y, Pellis T, Del Mestro E, Marzano B, Fanti G, Brodsky JB. Anesthetic management of morbidly obese and super-morbidly obese patients undergoing bariatric operations: hospital course and outcomes. Obes Surg. 2006; 16(12): 1563–1569.

[5] Collazo-Clavell ML. Bariatric surgery: important considerations for the primary care provider. Compr Ther. 2008; 34(3–4): 159–165.

[6] Fierabracci P, Pinchera A, Martinelli S, Scartabelli G, Salvetti G, Giannetti M, Pucci A, Galli G, Ricco I, Querci G, Rago T, Di Salvo C, Anselmino M, Vitti P, Santini F. Prevalence of endocrine diseases in morbidly obese patients scheduled for bariatric surgery: beyond diabetes. Obes Surg. 2011; 21(1): 54–60. doi: 10.1007/s11695-010-0297-6.

[7] Zimmerman M, Francione-Witt C, Chelminski I, Young D, Boerescu D, Attiullah N, Pohl D, Roye GD, Harrington DT. Presurgical psychiatric evaluations of candidates for bariatric surgery, part 1: reliability and reasons for and frequency of exclusion. J Clin Psychol. 2007; 68(10): 1557–1562.

[8] Bernstein DP. Cardiovascular physiology. In Morbid Obesity: Peri-operative Management, 2nd edition. Alvarez A, Brodsky JB, Lemmens HJM, Morton J (Eds.), Cambridge: Cambridge University Press, 2010. pp. 1–18.

[9] Vgontzas AN, Tan TL, Bixler EO, Martin LF, Shubert D, Kales A. Sleep apnea and sleep disruption in obese patients. Arch Intern Med. 1994; 154(15): 1705–1711.

[10] Koenig SM. Pulmonary complications of obesity. Am J Med Sci. 2001; 321(4): 249–279.

[11] Sahin M, Bilgen C, Tasbakan MS, Midilli R, Basoglu OK. A clinical prediction formula for apnea-hypopnea index. Int J Otolaryngol. 2014; 2014: 438376. doi: 10.1155/2014/438376.

[12] Dhonneur G, Combes X, Leroux B, Duvaldestin P. Postoperative obstructive apnea. Anesth Analg. 1999; 89(3): 762–767.

[13] Boushra NN. Anaesthetic management of patients with sleep apnoea syndrome. Can J Anaesth. 1996; 43(11): 599–616.

[14] Orlov D, Ankichetty S, Chung F, Brull R. Cardiorespiratory complications of neuraxial opioids in patients with obstructive sleep apnea: a systematic review. J Clin Anesth. 2013; 25(7): 591–599. doi: 10.1016/j.jclinane.2013.02.015

[15] Siyam M, Benhamou D. Difficult endotracheal intubation in patients with sleep apnea syndrome. Anesth Analg. 2002; 95(4): 1098–1102.

[16] Jones RL, Nzekwu MM. The effects of body mass index on lung volumes. Chest. 2006; 130(3): 827–833.

[17] Riley RW, Powell NB, Guilleminault C, Pelayo R, Troell RJ, Li KK. Obstructive sleep apnea surgery: risk management and complications. Otolaryngol Head Neck Surg. 1997; 117(6): 648–652.

[18] Kessler R, Chaouat A, Schinkewitch P, le Faller M, Casel S, Kreiger J, Weitzenblum E. The obesity hypoventilation syndrome revisited. A prospective study of 34 consecutive cases. Chest 2001; 120(2): 369–376.

[19] Kaw R, Hernandez AV, Walker E, Aboussouan L, Mokhlesi B. Determinants of hypercapnia in obese patients with obstructive sleep apnea: a systematic review and meta-analysis of cohort studies. Chest. 2009; 136(3): 787–796. doi: 10.1378/chest.09-0615

[20] Chung SA, Yuan H, Chung F.A systemic review of obstructive sleep apnea and its implications for anesthesiologists. Anesth Analg. 2008 Nov; 107(5): 1543–1563. doi: 10.1213/ane.0b013e318187c83

[21] Pelosi P, Croci M, Ravagnan I, Cerisara M, Vicardi P, Lissoni A, Gattinoni L. Respiratory system mechanics in sedated, paralyzed, morbidly obese patients. J Appl Physiol. 1997; 82(3): 811–818.

[22] Chalhoub V, Yazigi A, Sleilaty G, Haddad F, Noun R, Madi-Jebara S, Yazbeck P. Effect of vital capacity manoeuvres on arterial oxygenation in morbidly obese patients undergoing open bariatric surgery. Eur J Anaesthesiol. 2007 Mar; 24(3): 283–288.

[23] Neligan PJ, Porter S, Max B, Malhotra G, Greenblatt EP, Ochroch EA. Obstructive sleep apnea is not a risk factor for difficult intubation in morbidly obese patients. Anesth Analg. 2009; 109(4): 1182–1186. doi: 10.1213/ane.0b013e3181b12a0c.

[24] Karkouti K, Rose DK, Wigglesworth D, Cohen MM. Predicting difficult intubation: a multivariable analysis. Can J Anaesth. 2000; 47(8): 730–739.

[25] Gonzalez H, Minville V, Delanoue K, Mazerolles M, Concina D, Fourcade O. The importance of increased neck circumference to intubation difficulties in obese patients. Anesth Analg. 2008; 106(4): 1132–1136, doi: 10.1213/ane.0b013e3181679659.

[26] Illing L, Duncan PG, Yip R. Gastroesophageal reflux during anaesthesia. Can J Anaesth. 1992; 39: 466–470.

[27] Klein S, Burke LE, Bray GA, Blair S, Allison DB, Pi-Sunyer X et al. Clinical implications of obesity with specific focus on cardiovascular disease: a statement for professionals from the American Heart Association Council on Nutrition, Physical Activity, and Metabolism: endorsed by the American College of Cardiology Foundation. Circulation 2004; 110(18): 2952–2967.

[28] Arterburn D, Schauer DP, Wise RE, Gersin KS, Fischer DR, Selwyn CA Jr, Erisman A, Tsevat J. Change in predicted 10-year cardiovascular risk following laparoscopic Roux-en-Y gastric bypass surgery. Obes Surg. 2009; 19(2): 184–189. doi: 10.1007/s11695-008-9534-7.

[29] Afolabi BA, Novaro GM, Szomstein S, Rosenthal RJ, Asher CR. Cardiovascular complications of obesity surgery in patients with increased preoperative cardiac risk. Surg Obes Relat Dis. 2009; 5(6): 653–656.

[30] DeMaria EJ, Portenier D, Wolfe L. Obesity surgery mortality risk score: proposal for a clinically useful score to predict mortality risk in patients undergoing gastric bypass. Surg Obes Relat Dis. 2007; 3(2): 134–140.

[31] Kuruba R, Koche LS, Murr MM. Preoperative assessment and perioperative care of patients undergoing bariatric surgery. Med Clin North Am. 2007; 91(3): 339–351, ix.

[32] Poirier P, Alpert MA, Fleisher LA, Thompson PD, Sugerman HJ, Burke LE et al. Cardiovascular evaluation and management of severely obese patients undergoing surgery: a science advisory from the American Heart Association. Circulation. 2009; 120(1): 86–95. doi: 10.1161/CIRCULATIONAHA.109.192575.

[33] Narayan KM, Boyle JP, Thompson TJ, Sorensen SW, Williamson DF. Lifetime risk for diabetes mellitus in the United States. J Am Med Assoc. 2003; 290(14): 1884–1890.

[34] Mayer-Davis EJ, D'Agostino R, Karter AJ, Haffner SM, Rewers MJ, Saad M. et al. Intensity and amount of physical activity in relation to insulin sensitivity. The insulin resistance atherosclerosis study. J Am Med Assoc. 1998; 279(9): 669–674.

[35] Tuomilehto J, Lindstrom J, Eriksson JG, Valle TT, Hämäläinen H, Ilanne-Parikka P. et al. Finnish diabetes prevention study group. Prevention of type 2 diabetes mellitus by changes in lifestyle among subjects with impaired glucose tolerance. N Engl J Med. 2001; 344(18): 1343–1350.

[36] Arguedas JA, Leiva V, Wright JM Blood pressure targets for hypertension in people with diabetes mellitus. Cochrane Database Syst Rev. 2013; 10: CD008277. doi: 10.1002/14651858.CD008277.pub2. Review

[37] Sunahara KK, Sannomiya P, Martins JO. Briefs on insulin and innate immune response. Cell Physiol Biochem. 2012; 29(1–2): 1–8. doi: 10.1159/000337579. Epub 2012 Mar 1.

[38] Osar Z, Samanci T, Demirel GY, Damci T, Ilkova H. Nicotinamide effects oxidative burst activity of neutrophils in patients with poorly controlled type 2 diabetes mellitus. Exp Diabesity Res. 2004; 5(2): 155–162.

[39] Teegarden, D. Calcium intake and reduction in weight or fat mass. J Nutr. 2003; 133(1): 249S–251S.

[40] Sullivan FM, Donnan PT, Love T. Whole population secondary prevention of coronary heart disease in Scotland: the HEARTS database. Stud Health Technol Inform. 2004; 107(Pt 2): 1227–1229.

[41] Rosenbaum M, Leibel RL, Hirsch J. Obesity. N Engl J Med. 1997; 337(6): 396–407.

[42] Emerging Risk Factors Collaboration, Di Angelantonio E, Sarwar N, Perry P, Kaptoge S, Ray KK et al. Major lipids, apolipoproteins, and risk of vascular disease. JAMA. 2009; 302(18): 1993–2000. doi: 10.1001/jama.2009.1619.

[43] Collazo-Clavell ML, Clark MM, McAlpine DE, Jensen MD. Assessment and preparation of patients for bariatric surgery. Mayo Clin Proc. 2006; 81(10 Suppl): S11–7.

[44] Wong AB, Moore MS. Positioning of obese patients in out-of-operating room locations. Anesth Analg. 2007; 104(5): 1306.

[45] Warner MA, Warner ME, Martin JT. Ulnar neuropathy: incidence, outcome, and risk factors in sedated and anesthetized patients. Anesthesiology 1994; 81(6): 1332–1340.

[46] Sawyer RJ, Richmond MN, Hickey JD, Jarratt JA. Peripheral nerve injuries associated with anaesthesia. Anaesthesia 2000; 55(10): 980–991.

[47] https://www.asahq.org/resources/clinical-information/asa-physical-status-classification system

[48] DeMaria EJ, Murr M, Byrne TK, et al. Validation of the obesity surgery mortality risk score in a multicenter study proves it stratifies mortality risk in patients undergoing gastric bypass for morbid obesity. Ann Surg. 2007; 246: 578–82; discussion 83–84.

[49] Kohn M, Booth M. The World Wide epidemic of obesity in adolescents. Adolesc Med. 2003; 14: 1–9.

[50] Dindo D, Muller MK, Weber M, et al. Obesity in general elective surgery. Lancet 2003; 361: 2032–2035.

[51] Buckley FP, Robinson NB, Simonowitz DA, et al. Anaesthesia in the morbidly obese. A comparison of anaesthetic and analgesic regimens for upper abdominal surgery. Anaesthesia 1983; 38: 840–851.

[52] Dominguez-Cherit G, Gonzalez R, et al. Anesthesia for morbidly obese patients. World J Surg. 1998; 22: 969–973.

[53] Cullen A, Ferguson A. Perioperative management of the severely obese patient: a selective pathophysiological. Can J Anaesth. 2012; 59(10): 974–996.

[54] Bostanjian D, Anthone GJ, Hamoui N, Crookes PF. Rhabdomyolysis of gluteal muscles leading to renal failure: a potentially fatal complication of surgery in the morbidly obese. Obes Surg. 2003; 13: 302–305.

[55] Collier B, Goreja MA, Duke BE. Postoperative rhabdomyolysis with bariatric surgery. Obes Surg. 2003; 13: 941–943.

[56] Levitan RM, Kinkle WC, Levin WJ, Everett WW. Laryngeal view during laryngoscopy: a randomized trial comparing cricoid pressure, backward upward-rightward pressure, and bimanual laryngoscopy. Ann Emerg Med. 2006; 47(6): 548–555.

[57] Dixon BJ, Dixon JB, Carden JR, Burn AJ, Schachter LM, Playfair JM, et al. Preoxygenation is more effective in the 25 degrees head-up position than in the supine position in severely obese patients: a randomized controlled study. Anesthesiology 2005; 102(6): 1110–1115.

[58] Salome CM, King GG, Berend N. Physiology of obesity and effects on lung function. J Appl Physiol. 2010; 108(1): 206–211.

[59] Mandal S, Hart N. Respiratory complications of obesity. Clin Med. 2012; 12: 75–78.

[60] Rehder K. Postural changes in respiratory function. Acta Anaesthesiol Scand. 1998; 113: 13–16.

[61] Aono J, Ueda K, Ueda W, et al. Induction of anaesthesia in the lateral decubitus position in morbidly obese patients. Br J Anaesth. 1999; 83(2): 356.

[62] Pelosi P, Ravagnan I, Giurati G, et al. Positive end expiratory pressure improves respiratory function in obese but not in normal subjects during anesthesia and paralysis. Anesthesiology 1999; 91: 1221–1231.

[63] Brodsky JB. Positioning the morbidly obese patient for anesthesia. Obes Surg. 2002; 12(6): 751–758.

[64] Benedik PS, Baun MM, Keus L, Jimenez C, Morice R, Bidani A, Meininger JC. Effects of body position on resting lung volume in overweight and mildly to moderately obese subjects. Respir Care. 2009; 54(3): 334–339.

[65] Nguyen NT, Cronan M, Braley S, et al. Duplex ultrasound assessment of femoral venous flow during laparoscopic and open gastric bypass. Surg Endosc 2003; 17: 285–290.

[66] Mure M, Domino KB, Lindhahl SG, et al. Regional ventilation–perfusion distribution is more uniform in the prone position. J Appl Physiol. 2000; 88: 1076–1083.

[67] Brodsky JB, Oldroyd M, Winfield HN, Kozlowski PM. Morbid obesity and the prone position: a case report. J Clin Anesth. 2001; 13(2): 138–140.

[68] Lohser J, Kulkarni V, Brodsky JB. Anesthesia for thoracic surgery in morbidly obese patients. Curr Opin Anaesthesiol. 2007; 20(1): 10–14.

[69] Domi R, Laho H. Anesthetic challenges in the obese patient. J Anesth. 2012; 26(5): 758–765.

[70] Ogunnaike BO, Jones SB, Jones DB, Provost D, Whitten CW. Anesthetic considerations for bariatric surgery. Anesth Analg. 2002; 95(6): 1793–1805.

[71] Ezri T, Medalion B, Weisenberg M, Szmuk P, Warters RD, Charuzi I. Increased body mass per se is not a predictor of difficult laryngoscopy. Can J Anaesth. 2003; 50(2): 179–183.

[72] Nguyen NT, Ho HS, Fleming NW, Moore P, Lee SJ, Goldman CD, et al. Cardiac function during laparoscopic vs open gastric bypass. Surg Endosc. 2002; 16(1): 78–83.

[73] Lundstrøm LH, Møller AM, Rosenstock C, Astrup G, Wetterslev J. High body mass index is a weak predictor for difficult and failed tracheal intubation: a cohort study of 91,332 consecutive patients scheduled for direct laryngoscopy registered in the Danish Anesthesia Database. Anesthesiology 2009; 110: 266–274.

[74] Engelhardt T, Webster NR. Pulmonary aspiration of gastric contents in anaesthesia. Br J Anaesth. 1999; 83: 453–460.

[75] Sebbane M, El Kamel M, Millot A, Jung B, Lefebvre S, Rubenovitch J, Mercier G, Eledjam JJ, Jaber S, Hayot M. Effect of weight loss on postural changes in pulmonary function in obese subjects: a longitudinal study. Respir Care. 2015 Jul; 60(7): 992–999. doi: 10.4187/respcare.03668. Epub 2015 Apr 7.

[76] Miller PR, Croce MA, Bee TK et al. ARDS after pulmonary contusion: accurate measurement of contusion volume identifies high-risk patients. J Trauma 2001 Aug; 51(2):223–228; discussion 229-30..

[77] Huschak G, Busch T, Kaisers UX. Obesity in anesthesia and intensive care. Best Pract Res Clin Endocrinol Metab. 2013; 27: 247–260.

[78] Aldenkortt M, Lysakowski C, Elia N, Brochard L, Tramer MR. Ventilation strategies in obese patients undergoing surgery: a quantitative systematic review and meta-analysis. Br J Anaesth. 2012; 109(4): 493–502. http://dx.doi.org/10.1093/bja/aes338

[79] Cheymol G. Effects of obesity on pharmacokinetics implications for drug therapy. Clin Pharmacokinet. 2000; 39(3): 215–231.

[80] Ingrande J, Brodsky JB, Lemmens HJM. Lean body weight scalar for the anesthetic induction dose of propofol in morbidly obese subjects. Anesth Analg. 2011; 113: 57–62.

[81] Lemmens HJ. Perioperative pharmacology in morbid obesity. Curr Opin Anaesthesiol. 2010; 23(4): 485–491.

[82] Adams JP, Murphy PG. Obesity in anaesthesia and intensive care. Br J Anaesth. 2000; 85(1): 91–108.

[83] Cork RC, Vaughan RW, Bentley JB. General anesthesia for morbidly obese patients: an examination of postoperative outcomes. Anesthesiology. 1981; 54(4): 310–313.

[84] Arain SR, Barth CD, Shankar H, Ebert TJ. Choice of volatile anesthetic for the morbidly obese patient: sevoflurane or desflurane. J Clin Anesth. 2005; 17(6): 413–419.

[85] Torri G, Casati A, Albertin A, Comotti L, Bignami E, Scarioni M, Paganelli M. Randomized comparison of isoflurane and sevoflurane for laparoscopic gastric banding in morbidly obese patients. J Clin Anesth. 2001; 13(8): 565–570.

[86] Casati A, Putzu M. Anesthesia in the obese patient: pharmacokinetic considerations. J Clin Anesth. 2005; 17(2): 134–145.

[87] Lemmens HJ, Brodsky JB. The dose of succinylcholine in morbid obesity. Anesth Analg. 2006; 102(2): 438–442.

[88] Schwartz AE, Matteo RS, Ornstein E, Halevy JD, Diaz J. Pharmacokinetics and pharmacodynamics of vecuronium in the obese surgical patient. J Anesth Analg. 1992; 74(4): 515–518.

[89] Lemmens HJ, Ingrande J. Pharmacology and obesity. Int Anesthesiol Clin. 2013; 51(3): 52–66.

[90] Suzuki T, Masaki G, Ogawa S. Neostigmine induced reversal of vecuronium in normal weight, overweight and obese female patients. Br J Anaesth. 2006; 97(2): 160–163.

[91] Loupec T, Frasca D, Rousseau N, Faure JP, Mimoz O, Debaene B. Appropriate dosing of sugammadex to reverse deep rocuronium-induced neuromuscular blockade in morbidlyobese patients. Anaesthesia. 2016 Mar; 71(3): 265–272. doi: 10.1111/anae.13344. Epub 2015 Dec 19.

[92] Ingrande J, Brodsky JB, Lemmens HJ. Regional anesthesia and obesity. Curr Opin Anaesthesiol. 2009; 22: 683–686.

[93] Nielsen KC, Guller U, Steele SM, Klein SM, Greengrass RA, Pietrobon R. Influence of obesity on surgical regional anesthesia in the ambulatory setting: an analysis of 9,038 blocks. Anesthesiology. 2005; 102: 181–187.

[94] Schroeder K, Andrei AC, Furlong MJ, Donnelly MJ, Han S, Becker AM. The perioperative effect of increased body mass index on peripheral nerve blockade: an analysis of 528 ultrasound guided interscalene blocks. Rev Bras Anestesiol. 2012; 62: 28–38.

[95] Flores JC. Post-anesthetic care unit management. In Morbid Obesity: Peri-Operative Management. Alvarez AO (Ed). Cambridge: Cambridge University Press, 2004. pp. 339–346.

[96] Nightingale CE, Margarson MP, Shearer E, Redman JW, Lucas DN, Cousins JM. Perioperative management of the obese surgical patient 2015. Anaesthesia 2015; 70(7): 859–876.

[97] Bamgbade OA, Rutter TW, Nafiu OO, Dorje P. Postoperative complications in obese and nonobese patients. World J Surg. 2007; 31, 556–560.

[98] Wang TJ, Parise H, Levy D, D'Agostino RB Sr, Wolf PA, Vasan RS, Benjamin EJ. Obesity and the risk of new-onset atrial fibrillation. JAMA 2004; 292: 2471–2477.

[99] Chakravartty S, Sarma DR, Patel AG. Rhabdomyolysis in bariatric surgery: a systematic review. Obes Surg. 2013; 23(8): 1333–1340.

[100] Stein PD, Beemath A, Olson RE. Obesity as a risk factor in venous thromboembolism. Am J Med. 2005; 118; 978–980.

[101] Kranke P, Apefel CC, Papenfuss T, Rauch S, Lobmann U, Rubsam B, Greim CA, Roewer N. An increased body mass index is no risk factor for postoperative nausea and vomiting. A systematic review and results of original data. Acta Anaesthesiol Scand. 2001; 45(2): 160–166.

[102] Ziemann-Gimmel P, Hensel P, Koppman J, Marema R. Multimodal analgesia reduces narcotic requirements and antiemetic rescue medication in laparoscopic Roux-en-Y gastric bypass surgery. Surg Obes Relat Dis. 2013; 9(6): 975–980.

[103] Ventilation with lower tidal volumes as compared with traditional tidal volumes for acute lung injury and the acute respiratory distress syndrome. The Acute Respiratory Distress Syndrome Network. N Engl J Med. 2000; 342: 1301–1308.

[104] Dickerson RN. Hypocaloric, high-protein nutrition therapy for critically ill patients with obesity. Nutr Clin Pract. 2014; 29: 786–791.

[105] Stamou SC, Nussbaum M, Stiegel RM, Reames MK, Skipper ER, Robicsek F. Effect of body mass index on outcomes after cardiac surgery: is there an obesity paradox? Ann Thorac Surg. 2011 91 (1); 42–47.

Permissions

All chapters in this book were first published in AETM, by InTech Open; hereby published with permission under the Creative Commons Attribution License or equivalent. Every chapter published in this book has been scrutinized by our experts. Their significance has been extensively debated. The topics covered herein carry significant findings which will fuel the growth of the discipline. They may even be implemented as practical applications or may be referred to as a beginning point for another development.

The contributors of this book come from diverse backgrounds, making this book a truly international effort. This book will bring forth new frontiers with its revolutionizing research information and detailed analysis of the nascent developments around the world.

We would like to thank all the contributing authors for lending their expertise to make the book truly unique. They have played a crucial role in the development of this book. Without their invaluable contributions this book wouldn't have been possible. They have made vital efforts to compile up to date information on the varied aspects of this subject to make this book a valuable addition to the collection of many professionals and students.

This book was conceptualized with the vision of imparting up-to-date information and advanced data in this field. To ensure the same, a matchless editorial board was set up. Every individual on the board went through rigorous rounds of assessment to prove their worth. After which they invested a large part of their time researching and compiling the most relevant data for our readers.

The editorial board has been involved in producing this book since its inception. They have spent rigorous hours researching and exploring the diverse topics which have resulted in the successful publishing of this book. They have passed on their knowledge of decades through this book. To expedite this challenging task, the publisher supported the team at every step. A small team of assistant editors was also appointed to further simplify the editing procedure and attain best results for the readers.

Apart from the editorial board, the designing team has also invested a significant amount of their time in understanding the subject and creating the most relevant covers. They scrutinized every image to scout for the most suitable representation of the subject and create an appropriate cover for the book.

The publishing team has been an ardent support to the editorial, designing and production team. Their endless efforts to recruit the best for this project, has resulted in the accomplishment of this book. They are a veteran in the field of academics and their pool of knowledge is as vast as their experience in printing. Their expertise and guidance has proved useful at every step. Their uncompromising quality standards have made this book an exceptional effort. Their encouragement from time to time has been an inspiration for everyone.

The publisher and the editorial board hope that this book will prove to be a valuable piece of knowledge for researchers, students, practitioners and scholars across the globe.

List of Contributors

Teodoro Durá-Travé
Department of Pediatrics, School of Medicine, University of Navarra, Pamplona, Spain
Department of Pediatrics, Navarra Hospital Complex, Pamplona, Spain
Navarra Institute for Health Research (IdisNa), Pamplona, Spain

Leyre Lloreda-Martín
Department of Pediatrics, School of Medicine, University of Navarra, Pamplona, Spain

Alberto Ríos-Muñoz, Inés Niyubahwe, Ander Ernaga-Lorea and Fidel Gallinas-Victoriano
Department of Pediatrics, Navarra Hospital Complex, Pamplona, Spain

Mahmoud M. A. Abulmeaty
Clinical Nutrition Program, Department of Community Health Sciences, College of Applied Medical Sciences, King Saud University, Riyadh, KSA
Obesity Research and Management Unit, Department of Medical Physiology, Faculty of Medicine, Zagazig University, Zagazig, Egypt

Ashok Kumar and Kanika Gupta
Centre For Systems Biology & Bioinformatics, UIEAST, Panjab University, Chandigarh

Simona Negreş, Cornel Chiriţă, Andreea Letiţia Arsene, Denisa Margină, Elena Moroşan and Cristina Elena Zbârcea
University of Medicine and Pharmacy "Carol Davila", Faculty of Pharmacy, Bucharest, Romania

Maria Teresa Anselmo Olinto
University of Vale do Rio dos Sinos, São Leopoldo, Brazil
Department of Nutrition, Federal University of Health Science of Porto Alegre, Porto Alegre, Brazil

Heloísa Theodoro
University of Vale do Rio dos Sinos, São Leopoldo, Brazil
Department of Nutrition, University of Caxias do Sul, Caxias do Sul, Brazil

Raquel Canuto
Department of Nutrition, Federal University of Rio Grande do Sul, Porto Alegre, Brazil

Visith Chavasit, Wantanee Kriengsinyos and Prapaisri Sirichakwal
Institute of Nutrition, Mahidol University, Nakhonpathom, Thailand

Mayuree Ditmetharoj, Manasuwee Phaichamanan, Kangsadan Singsoong and Araya Rojjanawanicharkorn
Food and Drug Administration, Nonthaburi, Thailand

Hidetaka Hamasaki
Department of Internal Medicine, National Center for Global Health and Medicine Kohnodai Hospital, Chiba, Japan
Hamasaki Clinic, Kagoshima, Japan

Hülya Çakmur
Department of Family Medicine, School of Medicine, University of Kafkas, Kars, Turkey

Bruce M. King
Department of Psychology, Clemson University, Clemson, SC, USA

María Guillermina Zubiría, Ana Alzamendi and Andrés Giovambattista
Neuroendocrinology Laboratory, Multidisciplinary Institute of Cellular Biology (IMBICE, CICPBA-CONICET-UNLP), La Plata, Argentina

Luisina Ongaro
Department of Pharmacology and Therapeutics, Centre for Research in Reproduction and Development, McGill University, Montreal, QC, Canada

Eduardo Spinedi
Center of Experimental and Applied Endocrinology (CENEXA, UNLP-CONICET, PAHO/ WHO Collaborating Center for Diabetes), La Plata Medical School, National University of La Plata, La Plata, Argentina

Laura Mihaela Trandafir, Ileana Ioniuc and Ingrith Miron
Pediatric Department, University of Medicine and Pharmacy "Grigore T. Popa", Iasi, Romania

Paul H. Thibodeau
Department of Psychology, Oberlin College, Oberlin, OH, USA

Stephen J. Flusberg
Department of Psychology, Purchase College, SUNY, Purchase, NY, USA

Ismail Demirel, Esef Bolat and Aysun Yıldız Altun
Department of Anesthesiology and Reanimation, School of Medicine, Fırat University Elazığ, Turkey

Index